D1756871

Manipal Manu
Clinical Medicine

Second Edition

this book belongs to Kala Roopakumaresan.
11010/014

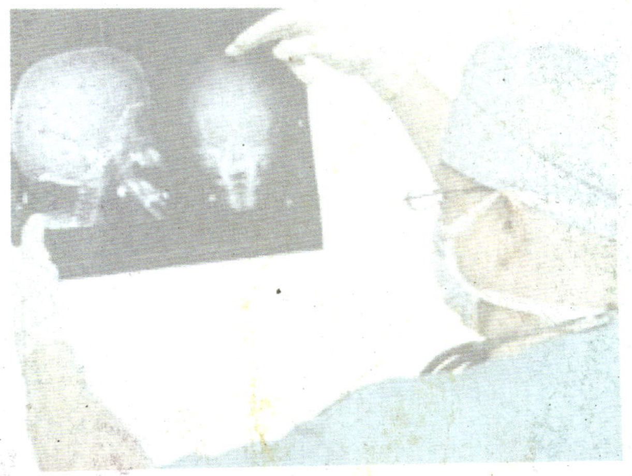

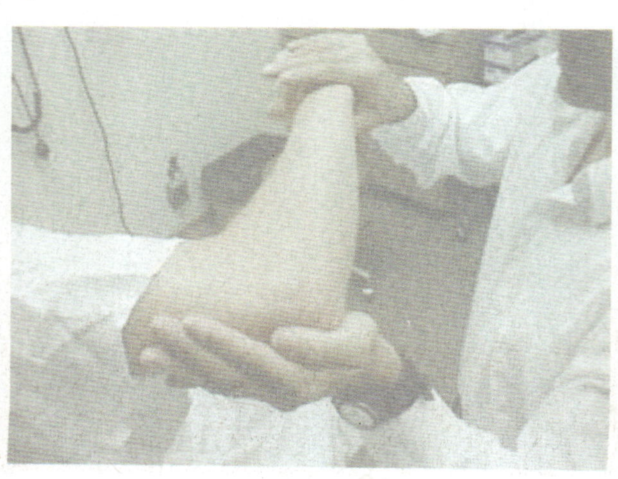

Manipal Manual of
Clinical Medicine

Second Edition

BA Shastry

Professor of Medicine and Consultant Physician
Kasturba Medical College and Hospital
Manipal, Karnataka, India

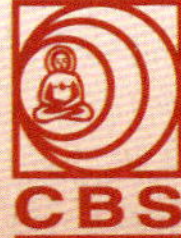

CBS Publishers & Distributors Pvt Ltd

New Delhi • Bengaluru • Chennai • Kochi • Pune
Hyderabad • Kolkata • Mumbai • Nagpur • Patna

Disclaimer

Science and technology are constantly changing fields. New research and experience broaden the scope of information and knowledge. The author has tried his best in giving information available to him while preparing the material for this book. Although, all efforts have been made to ensure optimum accuracy of the material, yet it is quite possible some errors might have been left uncorrected. The publisher, the printer and the author will not be held responsible for any inadvertent errors, omissions or inaccuracies.

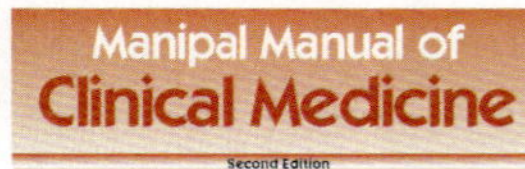

ISBN: 978-81-239-2265-2

Copyright © Author and Publisher

Second Edition: 2013

First Edition: 2004

All rights reserved. No part of this book may be reproduced or transmitted in any form or by any means, electronic or mechanical, including photocopying, recording, or any information storage and retrieval system without permission, in writing, from the author and the publisher.

Published by Satish Kumar Jain for

CBS Publishers & Distributors Pvt Ltd

4819/XI Prahlad Street, 24 Ansari Road, Daryaganj, New Delhi 110 002, India.

Ph: 23289259, 23266861, 23266867 Fax: 011-23243014 Website: www.cbspd.com
e-mail: delhi@cbspd.com; cbspubs@airtelmail.in

Corporate Office: 204 FIE, Industrial Area, Patparganj, Delhi 110 092

Ph: 4934 4934 Fax: 4934 4935 e-mail: publishing@cbspd.com; publicity@cbspd.com

Branches

- **Bengaluru:** Seema House 2975, 17th Cross, K.R. Road, Banasankari 2nd Stage, Bengaluru 560 070, Karnataka
  Ph: +91-80-26771678/79 Fax: +91-80-26771680 e-mail: bangalore@cbspd.com
- **Chennai:** 20, West Park Road, Shenoy Nagar, Chennai 600 030, Tamil Nadu
  Ph: +91-44-26260666, 26208620 Fax: +91-44-42032115 e-mail: chennai@cbspd.com
- **Kochi:** 36/14 Kalluvilakam, Lissie Hospital Road, Kochi 682 018, Kerala
  Ph: +91-484-4059061-65 Fax: +91-484-4059065 e-mail: kochi@cbspd.com
- **Pune:** Bhuruk Prestige, Sr. No. 52/12/2+1+3/2 Narhe, Haveli (Near Katraj-Dehu Road Bypass), Pune 411 041, Maharashtra
  Ph: +91-20-64704058, 64704059, 32342277 Fax: +91-20-24300160 e-mail: pune@cbspd.com

Representatives

- **Hyderabad** 0-9885175004
- **Kolkata** 0-9831437309, 0-9051152362
- **Mumbai** 0-9833017933
- **Nagpur** 0-9021734563
- **Patna** 0-9334159340

Printed at Manipal Technologies Ltd., Manipal.

to

____

my
family members

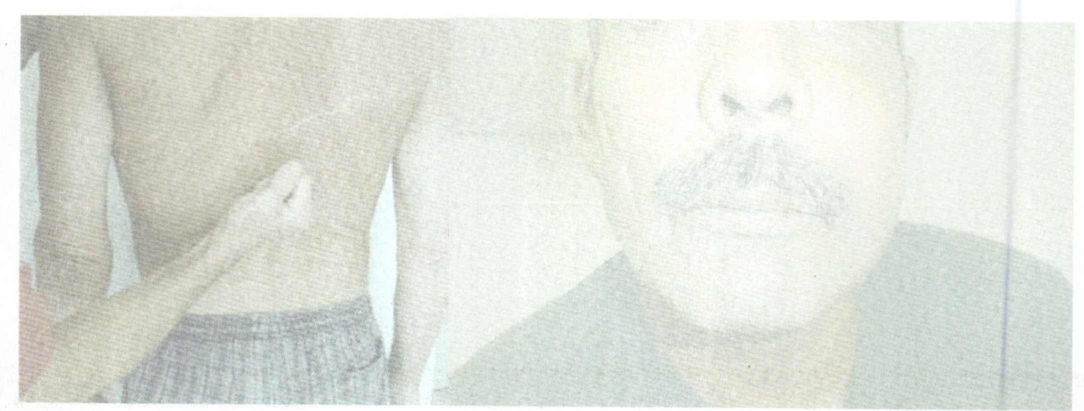

Foreword

It gives me great pleasure to pen this foreword for my esteemed colleague Dr. Shastry's book on clinical medicine.

This book is a comprehensive guide for undergraduate students on correct clinical methods and their interpretation, and is a ready-reckoner for use in bedside clinics. It has several illustrations depicting physical signs which make it easy for the student to comprehend what is being described in the text. The book covers all systems and gives the student a brief, simple but comprehensive idea of how to examine a patient with medical illness.

Modern medicine has moved on and investigations have become an essential part of diagnosis. Keeping this in mind, common chest X-rays have been compiled with care and made for easy understanding. The recent additions of chapters on ECG made for excellent introduction to this tough subject and will be an icebreaker for students to start reading routine ECGs. New chapters on drugs, emergencies and bedside procedure make this book very useful for students appearing for MBBS examination. No wonder it is very popular among students all over India and has found wide acceptance in teaching institutions.

On a personal note, Dr. Shastry has been an excellent teacher and has been the core of teaching faculty at Manipal for two decades. His knowledge and wisdom gleaned over the years have been crystallised in this book, which is being updated so regularly.

I congratulate him on his substantial contribution to clinical medicine and wish him all the very best in years to come.

Prof **Sudha Vidyasagar**
Professor and Head
Department of Medicine
Kasturba Medical College and Hospital
Manipal 576119
Karnataka, India

Preface to the Second Edition

Manipal Manual of Clinical Medicine has been written to help the students in medicine to prepare for the final examination.

Along with the chapters on clinical medicine, as in the first edition, certain chapters like medical instruments, bedside procedures, chapters on ECG, X-rays and drugs have been added to help the students in preparing for their examinations better. Additional clinical information has been added in chapters on cardiology and neurology for the benefit of postgraduate students in medicine.

I am extremely grateful for the support given to me by my departmental colleagues and friends and also for their suggestions.

I sincerely thank Mr SK Jain, Managing Director, CBS Publishers & Distributors Pvt Ltd, New Delhi, for the encouragements and support given to me while preparing the book.

I welcome any criticism and suggestion by the readers for improving the content and quality of the book.

BA Shastry

Preface to the First Edition

Teaching a large number of undergraduate and postgraduate students made me realise the need for a book in clinical medicine which is simple and precise. *Manipal Manual of Clinical Medicine* has been written to help the students in medicine to prepare for their final examination.

Keeping in view the vastness of clinical medicine, important topics have been covered in detail and smaller topics covered in brief. Standard textbooks of medicine and clinical methods have been used as reference in preparing this book.

I take this opportunity to express my gratitude to the staff of the Department of Medicine for their constant encouragement and suggestions.

I would like to thank Mr Umesh Acharya, artist from dental college, for his diagrams and photographs while preparing this book.

I am grateful to Ms Vijaya P Rao, Dr Ramkrishna and Mr Ganapathi Bhat for the initial preparation of manuscript and Vishu typewriters for the first phase of computer work.

I sincerely thank Mr SK Jain, Managing Director, CBS Publishers & Distributors Pvt Ltd, New Delhi, for the encouragement and support given to me while preparing the book.

I thank Prof NR Rau for his encouragement in preparing the material of this book and for having written the Foreword.

I welcome any criticism and suggestion by the students to improve the quality of this book.

BA Shastry

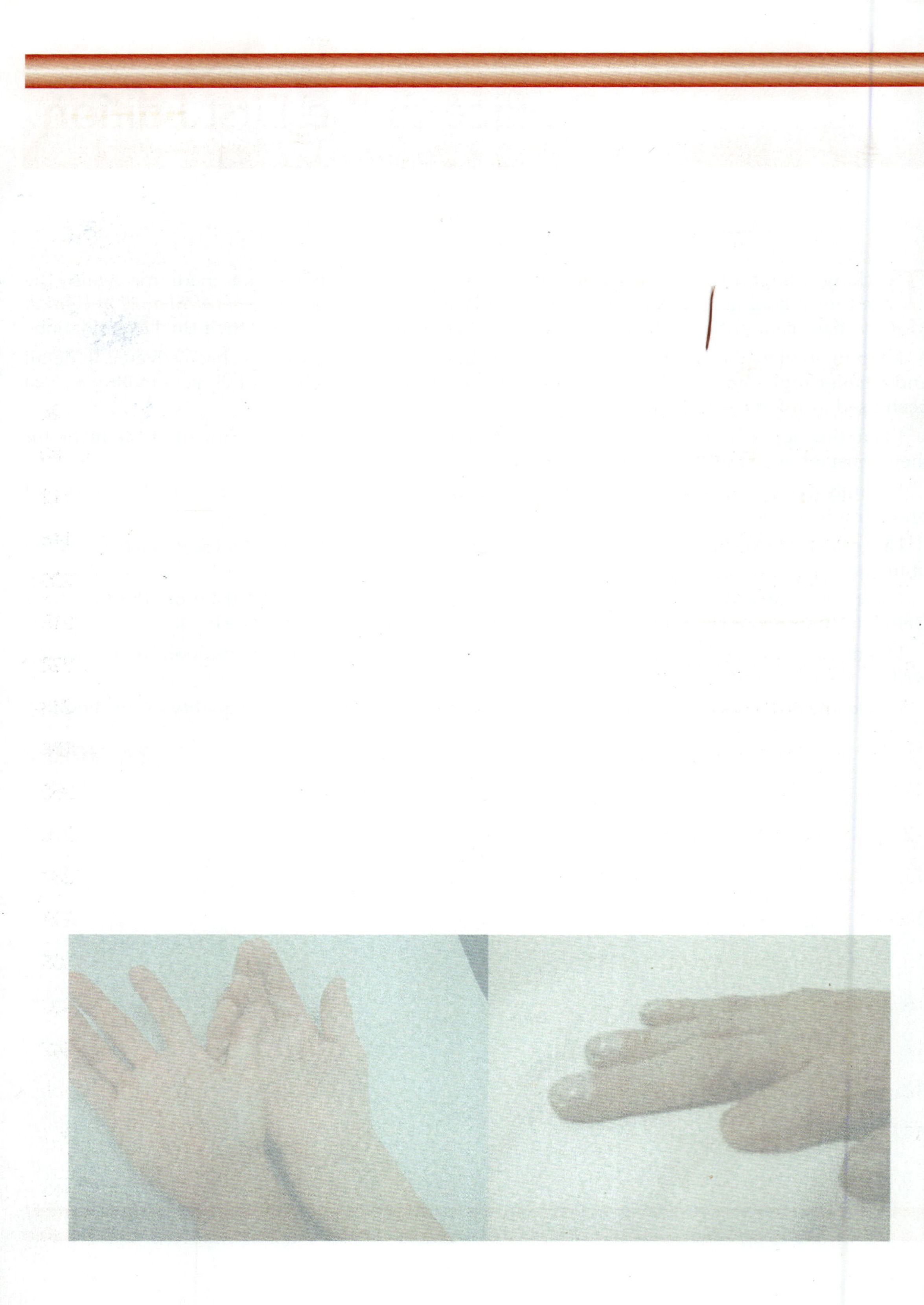

Contents

Foreword by Prof Sudha Vidyasagar vii

Preface to the Second Edition viii

Preface to the First Edition ix

1. **General Physical Examination** 1
2. **Cardiovascular System** 24
3. **Respiratory System** 80
4. **Gastrointestinal and Hepatobiliary System** 112
5. **Nervous System** 148
6. **Disorders of Muscle and Peripheral Nerves** 209
7. **Hematological Disorders** 218
8. **Renal and Urogenital System** 228
9. **Locomotor System** 238
10. **Endocrine Disorders** 253
11. **Unconscious Patient** 268
12. **Examination of the Eye** 278
13. **Common Radiological Abnormalities** 287
14. **Common Bedside Procedures in Medicine** 297
15. **Common Therapeutic Agents** 308
16. **Medical Emergencies** 332
17. **Instruments** 342
18. **ECG and Common ECG Abnormalities** 348
19. **Normal Laboratory Data** 361

Index 365

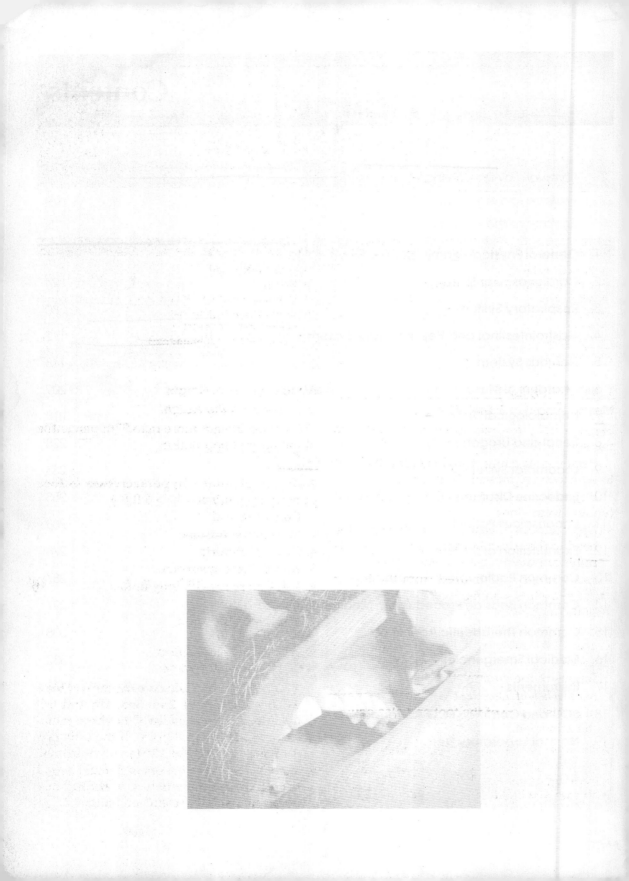

General Physical Examination

1

CHECKLIST FOR GENERAL PHYSICAL EXAMINATION

- Skeletal height
- Nourishment (nutritional status)
- Vital signs
- Pallor
- Icterus
- Cyanosis
- Clubbing
- Lymphadenopathy
- Edema
- Examination of hands and feet
- Examination of genitalia
- Examination of breast
- Examination of skin and hair

1. SKELETAL HEIGHT

Measurement of Skeletal Height

Skeletal height is measured from vertex to the sole of the foot.

Person is standing straight against the wall to which a vertical scale is attached.

Height is measured from the top of the head (vertex) to the foot.

- *Upper segment:* Measured from the top of the head to the upper border of the symphysis pubis or (total height—lower segment).
- *Lower segment:* Measured from the top of the symphysis pubis vertically to the sole of the foot (floor).
- *Arm span:* Stretch the upper limbs horizontally outwards and measure the distance between the tips of the middle fingers of the two outstretched hands.
- *Normal height:* Usually two times the length of pubis to sole of the foot and also equals the arm span.

Note: Measure the skeletal height while
- The person is standing erect
- Wearing only inner clothes
- Not wearing footwears

Abnormalities of Height

a. Increase in the Height

Tall stature: Height more than 97th percentile of the normal population.

Causes

Anterior pituitary hypersecretion before puberty (gigantism = ht > 6 ft 8").

- Constitutional
- Marfan's syndrome
- Homocystinuria
- Klinefelter's syndrome
- Tall thin built with long limbs
- Eunuchoidism
- Marfan's syndrome.

Clinical Signs Associated with Marfan's Syndrome

- *Metacarpal index:* Calculate the ratio of total axial length of the 2nd, 3rd, 4th and 5th metacarpals. Total width of the above metacarpals at their mid point. If the ratio is ≥ 8.4 it is suggestive of Marfan's syndrome.
- *Thumb sign:* Projecting out of thumb beyond the ulnar border when it is completely opposed inside the clenched hand.

- *Wrist sign:* Overlapping of the distal phalanges of the 1st and 5th digits of one hand when they are wrapped around the opposite wrist.

b. Decrease in the Height

Dwarfism (short stature): Standing height is below the 3rd percentile for children of similar age and ethnic group (decrease in height is more than 3.5 SD below the mean height).

Causes

- *Endocrine disorders*
  - Hypopituitarism
  - Primary hypothyroidism
  - Cushing's syndrome
  - Pseudo hypoparathyroidism.
- *Systemic illness*
  - Malabsorption syndrome
  - Chronic systemic disorder, e.g. cardiac/respiratory
  - Malnutrition.
- *Chromosome abnormalities,* e.g. Turner's syndrome
- *Other causes*
  - Intrauterine growth retardation
  - Constitutional dwarfism.

Causes of Arm Span More than the Total Height

1. Marfan's syndrome
2. Homocystinuria
3. Klinefelter's syndrome

Heel Pad Thickness

Calculate the distance at the lower most point (of the X-ray shadows) between the calcaneum and heel pad soft tissue.

Abnormal Heel Pad Thickness

- Males > 21 mm
- Females > 18 mm

Causes of Increased Heel Pad Thickness

- Acromegaly
- Conditions associated with obesity
- Conditions associated with edema.

2. NUTRITIONAL STATUS

Assessment of Nutritional Status

Nutritional status is assessed by

- Muscle bulk
- Subcutaneous fat
- Deficiency signs.

Note: Presence of edema should be considered while assessing the nutritional status.

Nutritional Assessment

Measure the muscle bulk and subcutaneous fat while assessing nutrition.

Subcutaneous Fat

Measure the triceps skin fold thickness of the left mid arm—measurement is ideally done by calipers (Lange's or Herpenden's).

Average adult measurement of triceps skin fold thickness

- Males 12.5 mm
- Females 16 mm

Muscle Bulk

Measure the left mid upper arm circumference.

Average measurements

- Males 25.5 cm
- Females 23 cm

3. FAT DISTRIBUTION AND ITS ABNORMALITIES

Localised deposition of fat results in lipomas.

Localised lipoatrophy may result due to insulin injection.

Progressive lipodystrophy—less fat in the upper part of the body with excess fat in the lower part.

Xanthomas

- Lipid containing nodules present in the soft tissues and tendons.
- Xanthomas may be associated with premature coronary atherosclerosis.

Different Types of Xanthomas and their Clinical Significance

Eruptive Xanthomas

- Associated with type I and II hyperlipidemias.
- Yellow coloured nodules distributed allover the body.

Tendon Xanthomas

- Associated with type II hyperlipidemia.
- Swelling in the region of tendons of elbow, tendocalcaneus, etc.

Palmar Xanthomas

- Associated with type III hyperlipidemia.
- Palmar creases will have yellowish discoloration.

Body Weight and Body Mass Index (Quatelet's index)

Body mass index (BMI): Measured by weight in kg divided by body height in meters square.

Assessment of body weight according to BMI

Normal weight	BMI 18 to 25
Overweight	BMI 25 to 30
Obesity	BMI 30 and above
Extreme (morbid) obesity	BMI 40 and above
Underweight	BMI less than 18

BMI less than 18 indicates undernutrition and requires nutritional supplementation.

Waist/Hip Ratio

Keep the patient erect.

- Measure the waist at the level equidistant between the costal margin and iliac crest.
- Measure the hip at the level of greater trochanter.

Significance: Normal waist/hip ratio: < 0.8

- Central abdominal obesity (apple shaped obesity): Waist/hip ratio > 0.9
- Gluteofemoral obesity (pear shaped obesity): Waist/hip ratio < 0.9
- If waist/hip ratio of > 0.9 in women and > 1 in men is abnormal and associated with more incidence of cardiovascular disease, diabetes mellitus, hypertension and insulin resistance.
- Waist measurement of > 102 cm in males and > 88 cm in females indicates high-risk abdominal obesity.

Cachexia: Severe wasting associated with pallor and wrinkled dry skin, e.g. malignant disorders, infections like tuberculosis and HIV disease, anorexia nervosa.

4. PALLOR

Pallor suggests the pale appearance of skin. Pale appearance depends on the skin pigmentation and skin thickness. Anemia suggests the colour of blood.

Note: Anemia and pallor are not synonymous terms.

Causes of pallor

- All anemic disorders.
- Hypopituitarism and hypogonadism (due to lack of pigmentation of skin).
- Left heart failure.
- Conditions associated with shock (due to decreased blood flow).
- Acute severe blood loss causes constriction of superficial blood vessels with dead white colour of the skin.

Anemia

See Chapter 7, on hematology.

Definition

Anemia is defined as the decrease in the hemoglobin level/RBCs or decrease in the oxygen-carrying capacity of the blood.

Examination of an Anemic Patient

Mucous membrane is the ideal site to look for pallor (oral mucosa and tongue).

- Conjunctival pallor: Turn down the lower eyelids on both sides simultaneously.
- Conjunctiva becomes pale when Hb% is < 8 gm/dl.
- Palmar crease is lighter in colour than the surrounding skin when Hb is < 8 gm/dl.

Severe pernicious anemia gives lemon or pale yellow tint to the skin and skin may become ashen grey in acute leukemias.

Sites to look for pallor

- Oral mucosa
- Tongue
- Conjunctiva
- Nail bed
- Palms and soles

5. ICTERUS

Definition: Yellowish discoloration of skin, sclera and mucous membranes due to excess of circulating bilirubin.

Causes of jaundice

1. Unconjugated hyperbilirubinemia:
   a. Due to increased production, e.g. hemolytic anemias, ineffective erythropoiesis.
   b. Due to defective uptake of bilirubin, e.g. Gilbert's syndrome.
2. Conjugated hyperbilirubinemia:
   a. Hepatocellular dysfunction
      - Acute and chronic hepatitis
      - Cirrhosis
      - Malignancy of liver
   b. Obstruction to outflow of bile from liver to duodenum, e.g. intrahepatic cholestasis, viral hepatitis, extrahepatic obstruction, gallstones, carcinoma head of pancreas.

Sites to look for jaundice

- Sclera
- Sublingual mucosa
- Oral cavity
- Palms and soles
- Skin

Jaundice is best appreciated in daylight.

Jaundice becomes clinically detectable when the bilirubin level is > 3 mg/dl.

Sclera

- Ask the patient to look downwards and look for the upper sclera for jaundice (Fig. 1.1).
- Sclera is the first structure to be involved in a patient with jaundice.

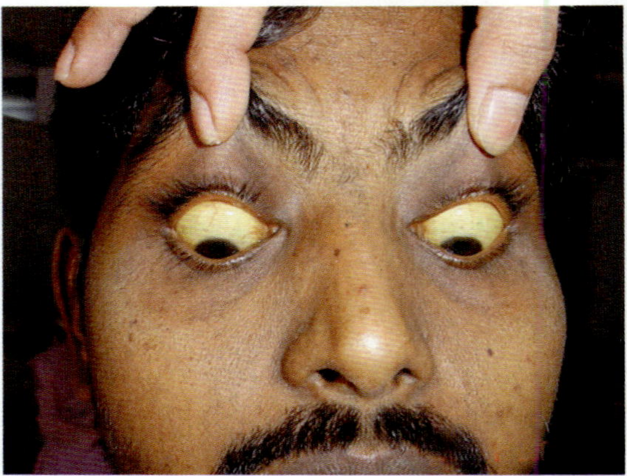

Fig. 1.1: Demonstration of jaundice

- Early involvement of the sclera is due to the high affinity of the elastic tissue to bilirubin.

Differences between Different Types of Jaundice (Table 1.1)

Latent Jaundice

Circulating level of bilirubin is more than normal (but less than 3 mg/dl) but clinically not detectable.

Causes of Yellowish Discolouration apart from Jaundice

a. Hypercarotenemia
b. Excessive exposure to phenols
c. Quinacrine intake

Hypercarotenemia

- Hypercarotenemia results from consumption of excess carotene-containing substances (e.g. carrots).

Key Points

- Skin becomes yellowish when the jaundice is severe.
- Sclera becomes lemon yellow in hemolytic jaundice.
- In obstructive jaundice sclera becomes dark yellow or greenish yellow.
- In long-standing jaundice sclera becomes greenish due to oxidation of bilirubin to biliverdin.

Table 1.1: Differences between different types of jaundice

Pre-hepatic	*Hepatic*	*Post-hepatic*	
Urine color	Initially normal, but on standing becomes darker due to conversion of urobilinogen to urobilin	Yellow	Deep yellow
Itching	–	–/+	++
Stool	Normal	Pale if cholestasis	Clay coloured
Anemia	Severe	+/–	+/–
Jaundice	Mild	Moderate/Severe	Moderate/Severe
Hepatomegaly	+/–	+	+/–
Splenomegaly	+	+/–	–
Gall bladder enlargement	–	–	+/–
Tests for hemolysis	+	–	+/–
Abnormal LFT	Only indirect bilirubin↑	Direct bilirubin↑ AST, ALT raise↑	Direct bilirubin↑ ALP raise

- Carotene becomes distributed in the subcutaneous fat and stains face, arms and soles yellow.
- Sclera does not become yellow in patients with hypercarotenemia.

Note: Patients with hypothyroidism will have yellowish appearance of face due to impaired metabolism of carotene.

6. CYANOSIS

Definition: Bluish discoloration of mucous membrane and extremities due to decreased oxygenation of blood.

Cyanosis occurs either due to increase in the desaturated hemoglobin or due to abnormal hemoglobins.

Cyanosis appears when the level of desaturated hemoglobin is > 5 gm/dl.

Types of Cyanosis (Table 1.2)

- Peripheral cyanosis
- Central cyanosis

Peripheral Cyanosis

Mechanism: Peripheral cyanosis occurs due to the decreased capillary blood flow allowing more time for the removal of oxygen by the tissues. For example:

1. Decreased cardiac output, cardiac failure/shock states.
2. Local vasoconstriction, e.g. cold exposure.
3. Arterial and venous obstruction.

Sites to look for peripheral cyanosis

Extremities fingers and toes/tip of nose.

Central Cyanosis

Excess of desaturated hemoglobin in the blood leaving the aorta causes central cyanosis.

Sites of central cyanosis: Tip of tongue and oral mucosa.

Etiology

a. Cardiac causes
   - Right to left shunting of blood, e.g. reversal of intracardiac shunts, cyanotic congenital heart disease

Table 1.2: Differences between central and peripheral cyanosis

Central cyanosis	*Peripheral cyanosis*	
Extremities	Warm	Cold
Warming the part	No effect	Cyanosis decreases
Breathing pure O_2 10 liters	May abolish cyanosis	No change occurs

- Peripheral AV communications
- Defective oxygenation of blood in lungs, e.g. left heart failure

b. Respiratory causes: Ventilation perfusion mismatch with defective oxygenation, e.g. pneumonia/COPD

c. Abnormal hemoglobins, e.g. sulfhemoglobin and methemoglobin

d. Carboxy hemoglobin: Carboxy hemoglobin gives a cherry red colour to the skin, e.g. CO poisoning.

Clinical Aspects of Cyanosis

- Left heart failure produces both central and peripheral cyanosis.
- Peripheral cyanosis and acutely developed central cyanosis are not associated with clubbing.
- Central cyanosis may appear only on exertion and peripheral cyanosis only on exposure to cold.
- Patient with central cyanosis will also have peripheral cyanosis with warm extremities, except in patients with heart failure (central cyanosis with cold periphery).

7. CLUBBING (Fig. 1.2)

Definition: Bulbous enlargement of distal segments of fingers and toes.

Causes

a. Cardiovascular:
- Cyanotic congenital heart disease
- Reversal of shunts (intracardiac)
- Infective endocarditis.

b. Respiratory:
- Suppurative lung disease: Bronchiectasis/lung abscess
- Malignant lung disease: Bronchogenic carcinoma
- Pleural disorders: Empyema thoracis/mesothelioma
- Interstitial lung disease

c. Gastrointestinal:
- Ulcerative colitis
- Crohn's disease
- Malabsorption syndrome

d. Hepatic: Cirrhosis of liver

e. Congenital and idiopathic clubbing.

Differential Diagnosis of Clubbing

- Hyperparathyroidism—due to resorption of terminal phalanx
- Psoriatic arthritis
- Vinyl chloride exposure
- Pachydermoperiostosis

Grades of Clubbing

Fluctuation: Nail bed becomes soft with redness around and floating of the nail in the nail bed. Minimal fluctuation is normal.

Elicitation of Fluctuation

- Examiner places the terminal phalanx of the patient's finger over the pulp of his two thumbs.
- Gentle pressure is applied with the tip of examiner's middle finger over the proximal phalanx of the patient's fingers for stabilising the terminal phalanx.
- Fluctuation is elicited over the patient's nail bed with the tips of examiner's index fingers.

Angle Obliteration

Normally there is an angle of about 15° (angle of Lovibond) between the nail and cuticle. In

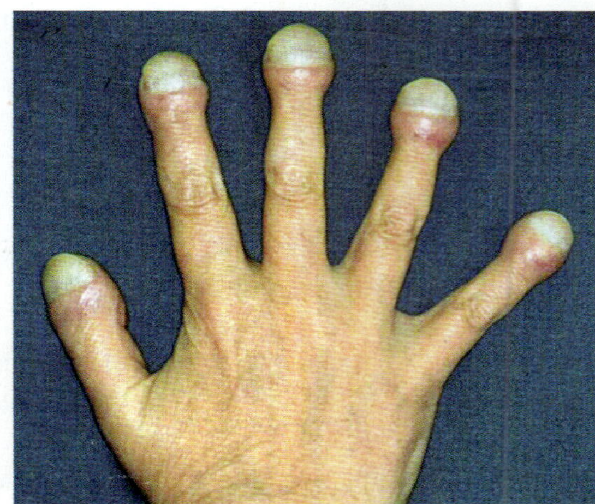

Fig. 1.2: Clubbing of fingers

patients with clubbing the angle is lost and may exceed 180°.

Shamroth's Sign

- Ask the patient to keep the two thumbnails opposing each other.
- Observe for the gap in between the nails.
- Reduction or loss of gap between the nails is a manifestation of clubbing.

Change in Curvature of the Nails

- Severe clubbing will be associated with increase in the longitudinal and lateral curvature of the nails.
- In extremely severe cases of clubbing distal phalanx will become bulbous with drumstick appearance.

Hypertrophic Osteoarthropathy

Commonly associated with severe clubbing.

Parts involved: Wrist and ankle with lower ends of long bones like radius, ulna, tibia and fibula.

Features

Wrist and ankle joint will have following features:

- Swelling
- Pain
- Stiffness
- Redness
- Rise of temperature
- Joint effusion
- Thickening of periosteum of long bones

Radiological Changes

Calcification of the subperiosteal region (separate from bone cortex).

Common Causes of Hypertrophic Osteoarthropathy

- Bronchogenic carcinoma
- Cystic fibrosis
- Bronchiectasis
- Cyanotic congenital heart disease

Pathogenesis of Clubbing

Neurogenic Theory

- Reflex vasodilatation of peripheral tissues and nail bed occurs due to brainstem stimulation.
- Brainstem stimulation may occur as a result of diseased lung and pleura generating impulses reaching the brainstem via the vagi and intercostal nerves.

Note: Features of clubbing and hypertrophic osteoarthropathy may disappear after resection of vagi and intercostal nerves.

Hormonal Theory

Proliferation of distal tissues occur due to hormone-like substances released by the deceased tissues.

Shunt Theory

AV shunting allows the substances to bypass the lung (normally these substances are degraded by the lung) which stimulate the distal tissue proliferation.

Proposed Vasoactive Substances in the Genesis of Clubbing

- Estrogen
- Ferritin
- Growth hormone
- Platelet derived growth factor (PDGF)

Growth Factor Theory

Platelet derived growth factor (PDGF) is released at the distal tissues by the circulating megakaryocytes which bypass the pulmonary circulation.

PDGF may activate fibroblasts, connective tissues and alter the endothelial permeability resulting in clubbing.

8. LYMPHADENOPATHY

Lymphatic system includes:

- Lymph nodes
- Lymphatic vessels
- Lymphatic tissues

Key Points
- Soft, flat lymph nodes of < 1 cm size are usually benign and require follow-up.
- Inguinal lymph nodes of less than 2 cm size are not abnormal.
- Lymph node size > 2 cm or size of 1.5 × 1.5 cm are significant and to be evaluated.

Lymphatic tissue includes tonsils, adenoids, spleen and Peyer's patches in the ileum.

Examination of Lymph Nodes

Check for the following details while examining a lymph node

- Number
- Size
- Site
- Consistency
- Discrete/Matted
- Mobile/Fixed
- Tenderness
- Fluctuation
- Surrounding skin
- Draining area

Characteristics of Different Types of Lymphadenopathy

Tuberculous Node

Soft, non-tender, matted nodes (attached to each other). Matting occurs due to peri-adenitis. Discharge, sinus or scar of previous suppuration of untreated cases may be present.

Tender Node

Signifies inflammatory or infective pathology with acute stretching of the capsule.

Lymphangitis

Superficial lymphatic vessels appear as red streaks running between the nodes and sites of original infection, e.g. filarial lymphangitis.

Fixity of Lymph Node

- Indicates inflammatory pathology.
- Deep fixity suggests malignancy.

Fluctuation of a Lymph Node

Suggests abscess forming conditions like sepsis or TB.

Lymphoma Node

- Discrete, mobile, non-tender, firm or rubbery (elastic) in consistency.
- May be symmetrical.
- Malignant lymph node
- Hard, non-tender fixed nodes which progressively enlarge.

Bubo

Inflammatory swelling of one or more lymph nodes in the inguinal region. Masses of lymph nodes may suppurate and drain pus, e.g. chancroid, lymphogranuloma venereum.

a. Localised Lymphadenopathy

Enlargement of lymph nodes in a single anatomical area.

Cervical Lymphadenopathy (Fig. 1.3)

Causes

- URTI
- Viral illness
- Oral or dental lesions
- Secondaries from primary head, neck, breast, lung and thyroid malignancy.
- Lymphoma and leukemias
- All causes of generalised lymphadenopathy.

Examination of Cervical Lymph Nodes

Examine from behind for sub-mental, tonsillar, submandibular, supraclavicular,

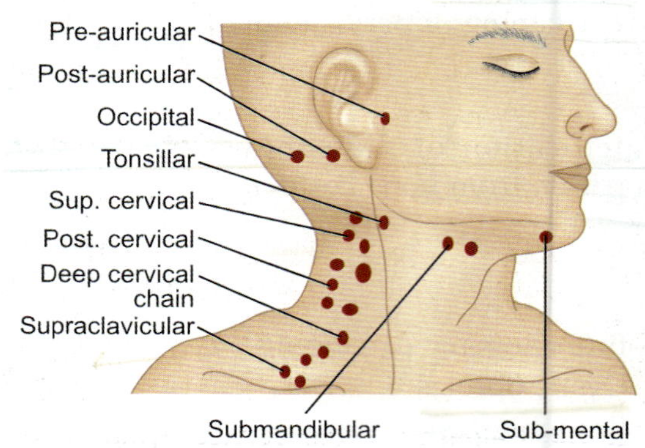

Fig. 1.3: Cervical lymphadenopathy

pre-auricular and deep cervical nodes (Figs 1.4 and 1.5).

Scalene Node

Node is present deep to sternomastoid muscle on the scaleneus anticus muscle.

Method of palpation: Finger is dipped through the clavicular head of sternomastoid behind the clavicle.

Significance: Secondary involvement of the lymph node due to bronchial carcinoma.

Jugulo-digastric Node

Most commonly enlarged lymph node, e.g. URTI and tonsillitis.

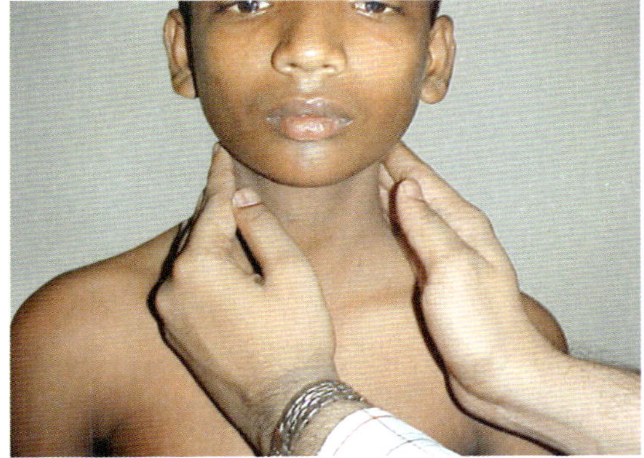

Fig. 1.4: Palpation of the cervical lymph nodes (anterior) from behind

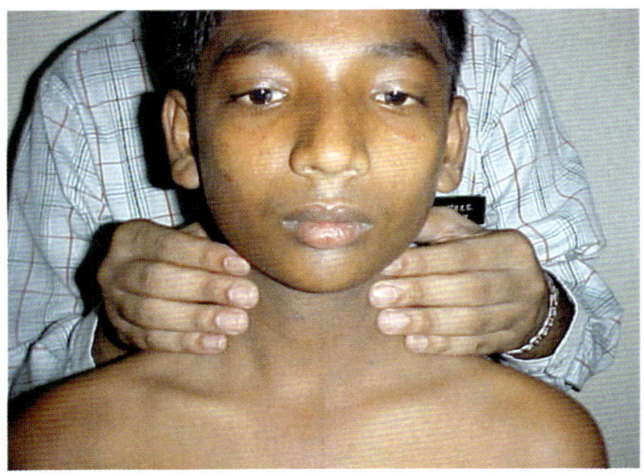

Fig. 1.5: Palpation of the cervical lymph nodes (posterior) from the anterior aspect

Palpate just posteriorly to the angle of the mandible.

Examine the posterior triangle of the neck up to the back for posterior auricular and occipital lymph nodes.

Waldeyer's Ring

Waldeyer's ring constitutes a group of lymphatic structures, which surround the opening of digestive and respiratory tracts.

Internal ring

- Adenoids (pharyngeal tonsil)
- Palatine tonsils
- Tubal tonsils
- Lingual tonsil

External Waldeyer's ring

- Occipital (posteriorly)
- Posterior auricular
- Pre-auricular
- Jugular and tonsillar
- Submandibular
- Sub-mental (anteriorly)

Significance: Waldeyer's ring adenopathy occurs with local disease or as a part of generalised lymphadenopathy especially in patients with non-Hodgkin's lymphoma.

Virchow's Node (Troisier's Sign)

Enlargement of left supraclavicular node occurs due to metastatic lesion from GIT or testicular malignancy (*see* also GIT).

Occipital lymphadenopathy: Occurs in scalp infection.

Pre-auricular lymph node: Enlargement can occur with conjunctival infection.

Axillary Lymphadenopathy

Causes

a. Infection or injury to the ipsilateral upper limb
b. Breast and chest wall disease
c. Lymphoma
d. Part of generalised lymphadenopathy

Method of examination (Figs 1.6 and 1.7)

Examiner sitting in front of the patient supports the patient's upper limb with his own, on the side to be examined.

Finger tips are inserted into the axillary vault (right finger tip for left axilla and vice versa) and anterior, posterior and medial walls are palpated in turn.

Epitrochlear Nodes

Causes of enlargement

- Infection and inflammation of ipsilateral hand

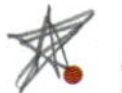

- Secondary syphilis
- Non-Hodgkin's lymphoma

Method of examination (Fig. 1.8)

Feel the epitrochlear node with the thumb.

Patient's elbow is partially flexed and grasped by the examiner's hand (right hand for right epitrochlear node and vice versa) while patient's wrist is supported by the examiner's non-examining hand.

Inguinal Nodes

Palpate (Fig. 1.9)

Horizontal nodes at just below the inguinal ligament.

Vertical nodes along the saphenous vein.

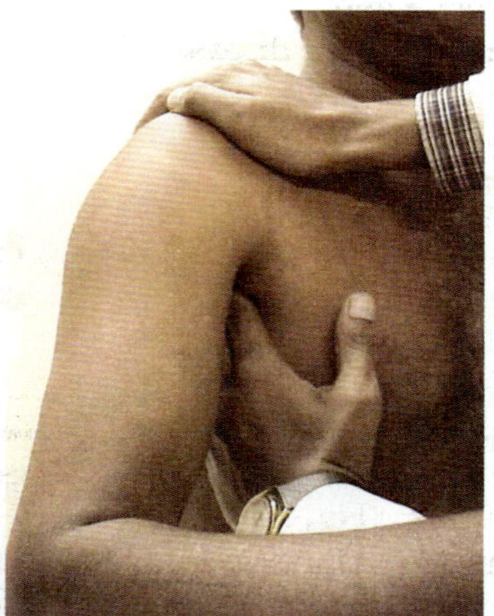

Fig. 1.6: Palpation of axillary lymph nodes (right side)

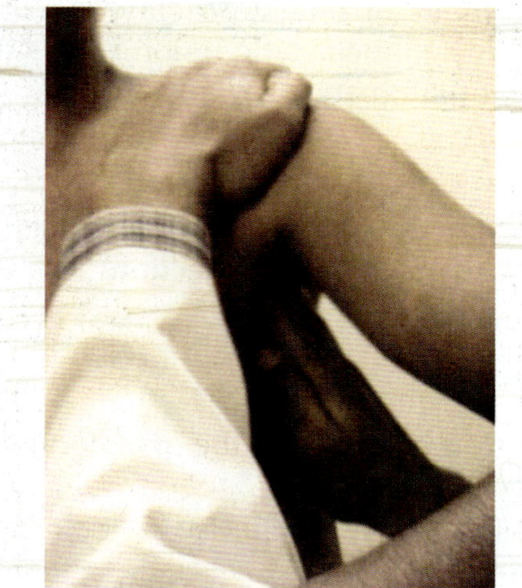

Fig. 1.7: Palpation of axillary lymph nodes (left side)

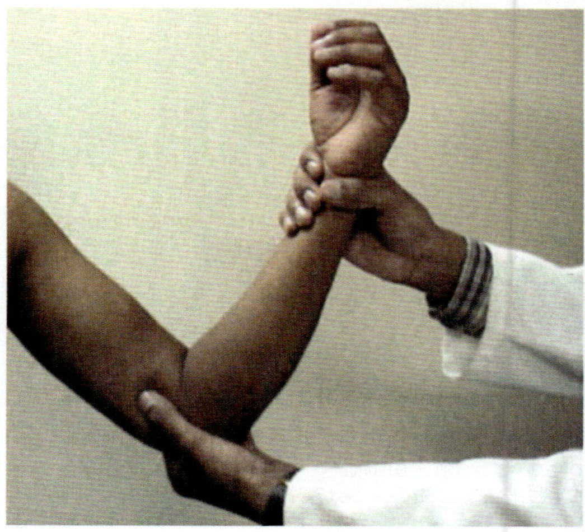

Fig. 1.8: Palpation of epitrochlear lymph node

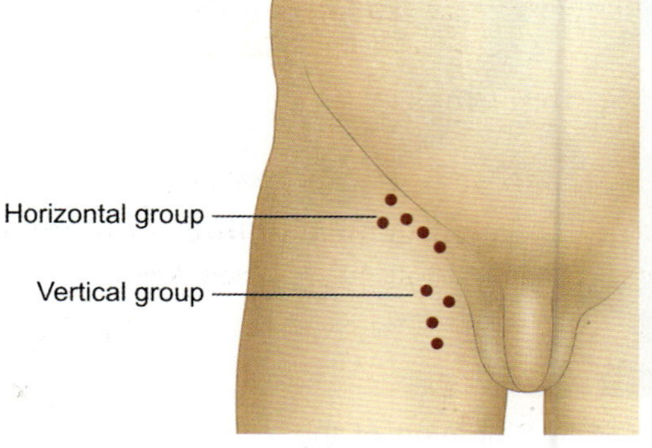

Fig. 1.9: Inguinal nodes

Causes of inguinal lymphadenopathy

- Infection trauma to the lower extremities
- Sexually transmitted diseases
- Lymphomas
- Metastatic cancer from primary in the rectum, genitalia and lower extremities.

Popliteal Glands

Palpate deeply into the popliteal fossa with both hands with the knee partially flexed.

Causes of enlargement of popliteal glands

- Knee joint disease
- Infection and trauma to the lower limb
- All causes of generalised lymphadenopathy.

Intra-abdominal nodes

Para-aortic nodes

Palpate deeply in the umbilical region along the aortic pulsation.

They are felt as round firm, confluent masses and are felt only when significantly enlarged.

Causes of intra-abdominal lymphadenopathy

- Tuberculosis
- Lymphomas
- Intra-abdominal malignant disorders
- Germ cell tumors

Intrathoracic Lymphadenopathy

Mediastinal and hilar lymphadenopathy.

Causes

- Bronchogenic carcinoma with secondaries
- Lymphomas
- Tuberculosis (usually unilateral)
- Sarcoidosis
- Histoplasmosis

B. Generalised Lymphadenopathy

Definition: Enlargement of three or more non-contiguous areas of lymph nodes.

Causes

Infection

- Viral infection
- Mononucleosis
- HIV infection
- Disseminated tuberculosis, histoplasmosis, etc.

Immunologic

- Rheumatoid arthritis
- SLE
- Sjögren's syndrome

Malignancies

- Hodgkin's and non-Hodgkin's lymphoma
- CLL
- ALL

Storage diseases

- Gaucher's and
- Niemann-Pick's disease

Endocrine disorders

Graves' disease

Drug-induced

For example, phenytoin sodium, carbamazepine, allopurinol.

9. PEDAL OEDEMA

Pedal oedema is due to excess collection of fluid in the interstitial tissues causing swelling of the tissues (Fig. 1.10).

Minimal swelling of the feet can normally occur at the end of day due to increased mean capillary pressure on standing.

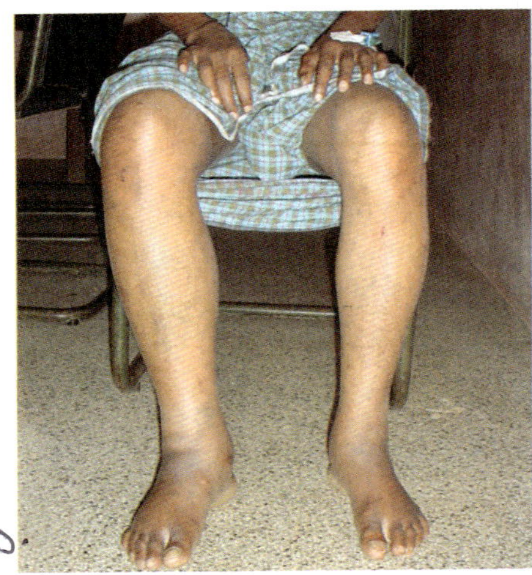

Fig. 1.10: Pedal oedema

Sites of Oedema

Site of oedema collection is predominantly determined by the gravity.

Common Sites of Oedema

- Legs, thigh, back, face and limbs.
- Sacral edema is common in bedridden patients.
- Abdominal wall edema can occur in patients with anasarca (pinch a fold of skin of abdominal wall and look for edema).

Elicitation of Oedema

Apply firm pressure over the lower part of the tibia (above the medial malleolus) or dorsum of feet for about 20–30 secs.

Observe for pitting nature of edema.

Pitting edema appears when the body weight increases by 10–15% due to fluid collection.

Causes

- Acute glomerulonephritis
- Nephrotic syndrome
- Cirrhosis of liver
- Congestive cardiac failure
- Hypoalbuminemia (nutritional)

Facial Oedema

- Loose subcutaneous tissue favours the accumulation of the fluid around the eyes.
- Periorbital puffiness occurs predominantly in the morning hours.

Causes of facial puffiness

- Acute glomerulonephritis
- Nephrotic syndrome
- Superior vena caval obstruction
- Angioneurotic edema
- Cushing's syndrome
- Myxedema

Non-pitting Oedema

Non-pitting oedema is characterised by the absence of pitting on applying pressure but with swollen tissues, e.g. chronic lymphedema, elephantiasis.

Myxedema is the collection of firm mucinous material in the subcutaneous tissues.

Different Types and Causes of Oedema

Oedema of upper part of the body can be caused by intrathoracic tumors.

Conjunctival Oedema (Chemosis)

Causes

- Graves' disease
- Superior vena caval obstruction
- Hypoalbuminemia

Localised Oedema

Causes

- Venous or lymphatic obstruction
- Allergic disorders
- Inflammatory disorders

Generalised Oedema (Anasarca)

Causes

- All causes of hypoalbuminemia
- Cirrhosis of liver
- Nephrotic syndrome
- Nutritional

Allergic oedema, angioneurotic edema usually involves face and lips and may affect glottis and larynx.

Unilateral Oedema

Causes

- Cellulitis
- Lymphatic obstruction
- Deep vein thrombosis

CNS lesion on one side can affect the vasomotor fibers on that side. Lymphatic and venous drainage is also affected on the affected side causing unilateral edema.

Lymphatic Oedema

Normally, lymphatics absorb small quantity of albumin filtered from the capillaries.

Lymphatic edema due to obstruction to the lymphatic flow.

Causes

- Recurrent filarial lymphangitis—limbs, breast and genitalia.
- After radical mastectomy
- Radiation for carcinoma breast
- Lymphatic obstruction due to mass lesion.

Milroy's Disease

Congenital hypoplasia of lymphatic vessels of legs associated with pedal edema.

VITAL SIGNS

- Pulse (*see* Chapter 2, cardiovascular system)
- Blood pressure (*see* Chapter 2, cardiovascular system)
- Respiratory rate (*see* Chapter 3, respiratory system)

Temperature

Usage of thermometer

Recording of Temperature

- **Conscious adults**: Record oral or axillary temperature.
- **Unconscious/collapsed/elderly**: Record the rectal temperature.
- **Children:** Record the axillary or rectal temperature.

Temperature can also be recorded in children in the groin with the thigh flexed over the abdomen.

Note: Rectal temperature is >0.5°C of oral temperature > 0.5° C of axillary temperature.

Key Points

- Thermometer must be accurate.
- Keep the thermometer for at least half a minute for temperature rise to occur.
- While recording the oral temperature, patient should breathe through the nose with lips tightly closed.
- Wash the thermometer with cold water and with antiseptic after usage.
- Shake the thermometer to bring the mercury column normal before recording the temperature.

- *Normal body temperature:* 36.6°C to 37.2°C or 98–99°F.
- Circadian variation—0.5°C.
- Normally evening temperature is higher than the normal.
- Lowest level of body temperature is at 6 a.m.
- Highest level of body temperature is at 4 to 6 p.m.

FEVER

Increase in the body temperature with a rise in the hypothalamic set point.

- Morning temperature > 37.2°C (98.9°F) or evening temperature > 37.7°C (99.9°F) is suggestive of fever.
- *Menstruating women:* Temperature becomes 1°F greater (after ovulation) in the morning hours and will remain till the starting of next menstrual cycle.

Hyperthermia

Increase in body temperature but hypothalamic thermoregulatory set point is not changed.

Temperature rise exceeds the body capacity for losing heat, e.g. heat stroke.

- Thyrotoxicosis
- Pheochromocytoma
- Neuroleptic malignant syndrome
- Malignant hyperthermia, e.g. succinylcholine administration.

Hyperpyrexia

Temperature greater than 41.6°C or 107°F.

Causes

- Falciparum malaria
- Pontine hemorrhage
- Thyrotoxic crisis
- Neuroleptic malignant syndrome
- Heat stroke

Hypothermia

Temperature less than 35°C or < 95°F.

Causes

- Head injury
- Near drowning
- Alcohol intoxication
- Drug overdose—sedatives and hypnotics
- Severe hypothyroidism

Fever (Different patterns)

- *Continuous fever:* Fever does not touch normal within 24 hours but fluctuation is less than 1°C.
- *Remittent fever:* Fever does not touch normal within 24 hours but fluctuation is more than 2°C, e.g. bacterial infections.
- *Intermittent fever:* Fever is present only in certain parts of a day.
- *Quotidian fever:* Paroxysms of intermittent fever occur daily, e.g. falciparum malaria.
- *Tertian fever:* Fever occurs on alternate day, e.g. vivax malaria.
- *Quartan fever:* Attacks of fever occur with afebrile periods of two days in between, e.g. malariae malaria.
- *Pel-Ebstein fever:* Fever increases and persists for few days (3–10 days) and followed by an afebrile period (3–10 days), e.g. Hodgkin's and other lymphomas.
- *Relapsing fever:* Few days of fever followed by days of afebrile state and then again fever relapses, e.g. *Borrelia* infection, rat bite fever.
- *Double quotidian fever (double spike):* Two spikes of fever in a day, e.g. visceral leishmaniasis.

Fever with chills and rigors

- For example, malarial paroxysms
- Pneumonias
- UTI
- Septic conditions
- ***Temperature and pulse association:*** Normally, for every one degree increase of temperature pulse rate increases by around ten/minute.
- ***Temperature and pulse dissociation:*** Relative bradycardia, e.g. typhoid, brucellosis, and leptospirosis. Relative tachycardia, e.g. myocarditis.

State of Hydration

Normal body water constitutes 60–65% of total body weight.

- Intracellular water—around 30 liters.
- Interstitial fluid—around 10 liters.
- Blood volume—around 5 liters.

Assessment of Hydration

Check for the following parameters while assessing the state of hydration:

- Skin elasticity
- Intraocular pressure
- Blood pressure recording
- Postural hypotension

Signs of Dehydration

a. *Dry tongue* (patients with mouth breathing can also have dry tongue).
b. *Skin elasticity:* Pinch a fold of skin, folded skin remains as a ridge which only subsides slowly. Fluid loss of 4–6 liters will result in dry, loose and wrinkled skin.
c. *Intraocular pressure:* Intraocular pressure decreases and the eyeball becomes soft in patients with dehydration.
d. Postural hypotension.
e. *Supine hypotension* (systolic BP less than 90 mm Hg).

EXAMINATION OF FACE, HEAD AND NECK

DIFFERENT TYPES OF FACIAL APPEARANCES

1. Endocrine Disorders

- *Hypothyroidism:* Dull appearance, facial puffiness
- *Thyrotoxicosis:* Prominent eyes, startled appearance
- *Acromegaly:* Prognathism, frontal bossing
- *Cushing's syndrome:* Moon face

2. Neuromuscular Disorders

- *Facial palsy:* Deviation of angle of mouth to one side.
- *Third nerve palsy:* Ptosis on the affected side.

- *Horner's syndrome:* Narrow palpebral fissure on the affected side.
- *Parkinsonism:* Expressionless, mask-like face.
- *Myotonic dystrophy:* Frontal baldness, ptosis, wrinkling of forehead, narrowing of lower half of the face (due to masseter atrophy).
- *Tetanus:* Risus sardonicus (sustained facial muscle contraction resulting in facial grimace).

Plethoric Appearance of Face

- Polycythemic disorders
- Cushing's syndrome
- Alcoholism

Mitral facies: Bluish appearance of face with malar flush.

Hemolytic anemia: Chipmunk face (frontal bossing, malar prominence, protuberant teeth).

Hippocratic facies: Found in patients with terminal stage of illness.

Characteristics: Sunken eyes, dry skin with flattening of cheek and temporal areas.

Other conditions which can be made out on examination of face:

- Butterfly rash of SLE
- Heliotrope rash of dermatomyositis
- Pallor, cyanosis and jaundice
- Wasting of muscles

EXAMINATION OF EYES (Table 1.3)

- Check for ptosis
- Squint
- Pupillary irregularity (for details *see* Chapter 5, nervous system).

Exophthalmos

Prominent eyeball with forward protrusion.

Causes of exophthalmos

- Bilateral: Hyperthyroidism

Table 1.3: Examination of different parts of eye in relation to general medical disorders

	Abnormality	*Associated disorder*
Conjunctiva	Suffused	Polycythemia
	Pallor	Anemic disorder
	Dryness	Sicca syndrome
		Vitamin A deficiency
	Hemorrhage	Leptospirosis
		Bleeding disorder
Sclera	Jaundice	Hepatobiliary disorder
		Hemolytic anemia
	Scleritis/Episcleritis	Connective tissue disorder
	Blue sclera	Osteogenesis imperfecta
Cornea	Opacity	Keratitis
	KF ring	Wilson's disease
Iris	Iritis	Inflammatory bowel disease
		Rheumatoid arthritis
		Infectious disorder
	Depigmentation of iris	Albinism
Lens	Cataract	Diabetes mellitus
		Hypocalcaemia
	Iridodonesis (tremulousness of iris due to subluxation of lens)	Marfan's syndrome

- Unilateral: Cavernous sinus thrombosis, intraorbital tumors
- Pulsatile: Caroticocavernous fistula

Enophthalmos

Inward movement of eyeball.

Causes

- Severe emaciation
- Extreme dehydration
- Horner's syndrome

Hypertelorism

Characteristics: Increased distance between the two eyes (distance between the two medial canthi is increased). There will be apparent broadening of the root of the nose.

Defect: Lesser wing of the sphenoid bone is overdeveloped with relatively smaller greater wings.

Significance: Associated with congenital defects/mental deficiency, e.g. Down's syndrome.

EXAMINATION OF LIPS, CHEEKS AND GLANDS OF THE FACE

Abnormalities of Lips

- *Cleft lip*: Usually congenital
- *Chelitis*: Inflammation at the line of closure or mucocutaneus junction of lips. Found in patients with riboflavin deficiency.
- *Angular stomatitis:* Inflamed and painful cracking at the corners of the mouth. Found in patients with iron and riboflavin deficiency.
- *Cold sores:* Vesicles over the lips due to infection with herpes simplex type I virus. Commonly associated with febrile states.
- *Thick lips:* Acromegaly, myxedema

Cheeks

Abnormalities	*Associated disorders*
• Puffiness	• Oedema states
• Malar flush	• Steroid therapy
• Butterfly rash	• SLE
• Mitral facies	• Mitral stenosis

Parotid and Lacrimal Glands

Parotid swellings: Present in front of the ear.

Causes

- *Unilateral*
  - Acute parotitis (associated with calculus and sepsis)
  - Occasionally mumps
- *Bilateral*
  - Mumps
  - Sarcoidosis
  - Sjögren's syndrome
  - Leukemias

Lacrimal Glands

- *Location*: Lacrimal gland lies beneath the lateral part of the upper eyelid visible on everting the eyelid.
- *Lacrimal sac*: Situated between the nose and medial canthus of the eye.
- *Abnormalities*: Damage to the lacrimal gland or lacrimal nerves causes dry eye due to decrease of tears.

Enlargement of Lacrimal Gland

Causes

- Mumps
- Sarcoidosis
- Lymphoma
- Carcinoma

Obstruction to the nasolacrimal duct causes: Acute dacryocystitis and lacrimal sac abscess.

> *Note:* Different abnormalities of movements of face can occur with nervous system disorders (*see* Chapter 5, nervous system).

EXAMINATION OF HEAD AND NECK

Hydrocephalus

Characteristics

- Increase in the size of the head compared to the body size.
- Protrusion of the forehead.
- Sunken, downward deviated eyes.

- Bulging of the frontanelles due to separation of sutures.
- Increase in the size of the head also occurs in patients with Paget's disease.

Frontal Bossing

Causes

- Chronic hydrocephalus
- Thalassemias
- Rickets

EXAMINATION OF NECK

Abnormalities

- Thyroid enlargement (goiter)
- Lymphadenopathy
- Neck veins
- Arterial pulsations
- Trachea
- Scar mark

Thyroid Enlargement (Goiter)

see Chapter 10 endocrine disorders

Characteristics

- Present in the region of the thyroid (anterior aspect of the neck).
- Swelling moves with deglutition.
- Swelling may be nodular or diffuse.
- Goiter may press over the trachea or may have intrathoracic extension.
- Hyperthyroidism is associated with bruit over the thyroid.
- Thyroid malignancy can involve the recurrent laryngeal nerve.

Palpation of the thyroid swelling

Person is comfortably seated and palpation of thyroid is done from standing behind.

Note: Any mass connected with thyroid will move with deglutition.

Minimal thyroid enlargement may be better seen than felt.

Torticollis (Wry neck)

Causes abnormal positioning of the neck:

- Due to spasmodic contraction of muscles supplied by the spinal accessory nerves.
- Head is drawn to one side with the chin pointing to the other side, e.g. congenital, dystonias, stiff and painful neck conditions.

Web neck: Occurs in patients with Turner's syndrome.

Scar mark: Look for the scar of previous lymph node biopsy or thyroid surgery.

EXAMINATION OF NOSE

Abnormalities

- Enlargement of nose
- Reddening of the nose
- Saddle nose (depressed nasal bridge)
- Destruction of nasal structures

Associated Disorders

- Occurs in acromegaly
- SLE with butterfly rash
- Alcoholics
- Lepromatous leprosy
- Congenital syphilis
- Wegener's granulomatosis
- Tuberculosis (lupus vulgaris)

Epistaxis (Bleeding from the nose)

Causes

- Local diseases of the nose
- Systemic bleeding and clotting disorders
- Occasionally in hypertensives

EXAMINATION OF EAR

Abnormalities

- Ear discharge–suggests ear infection
- Vesicles over the ear–herpes zoster infection
- Tophi–gouty arthritis
- Prominent crease seen over the ear lobule–associated with increased incidence of coronary artery disease
- Bluish appearance–peripheral cyanosis

Low Set Ears

Draw a line from the outer canthus of the eye to the pinna of the ear on the same side. If less than 1/3rd of the pinna is above the line drawn suggests low set ears.

Significance: Low set ears are usually associated with other congenital anomalies.

EXAMINATION OF BREAST

INSPECTION OF THE BREAST

Check for

- Symmetry of two breasts
- Presence of ulcers and any swellings

Inspect also the skin of the breast for

- Ulceration
- Reddening
- Peau d'orange appearance
- Dimpling of skin

Palpation

- Use the flat of the hand and palpate all the four quadrants of the breast tissue.
- Palpation should also be done with the patient keeping the hand under her head.
- Palpate also with the upper limbs above her head and also on leaning forward.
- Examine for any mass lesion. Define the size, shape, surface and fixity of the mass.
- Palpate also the axillary tail, axilla and local lymph nodes for any abnormality.
- Examine the nipple for any discharge (serous, milk or blood).
- Male breast should also be examined for abnormalities like gynecomastia.

Common Clinical Breast Abnormalities

Skin Changes

Dimpling of skin–simple and benign dimpling results in retraction of the skin which is mobile.

Key Points

- Explain the purpose of the examination and avoid unnecessary embarrassment to the patient, while examining the breast.
- Properly expose the pectoral girdle.
- Ask the patient to keep the hands on the waist for proper examination.

- With malignant infiltration of skin–tumor becomes fixed to skin.
- Peau d' orange appearance–orange-like appearance of skin.
  Skin is swollen in between hair follicles.
- Peau d'orange appearance is due to lymphedema caused by obstruction of the intramammary lymphatics by the tumour.

Lesions of Nipple

Nipple inversion

- *Benign:* Symmetrical slit-like appearance due to periductal inflammation.
- *Malignant:* Distorted asymmetrical inversion.

Discharge from nipples

- *Minimal clear fluid:* Normal on massaging the breast.
- *Blood stained:* Papilloma, carcinoma
- *Galactorrhea:* Milky discharge (hyperprolactinemia)

Breast abscess

- *Lactational* in breastfeeding mothers–peripheral abscess
- *Non-lactational* due to extension of periductal mastitis–abscess is at the edge of the nipple.

Fibrocystic disease

- Common before menstrual periods
- Irregular nodules of varying sizes found bilaterally.

Fibroadenoma

- Discrete mobile rubbery swellings in the breast.
- Common cause of lump in the breast in the young (< 35 yrs).

Carcinoma breast

- Firm or hard mass
- Usually fixed and irregular.

EXAMINATION OF HANDS AND FEET

CLINICAL ABNORMALITIES OF HAND

Colour Changes of Hand

- Nicotine staining of fingers–chronic smokers
- Severe pallor–anemic disorders

- Palmar erythema–liver disorders, polycythemic disorder
- Bluish discolouration–peripheral cyanosis

Temperature

- Cold hands–peripheral vasoconstriction
- Warm hands–hyperthyroidism, CO_2 retention

Size

- Large hands which are thick with spade-like fingers–acromegaly
- Thick hands–myxedema

Importance of Shaking Hands with the Patient

- Delayed relaxation of hand grip in patients with myotonic dystrophy
- Cold hands, sweating associated with tremulousness–anxiety neurosis
- Large hands with increased sweating–acromegaly
- Warm hands with increased sweating and tremulousness–thyrotoxicosis

Shape and deformities of Hands and Feet

Causes of deformities and different shapes of hands and feet

- Trauma
- Rheumatoid arthritis
- Arachnodactyly–Marfan's syndrome
- Short 4th and 5th metacarpals–pseudohypoparathyroidism
- Carpal spasm–tetany

Different Posture of Upper Limb

Flexed arms and hand on the affected side–hemiplegia

- *Wrist drop:* Radial nerve palsy
- *Ulnar deviation:* Rheumatoid arthritis
- *Claw hand:* Ulnar and median nerve palsy

Dupuytren's Contracture

Characteristics: Flexion deformities of 4th and 5th fingers due to thickening and shortening of palmar fascia, e.g. alcoholic liver disease, diabetes mellitus.

Table 1.4: Examination of nails

Different nail abnormalities	*Associated conditions*
Platynychia (flat nails)	• Iron deficiency anemia
Koilonychia (spoon-shaped nails)	• Iron deficiency anemia
Leuconychia (white nails)	• Hypoalbuminemia
Nail bed infarct	• Vasculitis syndromes
Onycholysis (separation of nail from bed)	• Idiopathic, lichen planus, thyrotoxicosis
Missing nail	• Nail–patella syndrome
Half and half nail (red brown distally and white proximally)	• CRF
Beau's lines (transverse ridges over the nails)	• Indicates stoppage of nail growth temporarily. Affects all nails and appear after few weeks of illness. As the nail grows ridges also move to the distal part.
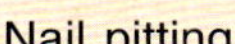 Nail pitting	• Psoriasis
Paronychia (swollen inflamed nail bed)	• Repeated trauma, working in wet conditions, diabetes mellitus, poor peripheral circulation
Discoloration of nails	• Anti-malarials, occupational, antibiotics, fungal infection, phenothiazines

Trophic Ulcers of the Hand

Causes

- Neurologic disease
- Vasculitic syndrome
- Raynaud's disease

EXAMINATION OF FEET (Table 1.5)

Bony abnormalities of lower limb

- Knock knees (genu valgum)–physiological up to 2 yrs of age
- Bow legs (genu varum)
  If persists after 2 yrs may be due to:
  - Rickets
  - Renal disease
  - Osteogenesis imperfecta
  - Rarely infection/trauma to the growth plate

Pes Cavus

Characteristics

- Increase in the arch of foot with fixed deformity.
- Foot is usually plantar flexed (equinus).
- Clawing of toes is usually associated.

Causes

- Familial SPFFa
- Peroneal muscular atrophy
- Friedreich's ataxia
- Syringomyelia

Rocker Bottom Feet

- Foot will be associated with protuberance of heel.
- *Significance:* Edward's syndrome (trisomy 18) with PDA.

EXAMINATION OF HAIR (*SEE* CHAPTER ON ENDOCRINOLOGY)

DEVELOPMENT OF HAIR AND DIFFERENT PHASES OF HAIR GROWTH

- *Lanugo hair*: Acts as a cover to the fetus. Fine hairs which are shed a month before birth.
- *Puberty*: Girls–hair development at pubis around the age of 11½ years.
  Boys–pubic hair develop around the age of 13 ½ years.
- Pubic hairs are coarser in nature and are under the control of adrenal androgens.
- *Axillary hair*: Appear after the pubic hair.
- *Body hair*: Develop and grow throughout the period of sexual maturity more in males.

Phases of Hair Growth

- *Anagen phase:* Growing phase of hair. Anagen phase of scalp hair lasts up to 5 years.
- *Telogen phase:* Resting or shedding phase may last up to 3 months.

Scalp Hairs

Total number is around 1 lakh. Check for the presence of nits, lice and dandruff over the scalp.

- *Nits:* Firmly adherent to the hair.
- *Dandruff:* Desquamatory lesions causing hair loss.

Table 1.5: Examination of feet

Abnormalities of feet	
Edema of feet	• Renal, cardiac, hepatic disorders • Hypoproteinemic states
Vascular changes: Chronic venous stasis	Pigmentation of lower part of legs and feet Eczematous changes and ulceration
Arterial ischemia	Pallor Loss of hair and sensation, ulceration
Neuropathic ulcers	• Painless ulcers develop over pressure points (diabetic ulcers)

Scalp Hair Loss

- Temporal recession of scalp hair occurs in males.
- Predominantly androgen dependant.
- *Alopecia areata:* Patchy scalp hair loss, e.g. local diseases of scalp–fungal infection and secondary syphilis.
- *Alopecia totalis:* Total loss of scalp hair

Causes of alopecia totalis

- Bacterial infection
- SLE
- Bums
- Radiation
- Fungal infections

Loss of Body Hair

Alopecia universals: Total loss of body hair.

Causes

- Anti-malignancy treatment, e.g. cyclophosphamide therapy
- Toxic illness
- Severe starvation
- Hypothyroidism

Flag Sign

- Brownish discolouration of hair interspersed with normal colour.
- It is a manifestation of protein energy malnutrition.

Loss of Sexual Hair

- Old age
- Hypopituitarism and hypogonadism
- Cirrhosis of liver

Excessive Hair Growth (Hypertrichosis)

- *Hirsutism:* Male pattern hair growth over the face, trunk and limbs in a female. Common after menopause.
- *Virilism:* Development of masculine features in a female.

May be a manifestation of excess androgen secretion.

Causes of excessive hair growth

- Familial
- Sexual precocity
- Adrenal hyperplasia/neoplasia
- Virilising adrenal tumors
- Drug-induced–androgens, minoxidil
- Polycystic ovary

EXAMINATION OF SKIN

DIFFERENT TERMINOLOGIES USED WHEN DESCRIBING SKIN LESIONS

- *Macule:* Flat and small lesions with altered texture and colour (< 2 cm).
- *Papule:* Solid elevated area of skin (< 0.5–1 cm).
- *Plaque:* Larger (> 1 cm) elevated area of skin.
- *Vesicle:* Small (< 0.5 cm) usually clear fluid–containing elevated lesions.
- *Pustule:* Small pus–containing lesions in the skin.
- *Bulla:* Large vesicle (> 1 cm).
- *Abscess:* Collection (> 1 cm in diameter) in the skin with significant depth.
- *Nodule:* Large (1–5 cm) solid lesion in the skin.
- *Wheal:* White compressible raised lesion produced by edema of dermis.

Localised pigmentation of skin

• Livedoreticularis	• Web-like lesions with reddish blue discoloration, e.g. autoimmune vasculitis
• Pellagra	• Pigmentation over the exposed parts of the body
• Erythema ab igne	• Due to long-standing sitting near the fire–with reticular appearance
• Café au lait spots	• See nervous system
• Rashes Fixed drug eruptions	• See next page

- *Angioedema:* Edema involving subcutaneous tissue producing a diffuse swelling.
- *Petechiae:* Bleeding spots (1–2 mm/pinhead size) in the skin.
- *Purpura:* Macular or papular collection of blood in the skin ($\geq$ 3 mm size).
- *Ecchymoses:* Large area of bleeding in the skin.
- *Hematoma:* Collection of blood in the skin with elevation.

Alteration of Skin Colour

- Pallor–*see* under pallor
- Flushed appearance of skin.

Generalised flushing of skin

Causes

- Febrile illness
- Hyperthyroidism
- Alcohol consumption
- Corticosteroid therapy
- CO_2 retention

Occasional attacks of flushing

- Menopausal syndrome
- Emotional outbursts

Pigmentation

Chloasma: Mask-like pigmentation of face, nipples, areola, etc. (e.g. pregnancy).

Characteristics of different types of pigmentation in different medical disorders

- *Addison's disease:* Bluish or brownish pigmentation

  Sites: Oral cavity, pressure points, bony prominences creases and scars.
- *Hemochromatosis:* Grey/grayish bronze colour of the skin
- *Acanthosis nigricans:* Thick brownish velvety appearance

  Sites: Axilla, sides of neck and groin

  Causes: Internal malignancy, insulin resistance
- *Xanthomas and xanthelasma: See* above.
- *Carotenemia and jaundice: See* jaundice

  Different skin lesions associated with general medical disorders

Autoimmune Disorders

- SLE Butterfly rash–*see* Chapter 9, locomotor system
- Systemic sclerosis–scarring and ulceration, acrocyanosis of fingers
- Dermatomyositis–edema of eyelids with heliotrope discoloration (*see* Chapter 9, locomotor system).

Inherited Disorders

- Peutz-Jeghers syndrome–lip and oral cavity pigmentation
- von Reclinghausen's disease–axillary freckling, café au lait spots
- Congenital ichthyosis–scaly skin

Systemic Disease

- *Erythema nodosum*: Reddish nodules, tender

  Site: Usually on the shin of tibia

  Causes: Tuberculosis, inflammatory bowel disease, sarcoidosis, leprosy, toxoplasmosis, sulfonamides
- *Depigmented macules:* Hansen's disease
- *Purpuric spots:* Bleeding/clotting disorders
- Pyoderma gangrenosum ulcerative colitis and skin ulcers rheumatoid arthritis.

Systemic Causes of Generalised Pruritus

- Diabetes mellitus
- Thyrotoxicosis
- Hepatic failure
- Obstructive jaundice
- Lymphomas
- Drug-induced
- Psychogenic

Drug-induced Skin Lesions

- Urticaria–penicillins
- Morbilliform rash–ampicillin
- Lichen planus like–gold and chloroquine
- Photosensitive–tetracyclines, sulphonamides
- Hair loss–cytotoxic drugs
- Erythema nodosum–sulphonamides
- Erythema multiforme–co-trimoxazole

Table 1.6: Hyperpigmentation of skin

Causes	
• Localised	Acanthosis nigricans Café au lait spots, nevus Fixed drug eruptions (recur in the same areas as circular areas of brown macules, e.g. analgesics, barbiturates, antimalarials).
• Generalised	Addison's disease Hemochromatosis Biliary cirrhosis Pellagra Megaloblastic anemia *Drugs:* Busulphan/Cyclophosphamide *Metals:* Arsenic/gold

Decreased Pigmentation of Skin

Types of Depigmentation and Associated Disorder

- *Albinism:* Total absence of pigmentation–congenital
- *Piebaldism:* Localised absence of pigmentation–congenital
- *Vitiligo:* Patches of depigmentation surrounded by hyperpigmentation, e.g. autoimmune disorders.
- *Tinea versicolor:* Localised hypopigmentation caused by pityrosporum
- *Post-inflammatory,* e.g. dermatitis/lupus disorders
  Hyperpigmentation of skin (Table 1.6).

SKIN LESIONS OF LEPROSY

Tuberculoid Leprosy

- Erythematous maculoanaesthetic patches.
- Lesions are few (single or 2 to 3 in number) and asymmetrical.
- Well-defined edges with central flattening.
- Hair growth is decreased with decreased sweating.
- Lesions will have few *Mycobacterium leprae*.
- Person reacts strongly to Lepromin test.
- Carries good prognosis.

Lepromatous Leprosy

- Multiple lesions, bilateral and usually symmetrical.
- Erythematous/hypopigmented patches with ill-defined edges.
- Patches may not have loss of sensation or loss of hair growth.
- May have papular, nodular lesions with thickening of skin.
- Lesions will have large number of Lepra bacilli.
- Lepromin test is negative and carries bad prognosis.

2 Cardiovascular System

CHECKLIST FOR GENERAL PHYSICAL EXAMINATION

- Symptoms and history of present illness
- Past history
- Family history
- Personal history
- Menstrual history and history of previous pregnancies
- Treatment history
- General physical examination
- External markers of cardiac disease
- Examination of peripheral cardiovascular system
- Examination of precordium

SCHEME OF HISTORY TAKING

Symptoms and History of Present Illness

- Dyspnoea
- Chest pain
- Palpitation
- Syncope
- Cough with expectoration and haemoptysis
- Cyanosis
- Right hypochondrial pain, swelling of feet and decrease in the urine output
- Gastrointestinal symptoms like anorexia, fullness of abdomen and vomiting
- Fatigability
- Fever
- Diabetes mellitus and hypertension

Past History

- Rheumatic fever
- Cyanotic spells
- Recurrent respiratory infections since childhood
- Detection of murmur/cardiac lesion at school going age
- Recent dental extraction, genitourinary instrumentation
- Hypertension, diabetes mellitus, ischaemic heart disease or any other significant medical illness.

Family History

- Hypertension
- Ischaemic heart disease
- Congenital heart disease
- Rheumatic heart disease
- Sudden death

Personal History

- Appetite
- Weight loss
- Disturbed sleep
- Bowel and bladder disturbances
- Habits–smoking and alcoholism
- Exposure to syphilis

Menstrual History and History of Previous Pregnancies

Significant in a female patient with cardiovascular disease.

Treatment History

- Penicillin prophylaxis for rheumatic fever
- Diuretics

- Anti-hypertensives
- Salt restriction
- History of taking sublingual medications
- History of taking drugs like aspirin, anti-coagulants, beta-blockers, digoxin, etc.

Specific History in a Patient of Suspected Congenital Heart Disease

1. History of heart disease, cyanosis and murmur in family members.
2. History suggestive of maternal rubella (fever with rash) during first 2 months of pregnancy (in patients with PDA, ASD, PS and tetralogy of Fallot).
3. Syncope, squatting episodes and attacks of cyanosis on straining (in patients with cyanotic heart disease).
4. Detection of murmur in infancy (usual in cases of VSD and PDA) and delayed developmental milestones.
5. Detection of murmur at school (school-going age) and restriction from physical activity at school and failure to thrive.
6. Recurrent attacks of respiratory infection and pneumonia since childhood (in large left to right shunts).
7. Consanguinity between parents.

APPROACH TO A PATIENT OF CARDIAC DISEASE

ANALYSIS OF PRESENTING SYMPTOMS

Dyspnoea

Definition: Abnormal awareness of breathing with discomfort.

- Dyspnoea is a significant manifestation of cardiac failure.
- Dyspnoea is more commonly due to left-sided cardiac failure than due to right heart failure.

Mechanism of Dyspnoea in a Patient of Cardiac Failure

Predominant factors contributing

1. Decreased lung compliance
2. Resistance to airflow
3. Excess respiratory stimulation and drive
4. Disturbed respiratory muscle function

1. *Decreased lung compliance is due to*
   Left heart failure causing pulmonary venous congestion and edema causing increased stiffness of lungs.
2. *Resistance to airflow is due to*
   Intrabronchial vessel congestion causing narrow airway caliber.
3. *Excess respiratory stimulation is due to*
   Stretch of J receptors (juxtacapillary) in the pulmonary interstitium, metabolic acidosis and hypoxia.
4. *Disturbed respiratory muscle function is due to*
   Decreased muscle blood flow, muscle fatigue, altered length and tension relation of the muscle fibers.

   Above mechanisms in combination will lead on to increased work of breathing and sensation of dyspnoea in a patient of cardiac failure.

Following details should be enquired with the patient while analyzing the symptom of dyspnoea

- Onset
- Duration
- Severity or grade
- Paroxysmal nocturnal dyspnoea
- Orthopnea
- Wheeze

Onset and duration

Acute or sudden onset of dyspnoea in a cardiac disease suggests:

Acute left heart failure (acute pulmonary edema), e.g.

- In patients with acute myocardial infarction
- Patients with mitral stenosis with atrial fibrillation

Non-cardiac Causes of Acute Onset Dyspnoea

a. *Respiratory causes*
   1. Acute attack of asthma
   2. Laryngeal edema
   3. Airway obstruction due to foreign body

4. Pulmonary embolism
5. Tension pneumothorax

b. Hysterical hyperventilation (dyspnoea is more at rest than on exertion)

Slowly Progressive Dyspnoea

Causes

1. Left heart disease with chronic left heart failure, e.g. left-sided valvular heart disease
   - Ischaemic heart disease
   - Hypertensive heart disease
   - Cardiomyopathy
2. Non-cardiac disorders like
   - Progressive anemia
   - Chronic bronchial asthma
   - Chronic obstructive pulmonary disease
   - Interstitial lung disease
   - Obesity

Severity (grading)

Functional grading of dyspnoea:

- *Grade I:* No limitation of any physical activity but dyspnoea occurs on more than ordinary (unaccustomed) exertion.
- *Grade II:* Dyspnoea on ordinary daily activity.
- *Grade III:* Dyspnoea on less than ordinary daily activities.
- *Grade IV:* Limitations of all activities (dyspnoea at rest).

PAROXYSMAL NOCTURNAL DYSPNOEA (PND)—CARDIAC ASTHMA

Significant Symptom of Left Heart Failure (Pulmonary venous congestion)

Description of an Attack of PND

- Patient goes to sleep without symptoms.
- Sudden awakening of the patient from sleep after about 2–4 hours of sleep.
- Associated with cough, wheezing and sweating with an attack of severe suffocation.
- Patient sits up and gasps for breath.
- PND is relieved by getting up and sitting upright usually requiring 15 mins. to half an hour (patient may not go back to sleep, as he is afraid of the next attack).

Mechanism of PND

Main factors contributing to pulmonary venous congestion.

After sleeping for 2–3 hours

- Shifting of fluid from the lower part of the body causing pulmonary venous congestion in patients with pre-existing left heart disease.
- Decrease in the lung expansion due to elevated diaphragm.

Other Mechanisms

- Decreased respiratory drive during sleep.
- Loss of sympathetic support to left ventricle during sleep.

All the above mechanisms will lead on to pulmonary venous congestion and onset of dyspnoea and suffocation resulting in PND.

Sometimes a PND-like attack can occur in a patient of chronic airflow obstruction. So it is necessary to differentiate between cardiac asthma (PND with wheezing) and bronchospasm due to airflow obstruction.

Differences between cardiac asthma and bronchospasm of chronic airflow, obstruction (Table 2.1)

Note: In bronchial asthma, maximum airway obstruction occurs between 2 AM and 4 AM

ORTHOPNOEA

Definition: Dyspnoea that occurs immediately on lying down.

Characteristics Features

- Usually occurs within minutes of assumption of recumbancy
- Occurs when the patient is awake.
- Indicates the presence of severe left heart failure (pulmonary oedema).
- Manifests later than PND. (In slowly progressive left heart disease.)

Table 2.1: Differences between cardiac asthma and bronchospasm of chronic airflow obstruction

Cardiac asthma	*Dyspnoea of chronic airflow obstruction*
a. Dyspnoea precedes cough	Long history of cough, sputum and wheeze Chronic smoking history may be present Cough with expectoration precedes dyspnoea
b. Symptoms of chest pain, palpitations are usually present	Usually not present
c. Getting up from sleep and sitting relieves dyspnoea	Dyspnoea is relieved by coughing out secretions (or by bronchodilators)
d. There may be evidence of cardiomegaly and murmurs	Rhonchi and crepitations may be detectable

Non-cardiac Causes of Orthopnea

Respiratory Causes

- Massive pleural effusion
- Tension pneumothorax
- Severe attack of asthma
- Emphysema
- Bilateral diaphragm paralysis

Abdominal Cause

Massive ascites

Mechanism of Orthopnea in Cardiac Failure

Main determining factor–pulmonary venous congestion.

On Assuming Recumbent Position

Pulmonary venous congestion occurs due-to-shift of fluid from lower part of the body to the lungs, which the failing left heart cannot accept. Raised diaphragm interferes with the lung expansion.

Above mechanisms in combination lead onto interstitial pulmonary oedema, decrease in the lung compliance with increased airway resistance resulting in dyspnoea.

Specific other Terminologies which are Used while Describing Dyspnoea

Platypnoea

Dyspnoea occurs on sitting (upright) rather than on lying down position. Example:

- Left atrial myxoma
- Left atrial ball-valve thrombus
- Pulmonary AV fistula

Trepopnea

Occurrence of breathlessness only when lying down in lateral position.

May be due to ventilation perfusion relationship alteration in certain body position. Trepopnea is usually associated with heart disease.

Wheeze

Suggests obstructions to the airflow in the medium-sized airways, can occur in patients of left-sided cardiac failure due to bronchial mucosal congestion.

Chest Pain

Chest pain of cardiac origin is predominantly due to myocardial ischaemia (ischaemic heart disease) because of coronary atherosclerosis.

Chest pain due to ischaemic heart disease is called angina pectoris (angina literally means choking).

Description of Angina Pectoris

Site

- Usually retrosternal.
- Sometimes occurs on both sides of the chest.

Type of Pain

- Specific character may be difficult to be described.

- Many patients describe it as a discomfort or an unpleasant sensation in the retrosternal area (while describing the pain, patient may keep his fist clenched over the precordial area Levine's sign).
- Sometimes the pain may be described as heaviness, squeezing, burning or constricting band across the chest.

Duration

- Usually 1 to 20 minutes.
- Unstable angina: Pain typical of angina but lasts for more than 10–15 mins and also pain may occur at rest.
- *Pain of myocardial infarction:* Prolonged angina-like pain persisting for more than few hours.
- If the pain lasts for less than 15 seconds, it is less likely to be angina pectoris.

Aggravating Factors

Exertion: Usually precipitates angina.

Pain of angina occurring at rest may be due to:

- Unstable angina
- Coronary spasm called Prinzmetal's angina.

Following Factors may also Precipitate an Attack of Angina

- Emotion and fright
- Cigarette smoking
- Exposure to cold
- Heavy meal

Relieving Factors

- *Taking rest:* Pain of angina characteristically subsides by taking rest.
- *Medication:* Taking coronary vasodilators like sublingual nitroglycerine.

Radiation of Pain

- Usually to the ulnar aspect of the left arm, wrist, epigastrium or left shoulder, neck and jaw.
- Rarely pain of angina can radiate to the right chest.

Associated Symptoms with an Attack of Angina

- Nausea, vomiting and sweating.
- Nausea, vomiting may be more likely associated with acute myocardial infarction.

Cardiac Causes of Precordial Pain apart from Angina Pectoris

- Pulmonary hypertension (due to right ventricular ischaemia or pulmonary artery dilatation).
- Pulmonary embolism
- Aortic dissection
- Mitral valve prolapse
- Pericarditis

Angina Equivalents

Some patients present with symptoms which may not be typical of angina but these symptoms indirectly suggest presence of coronary artery disease. These are called angina equivalents.

These may be:

- Dyspnoea—patient localises the site of origin of dyspnoea at the centre of chest (it is difficult to localise the actual dyspnoea).
- Discomfort felt in the lower jaw, left neck, shoulder and medial aspect of left arm and forearm.
- Dyspeptic symptoms like fullness of epigastrium, nausea and indigestion.

Patient with symptoms of angina equivalents may have other evidence of atherosclerosis like TIA, stroke and pain of vascular claudication.

Nocturnal Angina (Angina decubitus)

- Chest pain occurs in recumbent position.
- Resorption of fluid into the intravascular compartment in recumbent position results in increased myocardial oxygen demand causing chest pain (in patients with coronary artery disease).

Differential Diagnosis of Angina Pectoris

Even though many clinical conditions produce precordial pain, following conditions closely resemble angina pectoris and should be differentiated:

1. Costochondritis and myofascial pain
   - Pain is aggravated by movement of the chest and coughing.
   - There may be local costochondral and muscle tenderness over the precordium.
2. Acute pericarditis
   - Acute sharp pain and pain may last for hours.
   - Pain increases on breathing and decreases on sitting up and leaning forward.
3. Reflux oesophagitis GERD
   - Retrosternal/epigastric burning pain.
   - Pain increases on taking food and on assuming recumbent position.
   - No characteristic radiation of pain like angina pectoris.
   - Pain subsides on taking antacids or H_2 receptor blockers.

PALPITATION

Palpitation suggests awareness of heartbeat, which may be unpleasant.

Following details should be asked with the patient while analysing the symptom of palpitation

- Onset and duration
- Precipitating factors
- Relieving factors
- Description of palpitation
- Associated symptoms
- Post-palpitation diuresis

Onset and Duration

Palpitation which starts and terminates abruptly may be due to

- Paroxysmal supraventricular tachycardia (PSVT)
- Atrial fibrillation and atrial flutter. AF

Slow onset of palpitation with gradual termination of an attack may be due to

- Sinus tachycardia
- Anxiety states

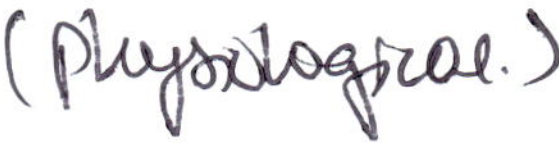

Precipitating Factors

- Palpitation on severe exertion is normal.
- Palpitation occurring on minimal exertion may be due to:
  - Anemia
  - Heart disease and heart failure
  - Atrial fibrillation
  - Thyrotoxicosis

Relieving Factors

- Holding the breath, induction of vomiting decreases the attack of palpitation in patient with PSVT.
- The decrease of palpitation may be due to the increase in vagal tone induced by these manoeuvres.
- Taking rest may relieve palpitation due to cardiac failure and anemia.

Periodicity and Description of Palpitation

Recurrent attacks of palpitation with absence of symptoms in between is common with

- Paroxysmal atrial tachycardia
- Intermittent atrial flutter and fibrillation

Palpitation may precipitate or aggravate cardiac symptoms like dyspnoea and angina, especially in patients with pre-existing heart disease. This may be due to:

Key Points

Palpitation may precipitate or aggravate cardiac symptoms like dyspnoea and angina, especially in patients with pre-existing heart disease. This may be due to:

1. Increased oxygen demand by the myocardium aggravating the underlying ischaemia causing the chest pain
2. Increased heart rate causes shortened diastole leading onto decrease filling of the left ventricle and pulmonary venous congestion leading onto dyspnoea.

1. Increased oxygen demand by the myocardium aggravating the underlying ischaemia causing the chest pain.
2. Increased heart rate causes shortened diastole leading onto decrease filling of the left ventricle and pulmonary venous congestion leading onto dyspnoea.

History of slow palpitation (due to slow heart rate) is found in patients with

- Complete AV block.
- History of forceful heart beat with throbbing sensation in the neck may be found in patients of aortic regurgitation or conditions associated with wide pulse pressure.
- If the patient feels irregular palpitation–skipped beats–it may be suggestive of a rhythm disorder like extrasystole or atrial fibrillation.
- Occasionally, patients may also give the history of feeling the sensation of the heart as stopped beating. This is due to the compensatory pause of extrasystoles.

Drug Induced Palpitation

Sympathomimetic amines, caffeine, smoking and vasodilators can cause palpitation. These medications should always be considered while approaching a patient of palpitation.

Associated Symptoms along with Palpitation

Occurrence of syncope following an attack of palpitation may suggest cardiac asystole/Stokes-Adams attack in a patient with complete heart block.

Stokes-Adams attack: Occurs in patients with complete AV block.

Characteristics

- Person loses postural tone
- Develops pallor and cyanosis
- Becomes flushed on recovery

Tingling and numbness of hands and feet, feeling of lump in the throat, hyperventilation along with palpitation occurs in patient with anxiety states.

Post-palpitation Diuresis

- Occurs usually after an attack of paroxysmal tachycardia.
- Due to the release of atrial natriuretic factor (stored in the atrial myocyte) due to atrial stretch.
- Suppression of ADH secretion may also play a role.
- Causes sodium and water excretion and diuresis.

SYNCOPE

Definition: Transient loss of consciousness with postural collapse.

Pre-syncope

A state of dizzy feeling with weakness and tendency to develop loss of postural tone. Consciousness is not lost.

Cardiac Causes of Syncope and Dizziness

Due to abnormal cardiac rhythms

Bradycardias:

- Carotid sinus syncope
- Sinus node disease
- Stokes-Adams attack
- Ventricular asystole

Tachycardias:

- Supraventricular tachycardia
- Ventricular tachycardias

Due to decreased cardiac output

- Massive myocardial infarction
- Cardiac tamponade
- LV outflow obstruction (severe AS, HOCM)
- RV outflow obstruction (severe PS, massive pulmonary embolism, severe pulmonary hypertension)
- Due to decreased venous return to the heart–atrial myxoma, ball-valve thrombus.

Differential Diagnosis of Syncope

1. Syncope which occurs on different body postures:
   a. As on standing for a long time
      - Vasovagal attack (common faint)

Note: Severe pain and emotional stress can also precipitate vasovagal attack.

   b. Immediately after getting up from the lying down position:
      - Due to postural hypotension.

      Causes
      - Antihypertensive drugs
      - Autonomic neuropathy
      - Volume depletion

   c. Onset of syncope on standing or bending and leaning forward–may also be due to left atrial myxoma and ball-valve thrombus.
   d. Syncope on movement of the head and neck may indicate:
      - Hypersensitive carotid sinus (especially in elderly)
      - Vertebrobasilar insufficiency (may be due to cervical spondylosis).
2. Syncope occurring at any body position may be due to:
   - Complete atrioventricular block
   - Hypoglycemia
   - Hyperventilation disorder
   - Epilepsy

Syncope on exertion: Significant symptom of severe aortic stenosis (AS).

Mechanism of Exertional Syncope in AS

During exertion there will be systemic vasodilatation. In patients with severe aortic stenosis, fixed cardiac output causes less blood supply to the brain causing cerebral ischaemia due to peripheral vasodilatation caused by exertion.

Other related mechanisms associated with syncope in a patient of severe AS:

- Transient arrhythmias
- Malfunctioning of baroreceptors.

Post-exertional Syncope

Syncope occurs after stopping the exertion.

- This is classically found in patients with hypertrophic obstructive cardiomyopathy.
- *Mechanism:* After exertion there will be pooling of blood in the lower limbs with decreased venous return to the heart. This leads to decrease in LV filling and LV volume causing more severe outflow obstruction in patients with HOCM.

Causes of Syncope Depending on the Onset

- Sudden onset of syncope: Stokes-Adams attack, ventricular tachycardia or may be a seizure disorder.
- Gradual onset of syncope:
  – Hyperventilation
  – Hypoglycemia

Symptoms along with Syncope

Following symptoms along with an attack of syncope may suggest the attack may be a seizure disorder rather than syncope:

- Clouding of consciousness for a longer time
- Incontinence
- Tongue biting and body injury
- Preceding aura

Significance of Associated Symptoms along with an Attack of Syncope

- Intake of insulin—hypoglycemia
- Intake of anti-hypertensives—postural hypotension
- Occurrence of chest pain—acute myocardial infarction, pulmonary embolism.
- Occurrence of neurological deficit—cerebrovascular disturbance
- Sudden getting up after micturition in elderly—micturition syncope.

Cough with Expectoration

Cough with sputum can occur in patients with cardiac disease under following circumstances:

- Dry, irritating nocturnal cough may be present in patients with pulmonary venous congestion secondary to left heart failure.
- Left heart failure results in pulmonary venous congestion and pulmonary edema-patient may bring out pink frothy sputum.
- Attacks of recurrent bronchitis are common with left heart disease (oedematous bronchial mucosa predisposes to recurrent infection).
- Patients with congenital shunt lesions like VSD, PDA, etc. can develop recurrent respiratory infection.

Following cardiac conditions may also present with cough with hoarseness of voice without upper respiratory infection:

- Aortic arch aneurysm
- Enlarged left atrium (severe mitral valve disease–Ortner's syndrome)
- Enlarged pulmonary artery (severe pulmonary hypertension).

Hoarseness of voice in above conditions is due to the pressure effect on the left recurrent laryngeal nerve.

HAEMOPTYSIS

Expectoration of blood with or without sputum can occur in a patient of cardiac disease.

Mechanism of Hemoptysis in a Cardiac Disease

a. Pink frothy sputum production in acute pulmonary edema.
b. Rupture of collaterals between bronchial venous and pulmonary system can occur in patients with mitral stenosis causing haemoptysis.
c. Edematous bronchial mucosa in patients with mitral stenosis may predispose to the development of chronic bronchitis with recurrent haemoptysis (winter bronchitis).
d. *Pulmonary infarction:* Due to congestive cardiac failure with mitral stenosis (late stages).

Pulmonary Apoplexy

This is the term used for the sudden severe haemoptysis which may be life-threatening.

Occurs in patients with early mitral stenosis.

Due to the rupture of thin-walled bronchial veins as a result of sudden rise of left atrial pressure.

CYANOSIS

History of cyanosis is relevant and may be present in the following cardiac conditions:

a. Cyanosis appearing in infancy indicates the presence of congenital cardiac anomalies with right to left shunt (e.g. Fallot's tetralogy).
b. Cyanosis beginning to appear after 6 weeks of age may be an indication of VSD with slowly progressive right ventricular outflow obstruction.
c. History of cyanosis in a suspected patient of congenital heart disease between the age of 5 and 20 years indicates reversal of left to right shunt (Eisenmenger's reaction).

Cyanosis predominantly occurring in the tongue suggests central cyanosis and can be due to:

a. Cyanotic congenital heart disease
b. Reversal of left to right shunt
c. Left heart failure

> *Note:* Cyanosis may not be present at rest and may appear only on exercise.

Bluish discolouration without cardiac disease can occur in patients with congenital methaemoglobulinaemia.

Arterial or venous obstruction, Raynaud's phenomenon can cause peripheral cyanosis.

Peripheral cyanosis can occur due to decreased cardiac output and cardiac failure

Pedal Oedema, Right Hypochondrial Pain and Decreased Urine Output

Presence of swelling of feet along with right hypochondrial pain suggest right ventricular failure (always associated with dyspnoea) in a patient of cardiac disease.

Swelling of Feet (Pedal oedema)

Right heart failure causes systemic venous congestion with increased hydrostatic pressure in the lower limb veins. This results in the transudation of fluid causing edema.

Ankle oedema is more common in ambulatory patients. Bedridden patients develop sacral edema.

Right Hypochondrial Pain

This is due to the enlarged and congested liver and stretching of its capsule.

Decreased Urine Output

In the presence of cardiac failure due to decreased cardiac output, renal blood flow decreases with decrease in the glomerular filtration rate. This causes decrease of urine output in patients with cardiac failure.

Edema of Cardiac Cause but not Associated with Cardiac Failure (Dyspnoea and orthopnea are absent)

- Tricuspid regurgitation
- Tricuspid stenosis
- Constrictive pericarditis
- Patient with advanced heart failure can also develop generalised edema of the body (anasarca).

Nocturia (More urine produced during night)

Due to increase of renal blood flow during recumbency and redistribution of intravascular blood volume. May be an early manifestation of heart failure.

Gastrointestinal Symptoms

Patient with right heart failure can have symptoms of anorexia, abdominal fullness and right hypochondria pain. This may be due to abdominal visceral congestion secondary to heart failure.

Occasionally patients of acute myocardial infarction and digitalis effect may also present with nausea and vomiting.

Fatigability

Many patients with chronic heart disease complain of easy fatigability.

It signifies impaired cardiac function and low cardiac output with impaired skeletal muscle blood flow.

Excessive use of diuretics in patients with CCF, severe reduction in the blood pressure and use of beta-blockers can also cause severe fatigue in patients with cardiac disease.

Fever

Fever may be the presenting symptom in patients with infective endocarditis, rheumatic fever or other systemic infections with cardiac disease.

Rheumatic Fever

Following history suggests an attack of rheumatic fever

- Usual age group involved 5–15 years.
- Symptoms of sore throat (pharyngitis) 2–3 weeks prior to the onset of joint pain.
- Joint pain
  - Migrating joint pain that involves major joints
  - Joints will be swollen, red and extremely painful
  - Joint pain will subside within 2–3 weeks (occasionally even without treatment) without residual deformities.

Symptoms of Rheumatic Carditis

Chest pain (due to pericarditis), dyspnoea and palpitation (due to myocarditis) suggest the presence of carditis.

Occasionally patients may present with symptoms of chorea (Sydenham's chorea) like involuntary movements and higher mental function abnormalities. Chorea may occur as a lone manifestation after about 3 months after the initial attack of rheumatic fever.

Symptoms and signs of rheumatic fever respond effectively to acetyl salicylic acid (aspirin).

Infective Endocarditis

Suspect infective endocarditis in any patient who has fever with cardiac murmur especially with recent history of undergoing dental extraction or genitourinary instrumentation.

Miscellaneous History

History of diabetes mellitus, hypertension and bronchial asthma should be enquired in all patients with heart disease.

- *Diabetes mellitus:* Predisposes to coronary artery disease and cardiac muscle abnormality.
- *Hypertension:* Can cause LVH, cardiac failure, coronary artery disease and aortic-valve disease.
- *Bronchial asthma:* Beta-blockers should be cautiously administered in a patient of bronchial asthma with hypertension. It may precipitate bronchospasm.

Past History

1. *Rheumatic fever:* Enquire about the previous illness suggestive of rheumatic fever or rheumatic chorea. 50% of patients with rheumatic valvular disease may not give the history of rheumatic fever, as it would have been sub-clinical.
2. Recurrent attacks of lower respiratory infections since childhood is common in adults with left to right intracardiac shunts.
3. Detection of murmur at school going age may be an indication of presence of cardiac lesion since childhood (e.g. congenital shunt lesions–VSD, PDA).
4. Enquire about the recent dental extraction or genitourinary instrumentation in patients with cardiac lesion and fever to rule out the possibility of infective endocarditis.
5. Previous history of angina should be elicited in patients presenting with myocardial infarction or CCF.
6. Previous history of diabetes mellitus and hypertension should be enquired because of their importance in causing coronary artery disease and heart failure.
7. Enquire attacks of cyanotic spells and squatting after exertion–common in patients with Fallot's tetralogy.

Squatting after Exertion

Child assumes squatting position after exertion. Squatting results in increased peripheral vascular resistance and decreased venous return and decreased right to left shunt and decrease of dyspnoea.

Cyanotic Spells

Child becomes bluish, hyperventilates and may develop syncope and convulsion usually after feeding or crying due to decreased pulmonary blood flow and increased right to left shunt.

Family History

Following cardiac diseases can affect more than one family members. Enquire the patient about these cardiac diseases in other family members.

- Essential hypertension and hypertensive heart disease
- Coronary artery disease
- Congenital heart disease
- *Rheumatic fever:* Rheumatic fever can manifest in more than one members of a family because of transmission of streptococci due to overcrowding or close contact.
- Sudden death of a first degree relative in a family–one should search for causes like hypertrophic obstructive cardiomyopathy, prolonged QT interval and coronary artery disease in other close family members.
- Marfan's syndrome can cause aortic regurgitation and dissecting aneurysm of aorta and can run in the family.
- Enquire also about the history of murmurs, cyanosis in other family members in a suspected patient of congenital heart disease.

Personal History

Appetite loss and fullness of the epigastrium are common in patients with CCF and on digitalis therapy.

- *Weight loss:* Severe weight loss is common in patients with chronic heart failure.
- *Sleep:* Sleep may be disturbed due to PND and orthopnea in patients with cardiac failure.
- *Smoking:* Enquire the duration and amount of cigarette smoking. Smoking is a significant risk factor for coronary artery disease.
- *Alcoholism:* Enquire the duration and the amount of alcohol consumption. Alcohol in large amounts can cause cardiomyopathy, CCF and cardiac arrhythmias.
- *Urine output:* Amount of urine passed should be enquired in all patients with cardiac disease (as discussed earlier).

Menstrual History and Previous Pregnancies

Menstrual flow may be decreased in female patients with chronic CCF.

Pregnancy and Heart Disease

Detailed history of previous pregnancies should be elicited in a female patient with cardiac disease.

Altered Hemodynamics during Pregnancy and its Effect on Cardiac Function

- Blood volume increases rapidly during pregnancy starting from 6th week of gestation up to mid-pregnancy. Thereafter, increase of blood volume occurs in a steady manner.
- Stress, labour pain and contractions of uterus alter haemodynamics during labour and delivery.
- Immediately, after delivery excess venous blood will be shifted to systemic circulation. Contraction of empty uterus and release of inferior vena caval compression (compressed by fetus) will also add to the blood volume.
- Patients with significant cardiac disease may not tolerate the pregnancy because of increase blood volume and altered haemodynamics and can develop cardiac failure.

Treatment History

1. Patients with previous attack of rheumatic fever may be taking long-acting penicillin (Benzathine Penicillin) once in 3 weeks suggesting the prophylaxis against rheumatic fever.
2. Taking sublingual nitrates may indirectly indicate the presence of ischaemic heart disease.
3. Detailed enquiry should be made about anti-hypertensive medications. These drugs may produce postural hypotension, fatigability and palpitation (due to tachycardia).
4. Drugs like sympathomimetics and digoxin can induce cardiac arrhythmias and beta-blockers may precipitate an attack of cardiac failure in susceptible patients.
5. Anti-neoplastic drugs like doxorubicin, cyclophosphomide can also induce LV dysfunction.
6. Details of previous cardiac interventions like angioplasty, coronary bypass and valve replacement should be enquired. (May be on anticoagulation with mechanical heart valves.)

EXAMINATION OF CARDIOVASCULAR SYSTEM

Scheme of Examination

General Examination

- Build
- Nourishment
- Pallor cyanosis clubbing
- Jaundice, pedal edema, lymphadenopathy

External markers of cardiac disease

Examination of

- Face
- Eyes

- Skin and mucosa
- Extremities

Vital signs
- Pulse
- Blood pressure
- Respiratory rate
- Temperature

Examination of the Peripheral Cardiovascular System

Radial pulse
- Rate
- Rhythm
- Volume
- Character
- Condition of vessel wall

Examination of
- Carotids
- Other peripheral pulses
- Jugular venous pulse and pressure
- Peripheral signs of wide pulse pressure (in relevant situations)
- Peripheral signs of infective endocarditis
- Peripheral signs of rheumatic fever

Examination of the Precordium

Inspection
- Precordial bulge
- Position of the apical impulse
- Pulsations in the
  - Left parasternal region
  - 2nd left intercostal space
  - 2nd right intercostal space
  - Epigastric pulsation
  - Suprasternal pulsation
  - Engorged veins over the chest
  - Spine (kyphoscoliosis)

Palpation
- Apical impulse–position and character
- Left parasternal heave
- Palpation of epigastric pulsation
- Thrills
- Palpable sounds

Percussion
- Right cardiac border
- Left cardiac border
- Left and right 2nd intercostal space.

Auscultation

Mitral, tricuspid, aortic, pulmonary and other additional areas for
- 1st and 2nd heart sounds
- Additional sounds
- Murmurs

Examination of Other Systems

- Respiratory system
- Gastrointestinal tract
- Central nervous system
- Musculoskeletal, endocrine, etc. (if necessary)

Examination of the Cardiovascular System

Build

Short stature and growth retardation can occur in children with severe congenital heart disease.

Tall Stature

Marfan's Habitus

Associated with aortic regurgitation, dissecting aneurysm of aorta and MVP (mitral valve prolapse).

Features of Marfan's Syndrome

- Long extremities
- Arm span more than the total height
- Longer lower segment than the upper segment
- Arachnodactyly (long, spider leg like fingers)
- High arched palate
- Iridodonesis (due to subluxation of lens)
- Abnormal metacarpal index (*see* Chapter 1, general physical examination).

Nourishment

Extreme degree of emaciation can occur in severe chronic heart failure due to:

a. Excess metabolic demand
b. Intestinal congestion causing decreased nutrient absorption.
c. Loss of appetite, nausea and vomiting occur due to hepatic congestion or digoxin therapy.
d. Protein losing enteropathy associated with severe right heart failure.
e. Excess concentration of tumour necrosis factor in the circulation.

Obesity (predominantly abdominal) can be associated with coronary artery disease (*see* Chapter 1, general physical examination).

Ear: Presence of crease in the pinna of the ear–associated with increased incidence of coronary artery disease.

Eyes: Exophthalmos—associated with thyroid heart disease.

Blue sclera: Osteogenesis imperfecta with aortic regurgitation.

Ophthalmic fundus: Look for
- Arteriosclerotic changes
- Hypertensive retinopathy
- Roth's spots (of infective endocarditis)
- Arterial pulsations in AR
- Corkscrew arteries—coarctation of aorta

Skin and mucous membranes: Look for
- Cyanosis, jaundice
- Bronze pigmentation (haemochromatosis with cardiomyopathy)
- *Xanthomas:* Fat-filled nodules found in the skin, tendon or soft tissues, associated with early coronary atherosclerosis (*see* Chapter 1, general physical examination).
- *Xanthelasma:* Deposition of lipid in the skin of eyelids—upper and lower eyelids (may be associated with hyperlipidemia).

Extremities:
- Arachnadactyly with long extremities:
  - Found in patients with Marfan's syndrome.
- Turner's syndrome:
  - Short statured female, cubitus valgus, medial deviation of extended forearm

Associated cardiac condition:
- Coarctation of aorta
- Bicuspid aortic valve
- Holt Oram's syndrome:
  - Thumb with an extra phalanx
  - Thumb lies in the same plane as other fingers
  - Radius and ulna may be deformed
  - Associated cardiac condition–ASD

General examination also includes the following signs

Pallor

Severe anemia may be associated with
- Chronic CCF
- Infective endocarditis

Severe anemia can itself cause—cardiac failure or aggravate the underlying heart disease

Patients with cyanotic congenital heart disease may have—polycythemia with suffused conjunctiva.

Table 2.2: Examination of face

Abnormalities	*Condition associated*
Following features may be indicative of underlying cardiac abnormality while examining the face	
• *Elfin facies*	
– Receding jaw, flared nostrils	Supravalvular aortic stenosis
– Pointed ears	
• *Mitral facies*	
– Malar flush	Mitral stenosis with decreased cardiac output and systemic vasoconstriction
– Pinkish purple patches over the cheek	
• High arched palate	Marfan's syndrome

Cyanosis

Central cyanosis occurs in the following cardiac conditions:

- Cyanotic congenital heart disease
- Reversal of left to right shunt
- Intrapulmonary right to left shunt
- Pulmonary edema (left heart failure)

Peripheral cyanosis occurs in

- Congestive cardiac failure
- Peripheral vascular disease

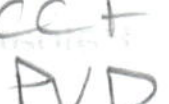

Differential cyanosis

Feet and toes are blue but hands and fingers are not cyanosed, e.g. PDA with pulmonary hypertension with reversal of shunt.

Reverse differential cyanosis

Fingers are more cyanosed than toes, e.g. transposition of great vessels with pulmonary hypertension with preductal coarctation with reversed flow through PDA.

Clubbing

Cardiac causes:

- Cyanotic congenital heart disease
- Reversal of left to right shunt
- Infective endocarditis

Cyanotic congenital heart disease may be associated with hypertrophic osteoarthropathy.

Jaundice

Following cardiac conditions may be associated with jaundice.

- Congestive cardiac failure with congestive hepatomegaly
- Cardiac cirrhosis
- Pulmonary infarction

Pedal oedema

Pitting edema of the feet can occur in:

- Congestive cardiac failure
- Constrictive pericarditis
- Tricuspid valve disease

Lymphadenopathy

Conditions associated with generalised lymphadenopathy may involve the cardiovascular system, e.g. lymphoma, SLE, etc.

Vital signs

- Pulse rate, rhythm, volume, character and condition of the vessel wall
- Blood pressure
- Respiratory rate
- Temperature

SYSTEMIC EXAMINATION OF CARDIOVASCULAR SYSTEM

Peripheral Vascular System

Pulse Definition

Waveform felt regularly over an artery due to expansion and elongation of the arterial walls passively produced by pressure changes during ventricular systole and diastole.

Radial Pulse *(Fig. 2.1)*

Compress the vessel against the lower end of the radius and feel the vessel with tips of fingers just lateral to the tendon of flexor carpi radialis.

Felt 80 millisecs after cardiac systole.

Brachial Artery

Feel the vessel immediately medial to the tendon of biceps by compressing the vessel against the humerus.

Felt 60 millisecs after the cardiac systole.

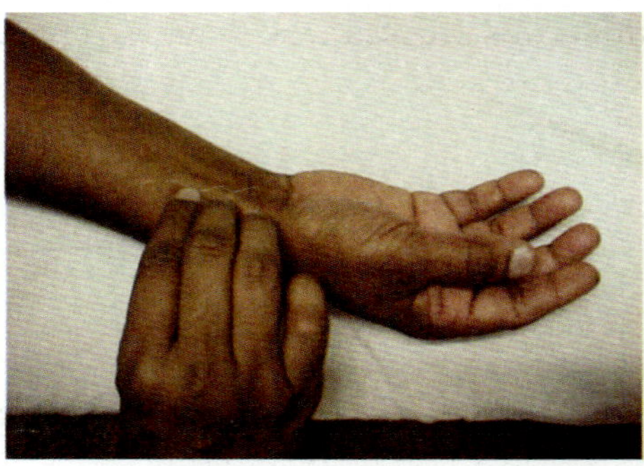

Fig. 2.1: Palpation of radial pulse at wrist

Carotid Artery

Press the thumb against the transverse process of cervical vertebra gently backwards. Feel the vessel at the medial border of the sternomastoid at the level of larynx. Right thumb is used for left carotid palpation and vice versa. Both carotids should not be palpated simultaneously.

- Careful palpation is required in patients with carotid atheroma or hypersensitive carotid sinus. (Elderly—palpate low down in the neck.)
- Carotid pulse is felt 30 millisecs after the cardiac systole.

Importance of Carotid Examination in Cardiac Disease

Carotid pulse should be examined for:

- Presence of thrill–associated with valvular aortic stenosis

Character of carotid pulse

- Slow upstroke–severe aortic stenosis
- Dancing carotids–severe aortic regurgitation
- Jerky carotids–obstructive cardiomyopathy

Femoral Artery

Feel the artery against the femur at a point midway between the iliac crest and the pubic ramus. Felt 75 millisecs after the cardiac systole.

Popliteal Artery

Feel the artery deep in the popliteal fossa with the fingertips pressed when the patient's knee is slightly flexed.

Posterior Tibial

Feel the artery behind the medial malleolus when the patient's foot is partially dorsiflexed.

Dorsalis Pedis

Palpate on the dorsum of the foot lateral to the tendon of extensor hallusis by compressing against the tarsal bones (Fig. 2.2).

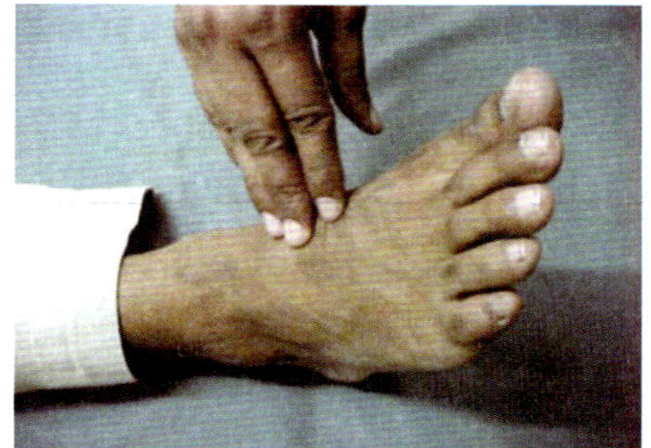

Fig. 2.2: Palpation of dorsalis pedis artery pulsation

Following parameters should be recorded while feeling for the pulse:

- Rate
- Rhythm
- Volume
- Character
- Condition of the vessel wall.

Rate: Normal rate–60 to 100/min.

Count at least for 30 seconds (ideally for one minute).

Abnormalities of the Pulse Rate

a. Bradycardia: Rate < 60/min

Causes

- Physiological—athletes
- Pathological
  - Complete AV block, beta-blocker therapy
  - Hypothyroidism

b. Tachycardia: Rate >100/min

Causes

- Physiological–exercise, anxiety
- Pathological
  - Supraventricular tachycardia
  - Tachyarrhythmias
  - Thyrotoxicosis
  - Sympathomimetic drug therapy, etc.

Rhythm

Normal: Regular sinus rhythm

Abnormal: Irregular rhythm.

Sinus Arrhythmia

Physiological acceleration of heart rate during inspiration and slowing at the beginning of expiration.

Common in young adults with increased vagal tone.

Sinus arrhythmia is abolished in patients with CCF and autonomic neuropathy.

Abnormal Rhythms of Pulse

Irregularly irregular causes

- Atrial fibrillation
- Extrasystoles (occasionally irregular)
- Paroxysmal atrial tachycardia, atrial flutter with varying block.

Regularly irregular pulse

- Pulsus bigeminus
- Pulsus trigeminus
- Paroxysmal atrial tachycardia and atrial flutter with fixed block.

Apex Pulse Deficit in Atrial Fibrillation

Count the pulse rate and heart rate for full one minute simultaneously. Note the difference between the heart rate and the pulse rate. In patients with atrial fibrillation heart rate will be significantly more than the pulse rate.

Mechanism of Apex Pulse Deficit

- There will be varying length of the LV diastole in patients with atrial fibrillation if there is shorter diastole (less of LV filling producing decreased stroke volume). Aortic pulse will be weak and may not be felt in the peripheral pulse.
- Longer diastole will lead onto increased LV filling with increased stroke volume resulting in stronger ventricular contraction causing peripheral pulse to be felt. This causes difference in the heart rate and the pulse rate causing pulse deficit.
- Varying length of the diastole is due to the varying refractory period of the AV node.

Differences between Multiple Ectopics and Atrial Fibrillation

Ectopics	*Atrial fibrillation*
1. Occasionally irregular	Irregularly irregular.
2. Pulse apex deficit minimum	Pulse deficit large.
3. Exercise abolishes ectopics	Exercise will not abolish irregularity.
4. 'a' wave is present in the JVP	'a' wave is absent in the JVP.

Tracing of a Normal Pulse Wave (Fig. 2.3)

- p–percussion wave
- n–dicrotic notch
- d–dicrotic wave
- p–percussion wave due to rapid rise of ventricular pressure and increased velocity of blood ejected from the ventricle.
- n–a sharp downward deflection related to the fall of aortic pressure due to backward flow of blood.
- d–dicrotic wave—small rise of pulse wave due to return of blood column due to closure of semilunar valves and also due to reflected waves from the periphery.

Special Characters of Pulse

Volume alteration in the pulse, e.g.

a. Anacroticus
 Alternans
b. Bisferiens
c. Collapsing
d. Dicroticus
e. Paradoxus
f. Parvus et tardus

Rhythm alteration in the pulse

1. Irregularly irregular pulse

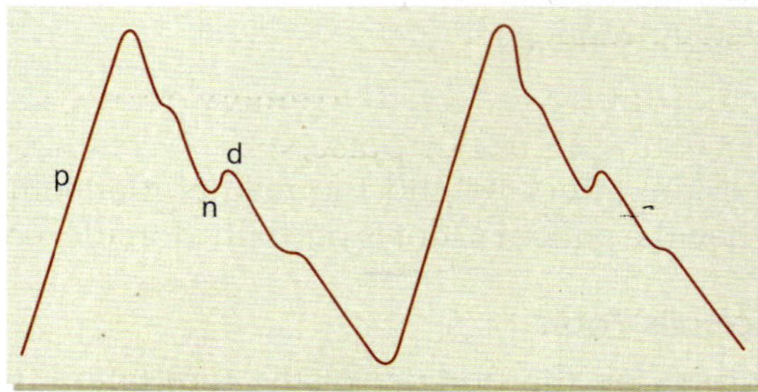

Fig. 2.3: Radial pulse tracing. p: Primary wave; d: Dicrotic wave; n: Dicrotic notch

2. Pulsus bigeminus
3. Pulsus trigeminus

Pulse Volume

Represents the degree of amplitude (expansion) of the pulse: Rough guide to indicate the stroke volume.

Volume Alternations in the Pulse

- High volume pulse (bounding), e.g. fever, anemia, AR and MR.
- Low volume pulse, e.g. state of shock, CCF and severe aortic stenosis.

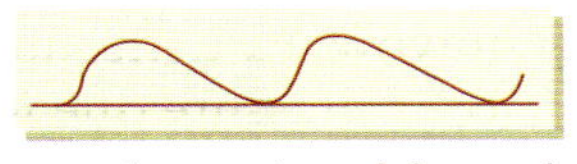

Low volume slow rising pulse

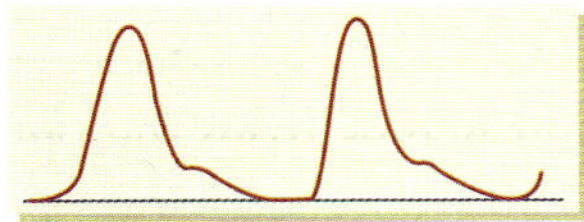

High volume collapsing pulse

Pulsus parvus et tardus

Low volume pulse with slow peaking, e.g.

- Aortic stenosis.
- Signifies fixed severe obstruction to the aortic out flow.
- Best appreciated in the carotids.

Collapsing pulse (Corrigan's or waterhammer pulse) (Fig. 2.4)

Rapid upstroke followed by precipitous fall (downstroke) of the pulse and made prominent by raising the patient's arm.

Waterhammer effect: Extremely rapid and forceful upstroke of pulse, e.g. of collapsing pulse: Severe AR, PDA, and large arteriovenous communication.

Mechanism of Rapid Upstroke

Due to greatly increased systolic pressure.

Large LV stroke volume ejected into the empty arterial system.

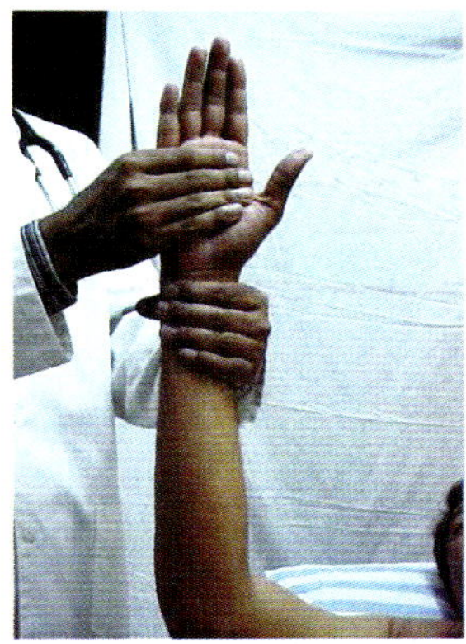

Fig. 2.4: Palpation of collapsing pulse

Rapid Downstroke

- Diastolic leak back into the left ventricle with sudden fall of aortic pressure.
- Peripheral vasodilatation and decreased peripheral resistance with rapid peripheral run-off of blood.

Note:

- Peripheral resistance may also decrease due to stretch of carotid and aortic sinus due to increased stroke volume.
- Patients of AR with CCF will have high diastolic pressure due to increased peripheral resistance.

Importance of Raising the Arm while Detecting the Collapsing Pulse

On raising the arm, peripheral run-off is better mechanism

- During rapid ejection of blood into the aorta at the peak of flow, sudden decrease of lateral pressure on the walls of ascending aorta occurs causing a sudden mid-systolic dip (Bernoulli effect–suction effect of rapid flow over a surface).
- Second wave on the upstroke—may be due to continued ventricular contraction and reflected waves from periphery.
- In patients with AS and AR mid-systolic dip represents decreased LV ejection due to maximum LV outflow obstruction at mid-systole.

Bisferiens Pulse

Pulse with 2 peaks (in systolic upstroke) separated by a dip (mid-systolic), e.g. in moderate AS with severe AR. In severe aortic regurgitation. Best appreciated in the carotids.

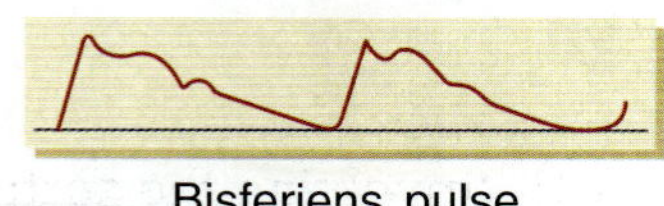

Bisferiens pulse

Mechanism

- During rapid ejection of blood into the aorta at the peak of flow sudden decrease of lateral pressure on the walls of ascen-ding aorta occurs causing a sudden mid systolic dip (Bernoulli effect–sudden effect of rapid flow over a surface).
- Second wave on the upstroke may be due to continued ventricular contraction and reflected waves from periphery.

Anacrotic Pulse

Slow raising pulse, peaking late in systole and will have a notch on the upstroke of carotid pulse "Anacrotic notch", e.g. patients with severe aortic outflow obstruction–severe AS.

Dicrotic Pulse

Pulse with two peaks, one in systole and other one in diastole.

Peak occurring in diastole is due to increased and palpable dicrotic wave occurring after the 2nd heart sound, best felt in the carotids.

Occurs in conditions with low cardiac output, soft elastic aorta and a high peripheral vascular resistance.

- For example, dilated cardiomyopathy and severe CCF
- Cardiac tamponade
- Young febrile patient without any other abnormality
- Hypovolemic shock

Pulses Alternans

Alternating large and small beats due to alternating strong and weak cardiac contractions.

- Occurs with regular rhythm and better appreciated with sphygmomanometer.
- Better felt in peripheral vessels (brachial/radial) it is ideal to hold the breath while checking for pulsus alternans, e.g. severe left ventricular failure.

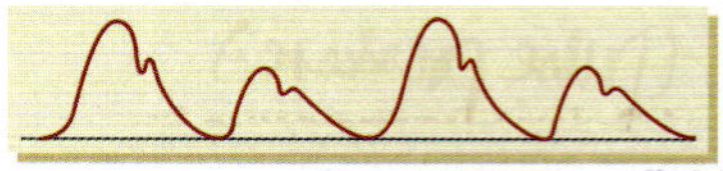

Pulsus alternans

Genesis of Pulsus Alternans

Represents significant impairment of LV function and contraction.

Weaker contraction is due to: Failure of some cells to contract (defective coupling).

Stronger contraction is due to participation of all cells after weaker contraction.

PULSES PARADOXUS

Felt as decrease in the pulse volume during normal inspiration due to accentuated fall in inspiratory systolic pressure, e.g. cardiac tamponade, constrictive pericarditis, severe airflow obstruction.

Normally, there is inspiratory decrease of systolic pressure of around 10 mm Hg.

In conditions like cardiac tamponade, severe airflow obstruction there is accentuated fall of systolic arterial pressure during inspiration.

This causes decrease of pulse volume or disappearance of pulse during inspiration.

Normal inspiratory fall in systolic pressure is due to:

1. Inspiratory decrease in the intrathoracic pressure causing pooling of blood in the pulmonary veins with decreased left ventricular flow and decreased LV stroke volume.
2. Inspiratory decrease in the intrathoracic pressure is reflected on the aortic pressure to drop.

Genesis of Pulsus Paradoxus in Pericardial Disorders

Inspiratory fall in BP: Due to reduced LV stroke volume.

During inspiration: There is increased RV filling causing bulging of interventricular septum and as LV cannot distend because of pericardial effusion and constriction, LV volume and filling decrease causing decrease of LV stroke volume and systolic blood pressure.

Genesis of Pulsus Paradoxus in Severe Airflow Obstruction

Following factors contribute to the genesis of pulsus paradoxus in severe airflow obstruction:

- Lung hyperinflation causes increase in pulmonary vascular resistance and marked decrease of intrapleural pressure especially on inspiration.
- Can also cause wide fluctuation in the intrathoracic pressure and decrease pulmonary venous return.
- Negative intrathoracic pressure can result in increased venous return to the right heart with increased RV volume and size. This can cause shift of interventricular septum to the left side causing decrease in the LV volume.

All the above factors contribute to the decrease in the LV stroke volume resulting in the inspiratory fall in the systolic pressure in patients with severe airflow obstruction.

Reverse of pulsus paradoxus, e.g. obstructive cardiomyopathy.

Alterations in the Rhythm of Pulse

Pulsus Bigeminus

Premature ventricular contraction occurring after each normal beat.

Premature beat is always followed by a short interval (pause), e.g. digitalis toxicity.

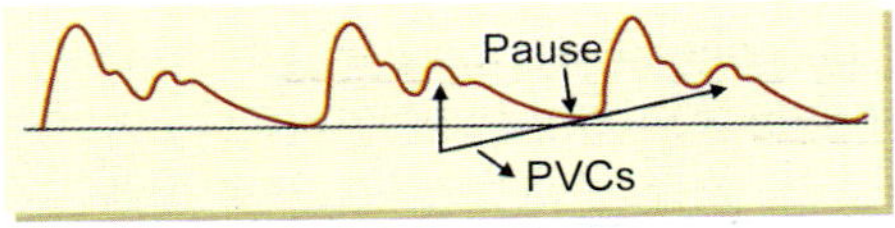

Bigemini pulse

Delay in the Femoral Pulse (Radio-femoral delay)

Delayed femoral pulse when compared to the appearance of right radial pulse occurs in a patient of coarctation of aorta. Delay of radial pulse:

Causes:

- Thoracic outlet obstruction.
- Aortoarteritis (involving the aortic arch).

Causes of radio-femoral delay

- Coarctation of aorta
- Aorto arteritis involving descending/ abdominal aorta
- Rarely atherosclerosis of aorta

Radio Radial Delay

- Thoracic outlet obstruction
- Aorto arteritis involving arch of aorta
- Supravalvular aortic stenosis
- Embolic occlusion of radial artery
- Aortic aneurysm

Condition of Vessel Wall

- Estimated by applying pressure with the fingertips over the artery or to roll the artery.
- Normal artery is not palpable (vessel wall merges with the surrounding tissues).
- In atherosclerosis the artery can be palpated and rolled with the fingers.
- Locomotor brachii: Dancing movement of thickened and tortuous brachial artery (arm is flexed at the elbow around 110° to make it easily visible). Indicates thickened vessel wall (e.g. atherosclerosis).

Importance of Examination of Peripheral Pulses in a Cardiac Disease

All peripheral pulses should be palpated. Start the palpation from peripheral pulse like dorsalis pedis and proceed towards the proximal pulses. Except for the occasional normal variation in their anatomical course, peripheral pulse may be feeble or absent in following conditions:

1. Conditions producing hypovolemic shock
2. Peripheral vascular disease

3. Embolic occlusion arising from the heart:
   - For example: Atrial fibrillation AF
   - Infective endocarditis IE
   - Left atrial myxoma
4. Coarctation of aorta–lower limb pulses are feeble.

BLOOD PRESSURE

Definition: Lateral pressure exerted by the blood on the vessel walls while flowing through it.

Measurement of blood pressure by cuff method.

BP Cuff Measurement

For the upper limb:

- In adults: Width 12 cm (should cover the 2/3 of the arm). Length of the cuff–25 cm
- Cuff width in obese–8 inches
- Cuff width for the lower limb—in adults 18 cm

Recording of Blood Pressure by Cuff Method

- Sphygmomanometer and observer's eye should be at the same level of the cuff on the patient's arm.
- Apply the cuff with its lower border I inch above the cubital fossa.
- Inflate the cuff to a pressure of 20–30 mm Hg above the level at which the radial pulse disappears. Place the stethoscope over the brachial artery.
- Reduce the cuff pressure 3 mm of Hg every second until the Ist sound is heard over the stethoscope (Korotkoff sound). Radial pulse becomes palpable. This indicates systolic pressure.

Key Points

- Patient should be in relaxed condition.
- All clothing should be removed from the upper arm before applying the BP cuff.
- Too narrow a cuff–BP estimation will be higher.

- Deflate the cuff until the sounds become faint (muffled) 4th phase of Korotkoff sound. Continue to reduce the pressure until the sound disappears (5th phase of Korotkoff sounds).

Diastolic Blood Pressure

The level of the pressure at which the Korotkoff sound disappear is taken as diastolic BP.

- If the Korotkoff sounds do not disappear even at zero mm Hg, then muffling of sounds (4th phase of Korotkoff) can be taken as diastolic BP. This is possible in conditions with extremely low diastolic BP such as severe AR.
- It is advisable to take 3 recordings (in basal conditions) a week apart to avoid anxiety associated hypertension (white coat hypertension) before defining the person as having hypertension.

If the diastolic BP increases on standing it is suggestive of essential hypertension.

If the systolic BP decreases on standing it may be suggestive of secondary hypertension (not on antihypertensive medication).

BP Recording in Patients with Atrial Fibrillation

Multiple recordings of BP and average of that are advisable in patients with atrial fibrillation.

- Systolic pressure: Level of blood pressure at which majority of Korotkoff sounds appear.
- Diastolic pressure: Level of blood pressure at which most of Korotkoff sounds disappear.

Key Points while recording blood pressure

- Record both supine and standing BP (2 minutes after standing) to rule out postural hypotension.
- Postural hypotension is said to be present when the systolic BP decreases by > 20 mm of Hg or the diastolic BP decrease by > 10 mm of Hg on standing. Postural hypotension can occur in patients with autonomic neuropathy or in patients on antihypertensive drugs.

Normal Blood Pressure

Systolic BP: 100–140 mm of Hg; diastolic BP: 60–90 mm of Hg.

Mean blood pressure

- Diastolic BP + 1/3rd of pulse pressure.
- Represents tissue perfusion pressure.

Pulse pressure: Difference between systolic and diastole pressure. Normal pulse pressure is around 40 mm of Hg.

Indications for Recording Lower Limb BP

1. If the pulse pressure is wide.
2. If the lower limb pulses are feeble.

Recording of Lower Limb Blood Pressure

- Patient is lying on his abdomen, BP cuff is applied above the knee around the thigh (cuff size 18 cm width).
- Auscultate over the popliteal artery in the same way as for recording of upper limb blood pressure.
- Normally, lower limb systolic BP is 10–20 mm of Hg higher than the upper limb (diastolic is identical).

Importance of Recording Lower Limb Blood Pressure

Lower limb blood pressure is decreased in patients with:

1. Coarctation of aorta
2. Aorto arteritis of the abdominal aorta
3. Aortic dissection

Lower limb systolic BP will be more than upper limb by 20 mm of Hg or more in patients with severe AR (Hill's sign).

Difference in the Blood Pressure in the Upper Limb

1. Supravalvular aortic stenosis: BP is higher in the right upper limb.
2. Subclavian steal syndrome: BP is reduced in the affected side.

White coat hypertension: Clinical or hospital recording of BP is higher than home recording.

Borderline hypertension: Initial diastolic blood pressure exceeds 90 mm of Hg, but repeated recordings will be below this level.

Annual checking of blood pressure is required.

Systolic hypertension: Usually defined as systolic blood pressure more than 140 mm of Hg with diastolic blood pressure less than 90 mm of Hg.

Causes

- Aortic regurgitation
- AV fistula
- Thyrotoxicosis
- Hyperkinetic circulation
- Beri beri
- Arteriosclerosis of aorta
- Patent ductus arteriosus

Accelerated Hypertension

Sudden rise of blood pressure above the previous recordings with fundal hemorrhages but without papilloedema.

Malignant Hypertension

Recording of diastolic blood pressure above 140 mm of Hg associated with papilloedema.

Pseudohypertension

- Condition characterised by high systolic and diastolic or mean BP measured indirectly by cuff method
- Direct intra-arterial recording of blood pressure is normal
- There is no evidence of hypertension induced target organ involvement (like retina, heart or kidney)
- It is due to sclerosis of arteries, e.g. elderly person, conditions like Monckeberg's arteriosclerosis.

Demonstration of Pseudohypertension

Inflate the BP cuff above the systolic pressure until the radial pulse has disappeared.

In patients with thickened arteries–radial/brachial artery will be felt even after the disappearance of pulse.

JUGULAR VENOUS PULSE AND PRESSURE (JVP)

JVP represents the pressure changes within the right atrium.

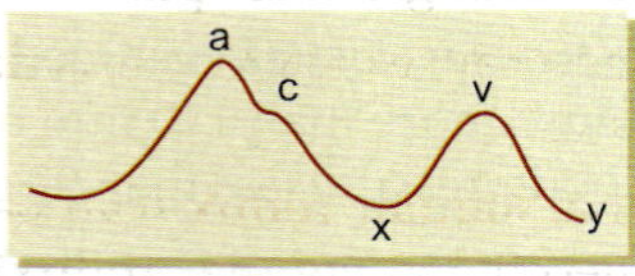

Normal JVP

Clinical Aspects of JVP

Internal jugular vein on the right side is preferred for examination of JVP as it is straighter than the left.

External jugular vein can also show the pulsations but less reliable than the internal jugular vein because of the following reasons:

1. It passes through fascial planes and extrinsic compression can alter the blood flow.
2. Because of the presence of venous valves, transmission of pressure can be interfered in the external jugular vein.

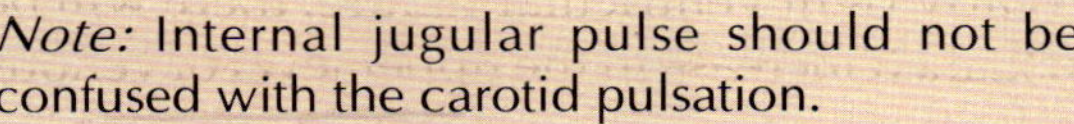

Note: Internal jugular pulse should not be confused with the carotid pulsation.

Normal Wave Pattern of Jugular Venous Pulse

Three positive waves (due to increased pressure in the right atrium).

- a–due to atrial systole
- c–movement of tricuspid valve into the right atrium during ventricular systole. (Carotid pulsation impact on the jugular vein may also contribute.)

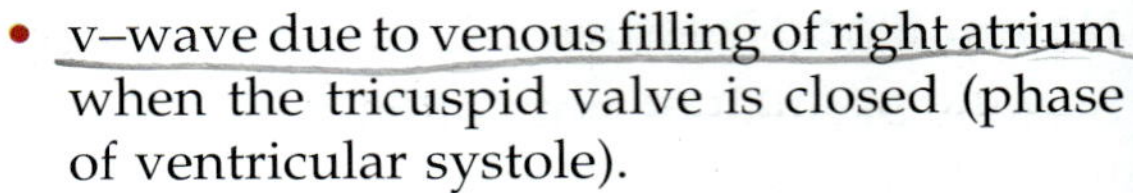

- v–wave due to venous filling of right atrium when the tricuspid valve is closed (phase of ventricular systole).

Two negative waves (due to decrease of pressure in the right atrium)

- X descent due to atrial relaxation and due to downward movement of the tricuspid valve during early right ventricular systole.
- Y descent due to tricuspid valve opening with right atrial pressure decrease.
- A wave usually precedes the carotid up stroke and v wave follows it. So waves of the JVP are timed with carotid upstroke.

Significance of Waves in the JVP

Prominent (Giant) 'a' wave represents forceful contraction of right atrium.

Causes

a. Conditions with stiff right ventricle:
   - RVH secondary to any cause.
   - Pulmonary hypertension.
   - Pulmonary stenosis

b. Tricuspid stenosis:
   - Prominent 'v' wave: Due to increased venous filling of right atrium, e.g. tricuspid regurgitation.
   - Prominent 'x' descent: ASD, RV volume overload, constrictive pericarditis.
   - Rapid 'y' descent: Constrictive pericarditis, tricuspid regurgitation.
   - Absence of 'a' wave: Atrial fibrillation cannon 'a' wave: Produced when the right atrium contracts against a closed tricuspid valve, e.g. regular cannon wave—atrial flutter with fixed block, junctional rhythm.

Table 2.3: Differentiating features between JVP and carotid pulse

	JVP pulse	*Carotid pulse*
Effect of posture	Varies with posture	Does not change
Effect of respiration	Changes with respiration	Does not change
Waveform	Present and better visible	Single upstroke better felt
Form of pulsation	Predominantly inwards	Predominantly outwards
Effect of finger pressure at the root of the neck	Abolishes the pulsation	No change and cannot be obliterated

- Irregular cannon wave: Complete heart block, premature ventricular beats.

Method of Examination of JVP

Patient should be comfortably lying in the bed at 45° position (for more effective examination 45° position is ideal. Keep the patient at 90° straight if venous pressure is very high).

- Neck can be slightly turned to the left side.
- Shine the torch tangentially across the neck
- Observe the lower part of the neck (at the medial border of the sternomastoid).
- Simultaneous palpation of the left carotid artery helps to differentiate between venous and arterial pulsations.
- Look for the waveforms.

Measurement of Jugular Venous Pressure (Fig. 2.5)

Patient is at 45° position.

1. Sternal angle is used as the reference point because the right atrium lies approximately 5 cm below the sternal angle at whatever body position.
2. Venous pressure (indirectly reflecting JVP) is measured from the centre of right atrium. Measure the vertical distance between the top of venous column and the level of the sternal angle. Normal distance is around 3–4 cm (cm of blood) which represents the normal jugular venous pressure.

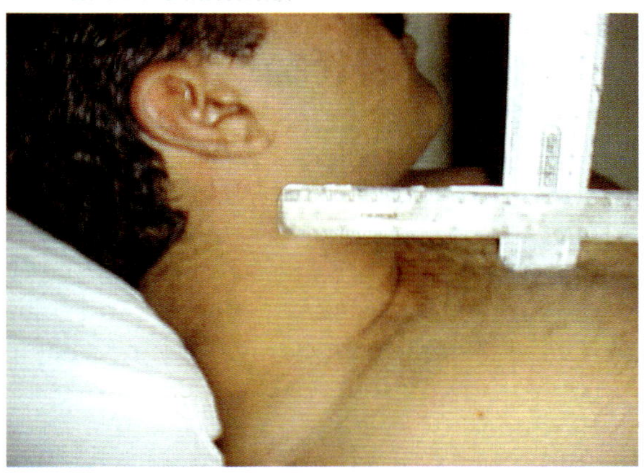

Fig. 2.5: Measurement of JVP

Normal central venous pressure is equal to 4 cm + 5 cm (depth of centre of right atrium from the sternal angle) = around 9 cm.

JVP is said to be raised if it is above 4 cm from the sternal angle at 45° patient's position.

Commonest cause of JVP raise is right-sided cardiac failure.

Abdominal jugular reflux (can be conventionally called hepatojugular reflux).

Helpful in detecting early right ventricular failure in patients who have normal JVP (at rest).

Technique of Elicitation

Apply firm pressure with the palm to the right upper quadrant of the abdomen for 10–30 secs while patient is breathing normally.

- Observe the jugular vein for any change in the level of pulsation.
- Normally, there is no significant change in the JVP.

Positive Test

In early right ventricular failure, there will be sustained increase in the upper level of venous pulsation (more than 4 cm). Can also be positive in a patient of tricuspid regurgitation. This test is negative in patients with hepatic outflow obstruction.

Causes of JVP Raise

1. Cardiac causes: Right ventricular failure.
   - Pericardial diseases, pericardial effusion
   - Constrictive pericarditis.
2. Congested states (no cardiac failure)—volume overload conditions.
3. Non-cardiac cause, superior vena caval obstruction (waveforms are absent in the JVP).

Note: Unilateral raise of JVP can occur in innominate vein occlusion.

Massive ascites and pleural effusion can also cause raise of JVP.

Kussmaul's Sign

Normally during inspiration upper level of the JVP decreases with negative intrathoracic pressure.

In a patient of constrictive pericarditis, there is increase in the upper level of JVP during inspiration. This is called Kussmaul's sign (due to interference with the blood flow to the right atrium during inspiration).

Causes of Kussmaul's Sign

- Constrictive pericarditis and CCF
- RV infarction

Peripheral Signs of Rheumatic Fever

1. *Arthritis:* Major joints—swollen, warm, tender.
2. *Erythema marginatum:* Red macular lesions with central pallor, non-itching and round margins found on trunk and proximal extremities.
3. *Subcutaneous nodules:* Nodule size—0.5–2 cm, non-tender and firm.

   Found over the extensor surfaces of knee, elbow and occiput.

Jaccoud's arthritis: Due to repeated attacks of rheumatic fever. Patient may develop marked ulnar deviation of the metacarpophalangeal joints due to subluxation.

In patients with collapsing pulse and wide pulse pressure, it is essential to look for other peripheral signs, e.g. in a patient of severe chronic AR.

Peripheral Signs of Chronic Severe AR

1. *Collapsing pulse* (waterhammer or Corrigan's pulse) already discussed.
2. *Corrigan's sign:* Dancing carotids (prominent carotid pulsation in the neck).
3. *Demusset's sign:* Nodding of head with each systolic pulsation.
4. *Quincke's sign:* Apply firm pressure on the nail tip. Observe for alternate flushing and blanching of the nail bed.
5. *Pistol shot sounds (Traube's sign):* Systolic sound is heard over the femorals when the stethoscope is placed on it.
6. *Duroziez's sign:* Systolic and diastolic murmur is heard over the femoral artery.
   - Proximal compression of the artery—systolic murmur is heard.
   - Distal compression of the artery—diastolic murmur is heard.
7. *Hill's sign:* Systolic pressure in the lower limb is more than the upper limb by more than 20 mm Hg. (Higher the pressure difference—more severe the AR.)

Other less prominent signs

- Pulsation of uvula—Müller's sign.
- Pulsation of the retinal artery—Becker's sign.
- Alternate blanching and flushing of face—Lighthouse sign.
- Pulsation of liver—Rosenbach's sign
- Pulsation of spleen—Gerhardt's sign.

Peripheral Signs of Endocarditis

In all patients with fever and underlying cardiac lesion check for the peripheral signs of infective endocarditis. These signs may not be present in all cases of endocarditis.

Signs of Endocarditis

1. Fever
2. Pallor
3. Clubbing
4. *Petechial hemorrhages:* Evidence of septic embolisation
5. *Splinter haemorrhage*
   - At the nail bed of fingers and toes
   - Flame-shaped or dark linear streaks
6. *Osler's nodes:* Tender subcutaneous nodules at pulp of fingers may be purplish red
7. *Janeway lesion:* Haemorrhagic or reddish macular lesions
   - Non-tender lesions over palms and soles
8. *Roth spots:* Pale centred oval haemorrhagic spots in the retina

Evidence of systemic embolisation and splenomegaly are other features of endocarditis.

EXAMINATION OF PRECORDIUM

Precordium: Area or part of the anterior chest wall which overlies the cardia (heart).

Important Anatomical Landmarks

1. *Midclavicular line:* Draw a line vertically downwards from the mid-point which is in between the suprasternal notch and tip of acromion.
2. *Anterior, mid and posterior axillary lines:* Draw vertical lines downwards along the anterior, mid and posterior axillary borders respectively.

Inspection and palpation can be suitably combined while examining the precordium. It is considered separately here in order to maintain the schematic presentation.

INSPECTION

Examiner can stand at the side of the bed or at the foot end for inspecting the precordium.

Precordial Shape

a. *Bulge (prominence):* Suggests cardiac enlargement before the occurrence of puberty.

b. *Pectus excavatum (sternal depression):* Pectus excavatum may be associated with ejection systolic murmur without any organic cardiac abnormality.

c. *Shield chest:* Present in patients with Turner's and Noonan's syndromes.

Characteristics of shield chest: Nipples are widely placed. Angle between the manubrium and body of the sternum is more than normal.

> *Note:* Well-built muscular chest with less developed lower extremities can be present in patients with coarctation of aorta.

APICAL IMPULSE

Definition: Outermost and lowermost definite cardiac impulse seen or felt.

Normal Apical Impulse

Seen when the patient lies supine or with the upper part of the body inclined to 30°. If not localized in supine position then patient can be made to sit and stoop forward (or patient laterally rotated to left).

Normal position: Left 5th intercostal space, 1 cm medial to the left midclavicular line or 9 cm lateral to the midsternal line on the left side.

Pulsations Over the Precordium

Look for the following pulsations over the precordium:

1. Left parasternal
2. Left 2nd space
3. Right 2nd space
4. Epigastric
5. Suprasternal pulsation

Details of these pulsations will be discussed under palpation.

Whole of precordium may pulsate under the following conditions:

- Severe aortic or mitral regurgitation
- ASD, VSD and PDA
- Hyperkinetic states (e.g. thyrotoxicosis).

> *Note:* Conditions like Fallot's tetralogy are associated with relatively quiet precordium.

Scar Mark

Observe for midline scar over the sternum

- Indicative of previous open cardiac surgery like coronary bypass graft or valve replacement.
- Left inframammary scar—closed mitral valvotomy done for mitral stenosis.

Spine: Look for kyphoscoliosis

- Severe kyphoscoliosis may lead to hypoxia and pulmonary hypertension.

Straight Back Syndrome

There will be absence of normal thoracic kyphosis in this condition.

Expiratory splitting of 2nd heart sound and parasternal mid-systolic murmur may be associated with it (may mimic findings of ASD).

- Diagnosis of straight back syndrome—mainly radiological
- Measure the intrathoracic transverse diameter just above the right dome of diaphragm.
- Measure the AP diameter from vertebrae to the back of sternum.
- If transverse: AP diameter ratio of 3 or more is suggestive of straight back.

PALPATION OF THE PRECORDIUM

Apical Impulse (Figs 2.6 and 2.7)

Palpation of Apical Impulse

- Patient is in the supine or sitting up position.
- Place the right hand over the left chest wall with the middle finger in the 5th intercostal space with its tip to locate the apex.
- Ideally patient should not be turned to the left lateral side for locating the apex, as cardia moves to a variable extent (around 0.5 to 1 cm) on turning to the left.

Normal Apex

- Normal apex is in the 5th intercostal space 1 cm medial to left MCL (midclavicular line), felt as a gentle tap and it is about 1 inch in diameter (up to 2.5 cm) and persists only up to 1/3 of systole.
- Apical impulse which is outside 10 cm to the left from the midsternal line is suggestive of cardiomegaly.

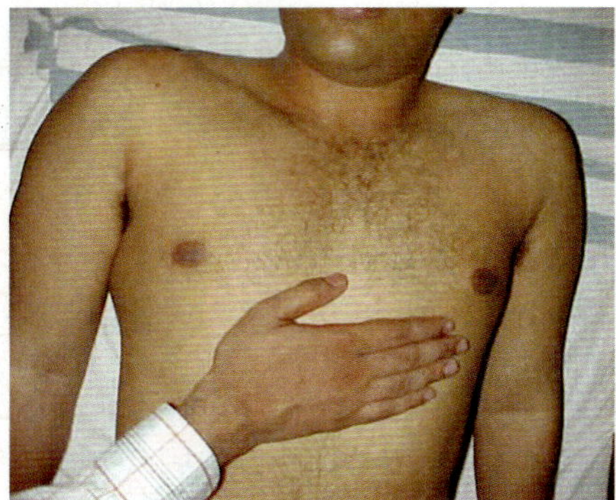

Fig. 2.6: Palpation of apical impulse

Key Points

1. Use fingertips for palpating sounds, distal palm or heads of metacarpals for palpating thrills and proximal palm for palpating heaves or lifts.
2. Time the palpatory events whenever necessary with simultaneous palpation of cardiac apex or carotid upstroke.
3. 2nd costal cartilage corresponds to the sternal angle from which the intercostal spaces can be counted for localisation of different cardiac areas.
4. Look for precordial tenderness (due to costochondritis) for the differential diagnosis of precordial pain.

- In patients with hypertrophic cardiomyopathy apical impulse will have two outward systolic movements (better seen than felt).

Dyskinetic Segment

This appears as a systolic bulge in patients with left ventricular aneurysm.

It is present about 1 or 2 intercostal spaces above and 1–2 cm medial to the apex.

Shifting of the cardiac apex occurs in following conditions

Cardiac cause: Cardiomegaly

Non-cardiac causes:

- Pleural or pulmonary disease
- Scoliosis
- Pectus excavatum

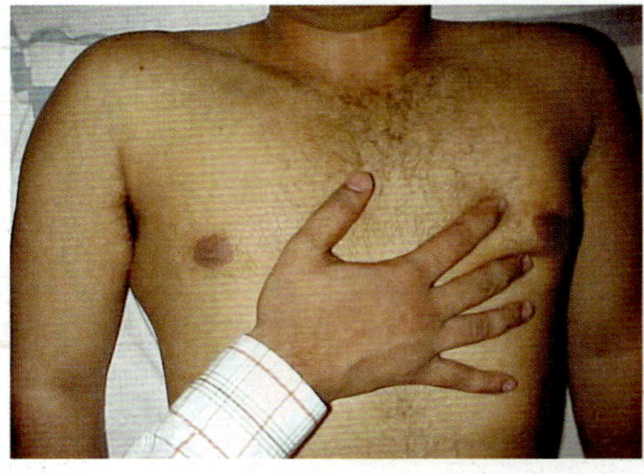

Fig. 2.7: Localising the cardiac apex with the finger (patient is supine)

- Conditions associated with elevated diaphragm (pregnancy, massive ascites).

Conditions wherein the cardiac apex may not be detectable

- Obesity
- Pleural or pericardial effusion
- Dextrocardia
- Emphysema

Congenital cardiac anomalies are more common with levocardia and dextrocardia than with situs inversus.

Different positions and characters of apical impulse

For detection of character of the apex, patient may be turned to the left (lateral side) (Fig. 2.8).

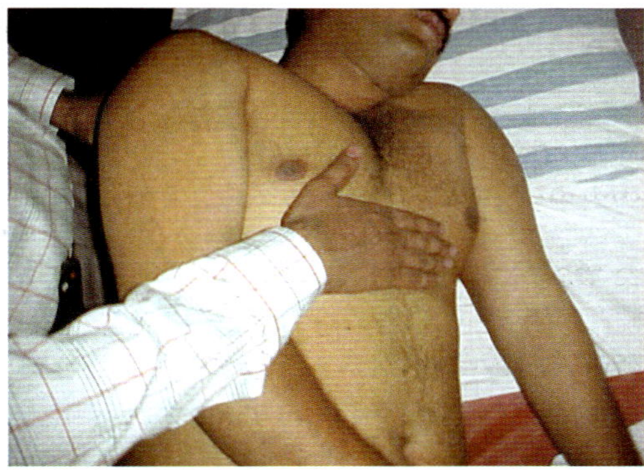

Fig. 2.8: Palpating the cardiac apex for the character (patient is in the left lateral position)

Tapping Apex

Felt as a hard-knock (like the knock on the other side of the closed door).

- Found in patient with mitral stenosis.
- It is the palpable loud 1st heart sound (closing snap).

Hyperdynamic Apex (Forceful)

- Apex is shifted outwards and downwards.
- With less sustained lift (more than 1/3 of systole but not throughout systole).
- Signifies left ventricular enlargement (volume overload).
- Apex is diffuse and may be more than 3 cm in diameter, e.g. AR and MR

Heaving Apex

- Sustained outward lift of the apex (duration more than 2/3 of systole).
- Position of the apex may not shift if it is concentric hypertrophy.
- Heaving apex suggests pressure overload of left ventricle (LV hypertrophy), e.g. AS and systemic hypertension.

Different Terminologies Used while Describing Cardiomegaly

- *Cardiac enlargement:* Suggests dilatation or increase in the chamber volume.
- *Cardiac hypertrophy:* Increase in the thickness of musculature and chamber volume is not increased.

Different positions of the heart in the thoracic cavity

1. *Situs solitus*	• Normal position Apex of the heart and stomach to the left side
2. *Dextrocardia*	• Heart and aorta are to the right side (stomach is on the left side)
3. *Situs inversus*	• Descending aorta, Left atrium, Cardiac apex, Stomach — are to the right side
4. *Levocardia*	• Position of the heart is on the left side (situs solitus) but stomach is on the right side
5. *Dextroversion*	• Aorta and stomach are on the left side, but apex of the heart is on the right, side (due to rotation)

Concentric Hypertrophy

- Uniform increase in the musculature with decrease in the cavity size.
- Dilatation may occur later.
- Occurs in conditions with LV pressure overload, e.g. systemic hypertension and aortic stenosis (severe).

Eccentric Hypertrophy

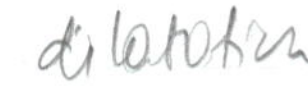

- Dilatation of the cardiac chamber with later occurrence of hypertrophy. Hypertrophy is not proportionate to dilatation.
- Occurs in conditions with LV volume overload, e.g. mitral regurgitation and aortic regurgitation.

Significance of other Pulsations over the Precordium

Left parasternal pulsations and heave:
Significance: Usually produced by the right ventricular enlargement or hypertrophy.

Method of Palpation

Patient is made supine and palpate during expiration. Best felt by the proximal part of the palm or fingertips kept over the left lower parasternal area. Appreciate the lift or heave.

Left parasternal lift (less sustained pulsation) signifies: Right ventricular volume overload conditions without hypertrophy, e.g. atrial septal defect and tricuspid regurgitation.

Left parasternal heave (sustained outward lift):

- Suggests right ventricular hypertrophy.
- Occurs in conditions with RV pressure overload, e.g. pulmonary artery hypertension and pulmonary stenosis.

In patient with emphysema—hyperinflated lungs intervene between the heart and chest wall, making it difficult to feel the left parasternal right ventricular pulsation. In such situations, it is ideal to appreciate the RV pulsation in the epigastrium.

Conditions Presenting with Left Parasternal Pulsation apart from RVH

Left 2nd intercostal space pulsation.

Occurs in conditions producing dilatation of pulmonary artery, e.g. severe pulmonary, artery hypertension, idiopathic dilatation of pulmonary artery, post-stenotic dilatation of pulmonary artery.

Technique of Palpation for Pulmonary Artery Pulsation

Patient is sitting and leaning forward. Press firmly with the finger over the left 2nd intercostal space.

Prominent systolic pulsation can be felt in the left 2nd intercostal space just to the left of sternum.

Suggests enlarged pulmonary artery pulsation. Sometimes only a palpable shock (sound) or tapping sensation felt which is due to loud pulmonary component of 2nd heart sound (P2).

This is found in patients with pulmonary artery hypertension.

Pulsation due to Massively Enlarged Left Atrium

Pulsation appears and ends later than the apex

- Felt at left of the sternum.
- Pulsation is due to—regurgitation of large volume of blood into left atrium.

Note: Pulsation due to RVH appears and disappears along with the apex.

Right Parasternal Pulsation

Occurs due to:

- Ascending aorta aneurysm
- Massively enlarged right atrium.

Rocking Movement of Ventricles

- LV hypertrophy produces lateral outward movement with left parasternal retraction.
- RV hypertrophy produces left parasternal outward movement with lateral retraction.
- Biventricular hypertrophy left parasternal and apical outward movement with inward movement of an area in between.

Subxiphoid (Epigastric) Pulsation

Causes: Right ventricular pulsation and prominent aortic pulsation.

- *Method of palpation:* Tip of the index finger or the thumb is inserted upwards and obliquely beneath (towards left) the xiphoid process with breath held in inspiration.
- *RV pulsation:* Pulsation is felt by the tip of the finger.
- *Aortic pulsation:* Felt by the pulp or beneath the pulp of the finger.

Suprasternal Pulsation

Causes

1. Unfolding of aorta or aneurysm of arch of aorta.
2. Hyperkinetic states.

Tracheal Tug

Demonstration of tracheal tug

- Hook the cricoid cartilage from behind with the fingers and apply upward pressure.
- Feel for the downward pull on the trachea with each pulsation (heart beat).
- Significance: Aortic arch aneurysm pulling over the left main bronchus.

Note: Patients with severe airflow obstruction will have tracheal descent instead of tracheal tug.

Pulsation of the Right Sternoclavicular Joint

Suggests: Anterior/right-sided aortic arch, e.g. Fallot's tetralogy.

Pulsation over the Posterior Chest Wall

Conditions: Coarctation of aorta due to dilated anastamotic channels over the surface of scapulae.

Method of examination for posterior chest wall pulsation

Patient will be standing and bending forward with arms hanging at sides. Inspect the patient's back around and between scapulae.

Pulsatile Liver

Palpate the liver bimanually. Hold one palm over the anterior surface of liver and the other palm its posterior lateral surface. Feel for the pulsation of the liver. (*see* also gastrointestinal tract).

Causes

- *Systolic pulsation:* Tricuspid regurgitation Aortic regurgitation
- *Pre-systolic pulsation:* Tricuspid stenosis

Thrills and Palpable Sounds

Thrills: Vibratory sensations (described as purring of cat) which are palpable manifestations of murmur.

Method of Palpation of Thrills

Best appreciated with the head of metacarpal bones (distal palm).

Significance of Thrills

- Suggests presence of a murmur.
- It localises the site of origin of a diffuse murmur.
- Favours (usually) presence of an organic valvular lesion.
- Thrills are more common with obstructive lesions with narrow orifice, thin chest wall and in conditions with rapid blood flow.
- In patients with valvular aortic stenosis thrill can be appreciated over the carotids.
- Diastolic thrill of mitral stenosis is better appreciated on turning the patient to left lateral side.
- Diastolic thrill in a patient of aortic regurgitation suggests severe AR.
- Continuous thrill is present in patients with PDA.

Sudden Appearance of Thrill

May occur in the following situations:

- Development of infective endocarditis causing valvular damage.
- Failure of prosthetic valve.

Palpable Sounds

Loud 1st sound of mitral stenosis: Felt as tapping apical impulse (closing snap).

Palpable 2nd Heart Sound

Palpable P2

- Palpable pulmonary component of 2nd heart sound.
- Felt as a tapping sensation in the left 2nd intercostal space (patient is upright and leaning forward).
- Due to forceful closure of pulmonary valve under abnormally high pressure.
- Found in patient with significant pulmonary arterial hypertension.

Palpable A2

- Palpable aortic component of the 2nd heart sound.
- Felt as a tapping sensation in the right 2nd intercostal space.
- Due to forceful closure of aortic valve under an abnormally high pressure.
- Found in patients with systemic hypertension.

Prominent 3rd and 4th Heart Sounds

Palpable as diastolic movement at the cardiac apex (left-sided 3rd and 4th heart sounds). Further details will be discussed under auscultation.

PERCUSSION

- Percussion gives less information in patients with cardiac disease.
- It is discussed here for completing the schematic presentation.

Key Points

- Always identify the area from where the thrill is felt.
- If the thrill coincides with the carotid upstroke it is systolic and if it does not, it is a diastolic thrill.

Percussion of Cardiac Borders

Right Cardiac Border

Define the upper border of the liver by percussing downwards in the midclavicular line from the right second intercostal space (normally upper border of the liver is in the right 5th intercostal space).

Percuss the intercostal spaces above the liver dullness in the midclavicular line moving towards the right sternal border.

- Observe for the change of percussion note (from the normal lung resonance to dull note).
- Normally the right cardiac border corresponds to the right sternal border.

Cardiac Causes of Dull Note Outside the Right Sternal Border

- Cardiomegaly
- Pericardial effusion

Percussion of the Right 2nd Intercostal Space

- Normally resonant
- In aneurysmal dilatation of the root of the aorta, right 2nd intercostal space becomes dull on percussion.

Percussion of the Left Cardiac Border

1. Find the apical impulse.
2. Start percussion from outside the apex in the 5th intercostal space (or from the mid-axillary line, if the apex is not felt) moving medially towards the left sternal border.
3. Percuss parallel to the left sternal border.
4. Observe for the changing percussion note from the normal lung resonance.
5. Percussion note changes to dullness when one reaches the left cardiac border (apex).
6. Repeat the percussion in the same way in the upper intercostal spaces above the apex till the change of note to delineate the left cardiac border (3rd and 4th spaces).

Normally in the adult male, left cardiac border is within 10 cm from the mid-sternal line in the left 5th intercostal space.

In the 3rd intercostal space if the left cardiac border is 4 cm from the midsternal line signifies cardiomegaly.

Conditions with Displacement of the Left Cardiac Border Outside the Normal Position

1. *Cardiomegaly:* Left cardiac border will be corresponding to the apex.
2. *Pericardial effusion:* Left cardiac border will be outside the apex (cardiac dullness outside the apex).

Percussion of the left 2nd Intercostal Space

Normally resonant

Cardiac Conditions Producing Dullness in the Left 2nd Space

1. Enlarged pulmonary artery.
2. Pericardial effusion.

Important Clinical Aspects of Cardiac Percussion

- Cardiac percussion is helpful in delineating the left border of the heart if the apex is not felt.
- In patients with emphysema cardiac dullness is reduced or absent due to hyperinflated lungs.
- Greatly enlarged right atrium can produce dull note in the right lower parasternal area.
- Cardiac malpositions can be detected by percussion (position of the heart can be compared with the position of the stomach).

AUSCULTATION

Important guidelines for proper cardiac auscultation

- Identify the different areas of auscultation correctly for detection of auscultatory events.
- Simultaneous palpation of the carotid artery is essential to time the event as systolic or diastolic.
- A good stethoscope and a quiet room are required for efficient auscultation.

Parts and Requirements of a Good Stethoscope

- Shallow bell
  - Useful in detecting low frequency sounds (3rd and 4th heart sounds) and low pitched murmurs. Should be applied lightly against the skin.
- Smooth thin diaphragm
  - For high frequency sounds and murmurs (1st heart sound, 2nd heart sound, opening snap and high pitched murmurs).
  - Diaphragm should be applied firmly against the skin.
- Tubing
  - Ideally should be 12 inches long, internally smooth and 4–6 mm in circumferential diameter.
  - It is better to have stethoscopes with double tubings for efficient auscultation.
- Ear tips
- Larger ear tips, which are slightly soft and made of rubbery material are ideal for use.

Auscultatory Areas (Fig. 2.9)

- *Mitral area:* Corresponds to the apex.

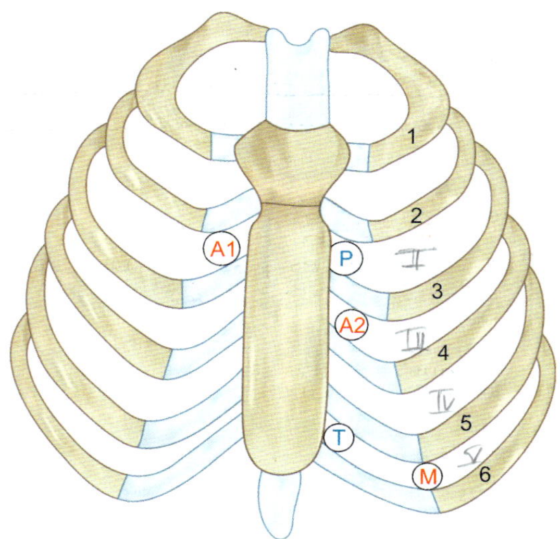

Fig. 2.9: Areas over the precordium over which different auscultatory areas of the heart are represented: A1–aortic area 1, A2–Erb's area, M–mitral area, T–tricuspid area, P–pulmonary area

- *Tricuspid area:* Left of the lower part of the sternum (4th and 5th intercostal space).
- *Aortic area:* Right of the sternum (in the 2nd intercostal space).
- *Pulmonary area:* Left of the sternum (2nd intercostal space).

Additional Areas of Auscultation

- *Left axilla:* For pansystolic murmur of mitral regurgitation (MR).
- Interscapular area for pansystolic murmur of MR.
- *Anterior chest:* 3rd intercostal space on the left side for the murmur of AR (Erb's area).
- Left infraclavicular area for:
  - MR murmur
  - PDA murmur
- Left 3rd and 4th intercostal space (sternal border) for murmur of VSD.

Sequence of Cardiac Auscultation

- Start from the apex.
- Proceed along the left sternal border below (tricuspid area) and pulmonary (above).
- Then auscultate the right 2nd space (aortic area).
- Auscultate additional areas whenever necessary.
- For auscultating aortic and pulmonary area—ask the patient to sit and stoop forward.
- Perform different auscultatory manoeuvres if required.

HEART SOUNDS

1st Heart Sound (Loud)

Produced by the closure of mitral M_1 and tricuspid T_1 valve simultaneously, so heard as a single sound.

1st heart sound indicates the onset of ventricular systole.

Method of Identification

- Heard as a Lub in (lub-dub) while auscultating for heart sounds.
- Immediately precedes/coincides with the apex or carotid pulse.
- Loudest at the apex.

Abnormality of 1st Heart Sound (S_1)

Causes of loud 1st Heart Sound

- Tachycardia
- Mitral stenosis
- Tricuspid stenosis
- Hyperkinetic states–thyrotoxicosis, severe anemia and febrile states.
- Indicates pliable anterior leaflet of the mitral valve.

1st heart sound can also be loud in ASD (due to loud tricuspid component).

Mechanism of Loud 1st Heart Sound in Mitral Stenosis

In patients with mitral stenosis mitral valve moves over a greater distance with higher velocity causing loud 1st heart sound due to:

1. High left atrial pressure causing the valve leaflets to be kept in a doomed position in LV cavity.
2. Valve closure occurs at a time when the LV pressure is very high.

Soft (Muffled) 1st Heart Sound

Causes

- Cardiac failure
- Bradycardia
- Mitral regurgitation, tricuspid regurgitation.

May also indicate calcified anterior mitral leaflet.

Key Points while auscultating heart sounds

- Sound intensity may be increased or decreased.
- Sounds may be abnormally split.
- Low frequency extra sounds may appear–3rd and 4th heart sounds.
- Additional sounds: Originating from the abnormal valves may be heard–clicks, snaps, etc.
- Decrease in the intensity of the heart sounds may be due to non-cardiac causes like obesity, emphysema and pericardial effusion.

Splitting of 1st Heart Sound

- Complete RBBB
- Pacing of left ventricle
- Ebstein's anomaly

Varying Intensity of 1st Heart Sound

- Beat to beat variation of the 1st heart sound occurs in atrial fibrillation.
- Cannon sound–intermittently loud 1st heart sound–in patients with complete heart block.
- Splitting of the 1st heart sound occurs in complete RBBB due to delayed tricuspid component.

2nd Heart Sound (Loud)

Genesis of 2nd Heart Sound

- Produced by the closure of aortic valve (A_2) and pulmonary (P_2) valves.
- Pulmonary valve closes later (due to lower pressure in the pulmonary artery) and aortic valve closes earlier due to early raise of left ventricular pressure and early activation of the LV.
- As a result 2nd heart sound is heard as 2 components, A_2 (Aortic component) and P_2 (pulmonary component).

Method of Identification

- Heard as dub (in lub-dub) while auscultating for the heart sounds.
- Follows the apical impulse and carotid pulse.
- Better heard at the pulmonary and aortic areas.

Splitting of the 2nd Heart Sound

Normal (Physiological) Splitting

- 2nd heart sound is heard as A_2 (aortic) and P_2 (pulmonary) component as a split.
- Split increases during inspiration (normal split–0.06 secs) with P_2 moving away from A_2.
- Split decreases during expiration (0.02 secs).
- Physiological split is common in children and young adults.
- Split is best appreciated in the pulmonary area.
- A_2 Aortic component can be heard in all areas.
- P_2 pulmonary component is best appreciated in the pulmonary area.
- P_2 Heard loud at the apex may be suggestive of pulmonary hypertension.

Mechanism of Physiological Split of 2nd Heart Sound

During inspiration 1: Due to negative intrathoracic pressure, there is increased return of the blood into the right ventricle. This results in delayed right ventricular ejection time with later closure of pulmonary valve–P_2 delayed.

During inspiration 2: There is increase in the capacitance of pulmonary vascular bed (decrease in the pulmonary vascular resistance). This results in the delay in the raise of pulmonary artery pressure, so as to equalise the right ventricular pressure to close the pulmonary valve. This time taken for the raise of pressure is called hangout interval. Because of this delay, pulmonary valve closure is delayed–P_2 moves away from A_2.

Abnormality of the 2nd Heart Sound

Loud 2nd heart sound

- *Loud aortic component (A_2):* Due to forcible closure of the aortic valve, e.g. systemic hypertension. Aortic root dilatation (aorta is closer to the chest wall).
- *Loud pulmonary component (P_2):* Due to forcible closure of the pulmonary valve, e.g. pulmonary artery hypertension.

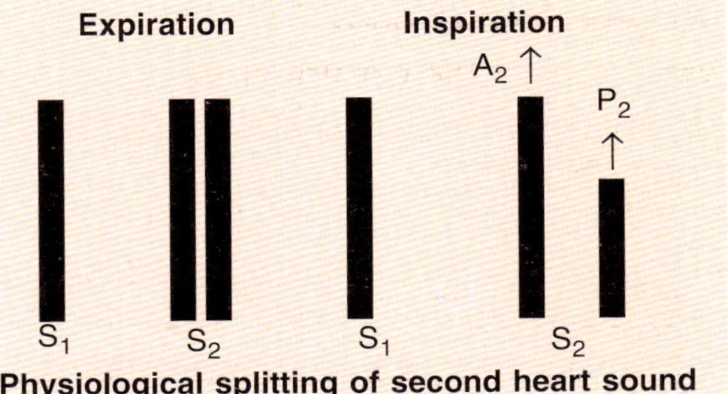

Physiological splitting of second heart sound

Causes of Loud P_2 without Pulmonary Hypertension

- ASD
- Straight back syndrome
- Idiopathic dilatation of pulmonary artery

Muffled (Soft) 2nd Heart Sound

- *Due to muffled aortic component (A_2):* Severe AS or aortic atresia (only pulmonary component is heard as a single sound).
- *Due to muffled P_2 (pulmonary component):* Severe PS or pulmonary atresia (only aortic component is heard)–Fallot's tetralogy.

Abnormal Splitting of 2nd Heart Sound

Persistent (wide) split → Not fixed / Fixed

Paradoxically split

Narrow split

Persistent (wide) split: Not a fixed split.

Split is audible in both inspiration and expiration but duration is not fixed, e.g. due to delay in the pulmonary component–RBBB and LV ectopic beat.

- Due to early timing of aortic component - severe MR
- Due to prolonged RV contraction pulmonary embolism/pulmonary stenosis. PAPVC (partial anomalous pulmonary venous connection).

Wide and Fixed split of 2nd Heart Sound

A_2 and P_2 are audible in both the phases of respiration and the duration of the split is fixed, e.g. uncomplicated osteum secundum ASD.

Mechanism of Wide Splitting in ASD

- Right heart receives additional volume of blood due to interatrial shunt.
- RV ejection time is prolonged due to additional volume of blood in the RV due to interatrial shunting causing delayed P_2 (pulmonary valve closure).

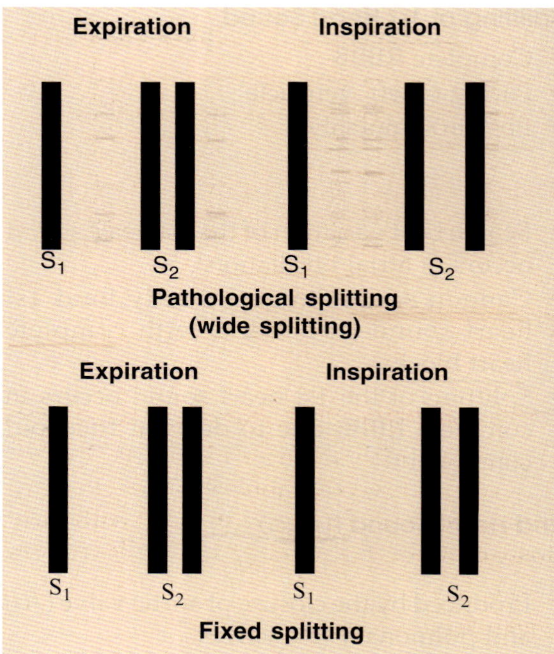

- Increased pulmonary capacitance in ASD causes increased pulmonary hangout interval with delaying of P_2"
- Above 2 mechanisms result in widening of the split.

Fixed Splitting of the 2nd Heart Sound in ASD

Free communication between right atrium and left atrium causes equal amount of blood flowing to RV and LV both during inspiration and expiration causing fixed time for valve closure.

Paradoxically Split (Reverse split)

- Pulmonary component occurs before the aortic component.
- On inspiration A_2 and P_2 gap narrows.
- On expiration split audible with separation of A_2 and P_2, e.g. LBBB and severe AS.

LBBB causes early right ventricular septal repolarisation with early P_2 and delayed A_2.

Severe AS: Causes prolonged LV ejection delaying A_2.

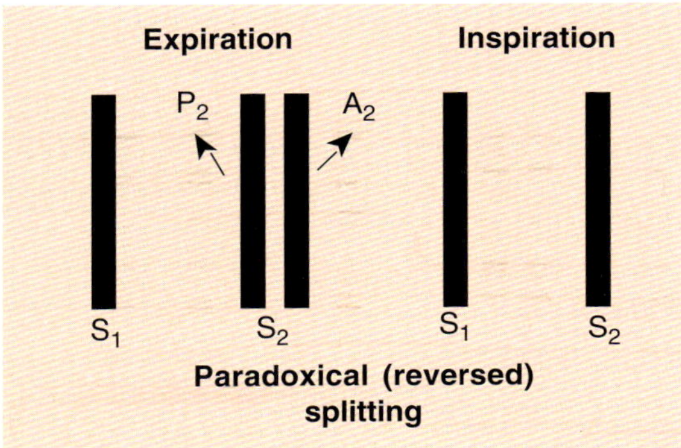

Paradoxical (reversed) splitting

Narrow Splitting of the 2nd Heart Sound

In patients with severe pulmonary hypertension increased pulmonary artery pressure causes decrease of hangout interval with early closure of the pulmonary valve (P_2 occurs early).

Single 2nd heart sound

- Due to absent A_2—severe AS
- Due to absent P_2—severe PS
- Fallot's tetralogy

3rd Heart Sound (S_3)

Genesis of 3rd Heart Sound

Sound is produced due to the rapid filling of the ventricle during early diastole leading to sudden limitation of expansion of the ventricle causing vibrations. 3rd heart sound can be physiological under following circumstances:

- Healthy young adults
- Athletes
- Pregnancy
- Fever

Characteristics of 3rd Heart Sound

Low frequency sound, heard better with the bell of the stethoscope. Heard in diastole–(early part of diastole)–protodiastolic during maximum (rapid) filling phase of ventricular filling (0.15 secs after 2nd heart sound).

Abnormal (Pathological) S_3

- S_3 occurring after the age of 40 years is always abnormal.
- Occurs due to altered physical property of left ventricle.
- 3rd heart sound occurs whenever there is increased rate and volume of flow across the atrioventricular valve and raised end diastolic pressure of the ventricle.

Pathological 3rd Heart Sound

Causes

- Left-sided/right-sided cardiac failure
- Mitral regurgitation/tricuspid regurgitation/aortic regurgitation
- Hyperdynamic circulation
- VSD and PDA–left-sided S_3
- ASD–right-sided S_3

4th Heart Sound

(Presystolic gallop)

Characteristics

- Low frequency sound.
- Heard in the later part of the diastole (presystolic) in patients with sinus rhythm.
- Better felt than auscultated.
- Disappears in patients with atrial fibrillation.

Genesis of 4th Heart Sound

- In conditions with decreased ventricular compliance there will be increased atrial contraction producing ventricular distension causing the sound during the presystolic phase.
- 4th heart sound occurs during the atrial filling phase of the ventricular diastole.

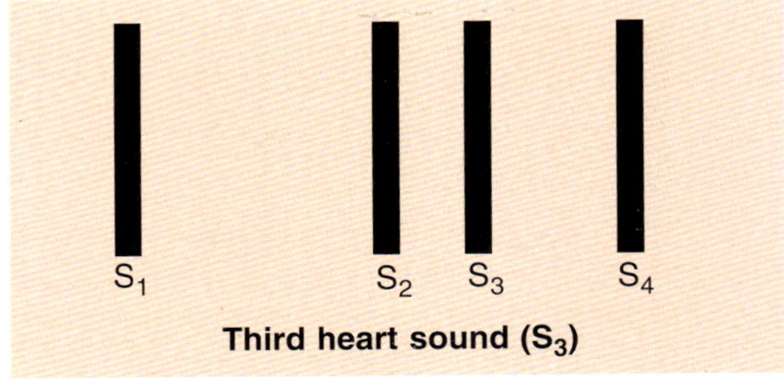

Third heart sound (S_3)

Characteristics of 4th Heart Sound

- They can be produced either from the right or left side of the heart.
- Better felt than auscultated.
- Low frequency sounds and are better heard with the bell of the stethoscope.
- Occurs in conditions with freely communicating atrioventricular orifices.
- Left-sided 3rd and 4th heart sounds are better heard:
  - At the apex
  - Left lateral position
  - During expiration

Right-sided 3rd and 4th heart sounds are better heard: At the lower left sternal border (tricuspid area) during inspiration.

Causes of 4th heart sound: Conditions associated with LVH and RVH.

4th Heart Sound (S_4)

Causes of pathological S_4

Left-sided S_4

- Severe aortic stenosis
- Systemic hypertension
- Hypertrophic obstructive cardiomyopathy
- IHD

Triple Rhythm

Combination of first heart sound–second heart sound and third or fourth heart sounds.

Gallop Rhythm

In patients with tachycardia. diastole becomes shortened. This causes 3rd and 4th heart sounds to coincide. This results in increase in the amplitude of the heart sounds making it easily detectable.

This type of summation of sounds results in summation gallop. Presence of S_1 S_2 and S_3 or S_4 together with tachycardia produces a gallop rhythm.

Additional Sounds

Ejection clicks: Occurs due to sudden opening of semi-lunar valves with their forward movement.

Aortic Ejection Click

- Occurs after the 1st heart sound.
- Indicates abnormality of the aortic valves, e.g. valvular aortic stenosis.
- Absent in supra- or sub-valvular aortic stenosis.
- In patients with bicuspid aortic valve, there can be only click without murmur.
- In calcified aortic valve ejection click will be absent.

Pulmonary Ejection Click

Present in patients with valvular pulmonary stenosis (e.g. congenital pulmonary stenosis). Only auscultating event occurring in the right side of the heart which is better heard on expiration. Becomes soft on inspiration.

Respiratory Variation of Pulmonary Ejection Click

Mechanism

On inspiration: Forward movement of the pulmonary valve occurs due to the trans-

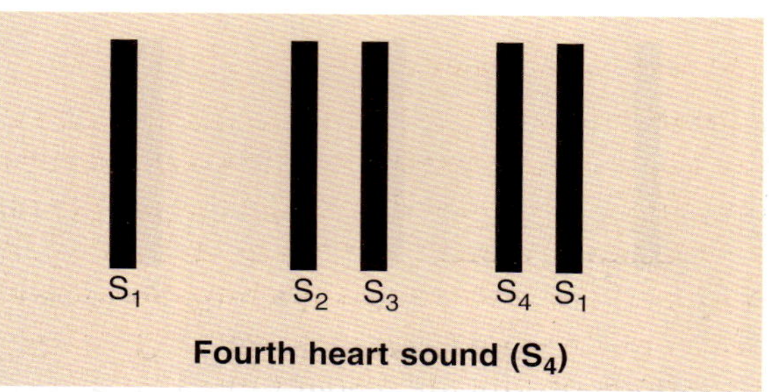

Fourth heart sound (S_4)

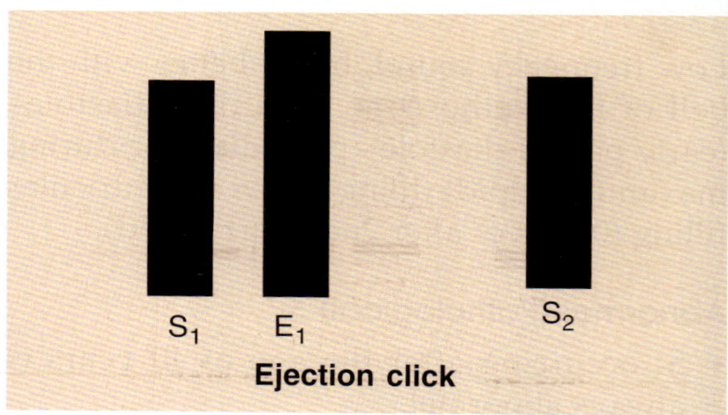

Ejection click

mission of high force of right atrial contraction to right ventricle and pulmonary valve. This leads to minimal forward movement of the valve on systole causing decreased intensity of ejection click on inspiration.

Non-ejection Mid-systolic Click

- Occurs in patients with mitral valve prolapse.
- May be associated with late systolic murmur.

Genesis of Mid-systolic Click of MVP

Occurs due to the vibrations produced by the sudden tensing of redundant leaflet of the valve when they prolapse into the atrium.

Ejection Sound of Dilated Arteries

Occurs in patients with dilated aorta or pulmonary arteries.

- Aortic ejection sound in patients with dilated aorta and systemic hypertension.
- Pulmonary ejection sound in patients with dilated pulmonary artery with severe pulmonary artery hypertension.
- Ejection sounds are due to semi-lunar valve opening producing resonation in the dilated artery.
- Sounds produced by wall of the dilated arteries.

Tumour Plop Sound

Occurs in cases of atrial myxoma. Myxomas are usually mobile with attachment to the atrial septum by a long stalk. Plop occurs when myxoma maximally descends towards AV orifice during diastole.

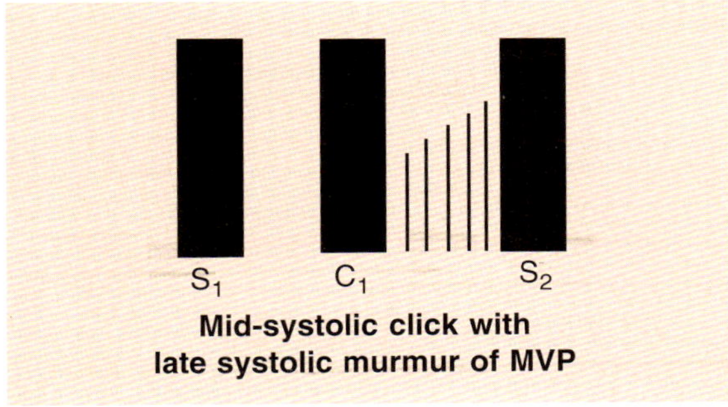

Mid-systolic click with late systolic murmur of MVP

Prosthetic Valve Sounds

- Both opening and closing sounds are produced by mechanical prosthetic valves.
- Closing sounds are louder compared to the opening sound.
- Metallic type first heart sound–produced by mechanical mitral valve.
- Metallic type of second heart sound–produced by mechanical aortic valve.
- Bioprosthetic valve sounds–sounds are similar to normal heart sound.
- Diminished intensity of prosthetic valve sound indicates:
  - LV dysfunction
  - Arrhythmias
  - Malfunctioning of valves.

Opening Snap (OS)

Produced due to sudden opening of mitral or tricuspid valve.

Characteristics

- High pitched sound.
- Occurs in diastole after the 2nd heart sound.
- Indicates thickened mobile valve leaflets.
- Disappears with the calcification of valves, e.g. mitral stenosis and tricuspid stenosis.

Opening Snap of Mitral Stenosis

- Better heard medial to the apex.
- It may radiate to the base of the heart.
- Interval between the 2nd heart sound and the opening snap (0.04 to 0.12 secs); varies inversely with severity of mitral stenosis.

Genesis of Mitral Opening Snap

In patients with mitral stenosis left atrial pressure is increased. This leads to abrupt opening of mitral valve. But because of the commissural fusion the valve cannot open fully and the valve stops opening suddenly. This sudden stoppage of opening causes vibrations producing a snapping sound.

Differentiation between Split 2nd Heart Sound and 2nd Heart Sound with Opening Snap

Sometimes opening snap may be heard over the pulmonary area and one may mistake the opening snap for the split 2nd heart sound.

In such situations: It is better to make the patient stand and auscultate.

On standing, 2nd heart sound OS interval increases—due to decreased venous return and decreased left atrial pressure.

On standing, split 2nd heart sound (A_2–P_2) gap decreases—due to decreased venous return to right heart.

MURMURS

Genesis of Murmurs

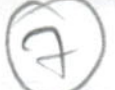

Murmurs are due to the vibrations produced by the turbulent flow at

1. The region of the valve
2. Near the valve
3. Abnormal communication within the heart

Mechanisms such as formation of sound currents due to sudden decrease of pressure may also play a role in the genesis of murmurs.

Following points should be noted while auscultating for a murmur

1. *Timing with the cardiac cycle:* Systolic/diastolic.
2. *Behavior with respiration:* Better heard on inspiration or expiration.
3. Low pitched or high pitched.
4. *Character:* Soft, blowing, rumbling, etc.
5. Presence of thrill.
6. Point of maximum intensity and direction of selective propagation.
7. Any specific manoeuvres or body positions which make the murmur more prominent.
   - Murmur may be systolic, diastolic or continuous.
   - Systolic murmurs coincide with the carotid upstroke.
   - Diastolic murmurs follow the carotid upstroke.

Systolic Murmurs

Mechanism of production of systolic murmurs

1. Increased flow through a normal valve, e.g. flow murmurs
2. Normal or decreased flow through the stenotic valve, e.g. aortic/pulmonary stenosis
3. Systolic leak from high to low pressure chambers, e.g. MR, TR and VSD.

Different types of systolic murmurs are as follows

- Early systolic
- Ejection systolic
- Late systolic
- Pansystolic or hollow systolic.

Early Systolic Murmur

Murmur begins with the 1st heart sound and diminishes in intensity and stops well before the 2nd heart sound (before mid-systole), e.g. acute MR, acute TR, small VSD and VSD with severe pulmonary hypertension.

Ejection (Mid-systolic) Murmur

Characteristics

- Commences after the 1st heart sound
- Peaks in mid-systole
- Stops before the 2nd heart sound
- There will be a definite gap in between the murmur and the 1st and 2nd heart sound
- Phonocardiogram records the murmur as diamond-shaped.

Following circumstances produce ejection systolic (mid-systolic) murmur

- Obstruction to the ventricular outflow, e.g. aortic stenosis and pulmonary stenosis.
- Due to ejection of blood into the dilated aorta or pulmonary arteries, e.g. ejection.

Key Points

- Murmurs which are produced on the right side of the heart are more prominent on inspiration
- Murmurs which are generated on the left heart vary with respiration less significantly when compared to right heart murmurs.

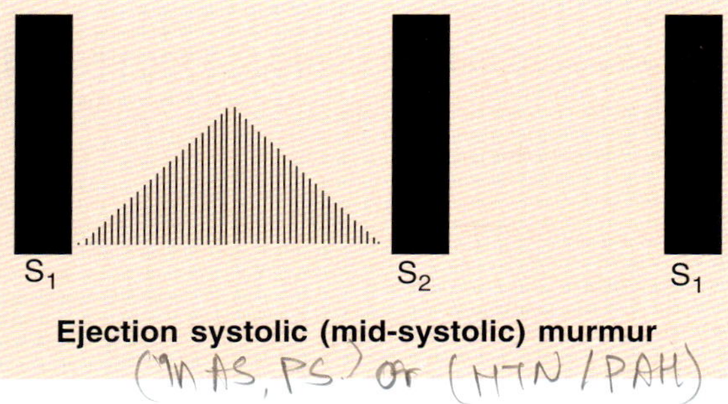

Ejection systolic (mid-systolic) murmur

systolic murmur in patients with AR and PR.

- Accelerated systolic flow into the aorta and pulmonary arteries: e.g. ejection systolic murmur which occurs in patients with systemic and pulmonary hypertension.

Note: Ejection systolic murmurs depend on the forward flow of blood. So in patients with irregular rhythm they vary from beat to beat in contrast to pansystolic murmurs.

Late Systolic Murmur

Murmur begins well after the 1st heart sound (clear gap between the murmur and the 1st heart sound) and continues up to the 2nd heart sound, e.g. mitral valve prolapse and papillary muscle dysfunction.

Pan (Holosystolic) Murmurs

Murmur begins with the 1st heart sound and ends with the 2nd heart sound or its component (A_2 or P_2).

1st heart sound is usually muffled; intensity of the murmur is uniform throughout the systole, e.g. MR, TR and VSD.

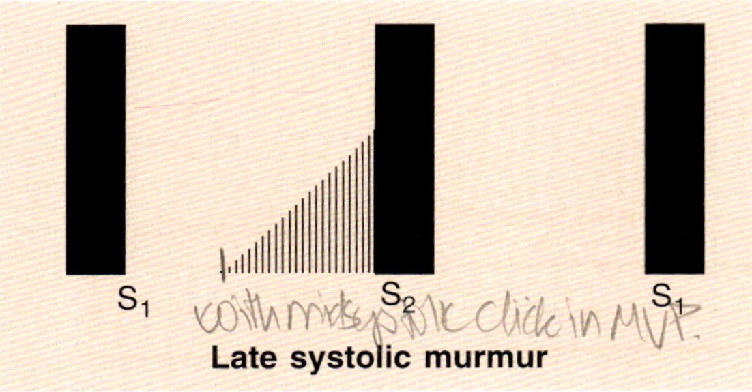

Late systolic murmur

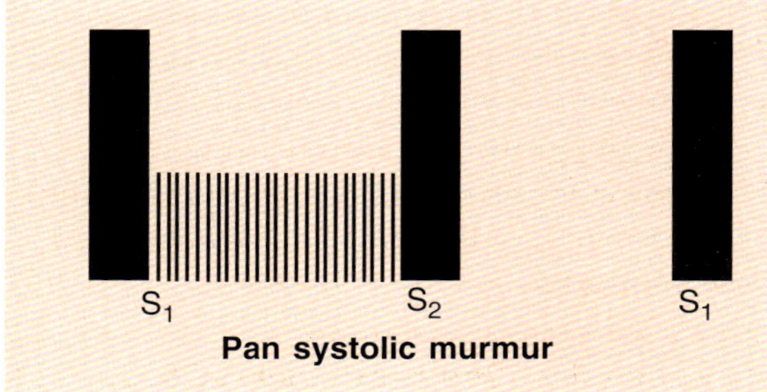

Pan systolic murmur

Genesis of Pansystolic Murmur

Generated whenever pressure difference between the two chambers or vascular bed is high throughout the systole and blood flow becomes turbulent.

Grading of Murmurs

Systolic murmurs are graded as follows:

Grades

1. Heard with great difficulty under ideal conditions.
2. Easily detectable.
3. Loud without a thrill.
4. Murmur is associated with thrill.
5. Very loud, heard over wide area or can be heard with the edge of the chest piece of the stethoscope applied to the chest wall.
6. Extremely loud, heard without the stethoscope or with the chest piece of the stethoscope just held away from the chest wall.

Innocent Murmurs

These murmurs are present in persons with normal cardiovascular system and normal carotid, brachial and femoral arteries.

- There is no physiological or structural abnormality in the cardiovascular system.
- They are ejection systolic in nature, less than grade 3 in intensity.
- Murmur varies in relation to change in body position, level of activity, examination to examination.
- They are not associated with thrill, not conducted to axilla or carotids.

- They arise from flow across a normal LV or RV outflow tract, e.g. young children (3–8 yrs): Vibratory systolic murmur—Still's murmur.

  Adult > 50 yrs—ejection systolic murmur.

Flow Murmurs

These murmurs are produced due to the altered physiological state and they are flow related and are usually associated with increased stroke volume.

Characteristics

- Usually mid-systolic (ejection systolic) in pattern.
- Predominantly heard at the pulmonary area.
- Intensity of the murmur increases by the manoeuvres that increase cardiac output.

Genesis of Flow Murmurs

a. Due to abnormally rapid flow of blood through a normal valve or ejection of blood into a dilated vessel, e.g. anemia, thyrotoxicosis and hypertension.

b. Due to increased transmission of the sound across a thin chest wall, e.g. systolic murmur heard in patients with straight back syndrome.

> *Note:* Systolic flow murmurs can also be heard in children and in pregnancy.

To and Fro Murmurs

In this situation both systolic and diastolic murmurs are heard but the 2nd heart sound is well heard (murmur does not envelope the 2nd heart sound).

In contrast to continuous murmur (where the blood flow is in one direction throughout systole and diastole), in cases of to and fro murmurs, blood flow in systole and diastole will be in opposite directions, e.g. ejection systolic murmur due to AS and early diastolic murmur of AR.

Diastolic Murmurs

Diastolic murmurs are heard after the 2nd heart sound and before the subsequent 1st heart sound.

Types of Diastolic Murmurs

Early Diastolic Murmur

Murmur starts just after the 2nd heart sound and gradually decreases in intensity (persists up to the opening of mitral and tricuspid valves), e.g. aortic regurgitation, pulmonary regurgitation (Graham Steell's murmur of pulmonary hypertension).

Mid-diastolic Murmur

Murmur begins well after the 2nd heart sound and may persist up to the next 1st heart sound (during passive ventricular filling), e.g. mitral stenosis, tricuspid stenosis, Austin Flint murmur and Carey-Coombs' murmur.

Mid-diastolic Flow Murmurs

Austin Flint murmur

Soft mid-diastolic murmur heard at the apex, in patients with severe AR.

Genesis of Austin Flint Murmur

In patients with severe AR, left ventricle fills from the regurgitant flow of blood from the aorta and also from the left atrium during diastole.

Blood leaking from the aorta will be jetting over the anterior mitral leaflet.

Both of the above events together will result in relative approximation of mitral leaflets

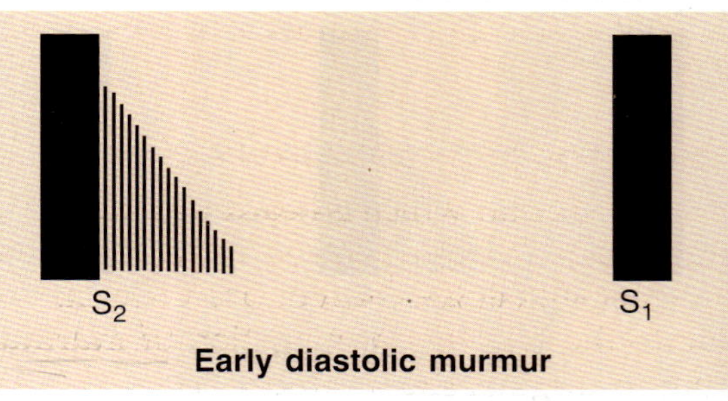

Early diastolic murmur

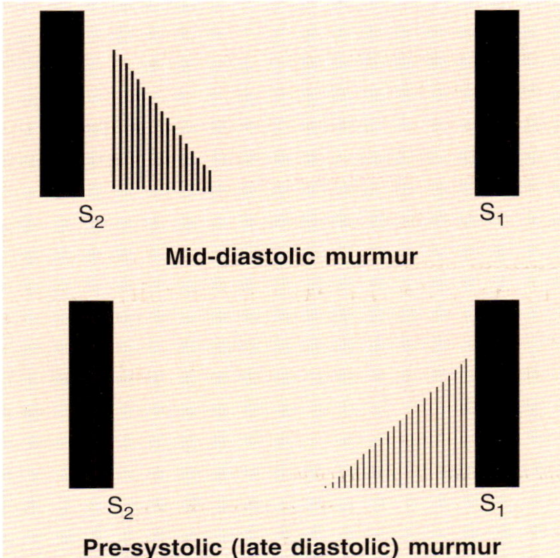

Mid-diastolic murmur

Pre-systolic (late diastolic) murmur

causing turbulence and vibrations producing a mid-diastolic murmur.

Carey-Coombs' Murmur

Mid-diastolic murmur which is heard in patients with acute rheumatic fever.

Murmur occurs due to inflammation of the mitral valve cusps in acute rheumatic valvulitis with turbulence of flow.

Miscellaneous Mid-diastolic Flow Murmurs

Due to increased volume and velocity of blood flow across a normal atrioventricular valve during diastole, e.g. MDM across the mitral valve: In patients with mitral regurgitation, VSD and PDA.

MDM across the tricuspid valve: Tricuspid regurgitation and ASD.

Mid-diastolic flow murmurs may be associated with S_3 in contrast to organic mitral stenosis.

Conduction and Radiation of Murmurs

It is the murmur which is heard with the same intensity or with decreased intensity at the different area of the chest or precordium. It is due to the selective propagation of murmur from its original site of production.

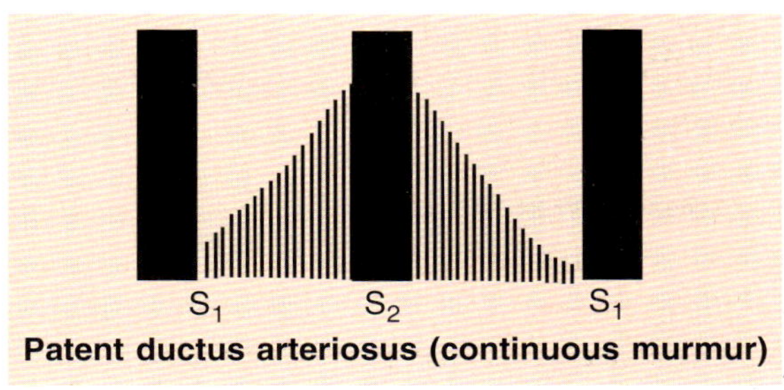

Patent ductus arteriosus (continuous murmur)

Examples of Murmur Conduction

Murmurs	Areas of conduction
• Aortic stenosis	• Right sternal edge • Neck (carotids)–apex
• Aortic regurgitation	• Left sternal border and right sternal border
• Mitral regurgitation	• Axilla and interscapular area Left and 2nd intercostal space
• Mitral stenosis	• Localised to the apex (conduction unusual)

Continuous Murmurs

Characteristics

Murmur begins in the systole (after the 1st heart sound) and continues without interruption through the 2nd heart sound (2nd heart sound is not heard) into all or part of the diastole.

Genesis of Continuous Murmurs

Blood flows without interruption from a vascular bed of higher resistance into a vascular bed of lower pressure or resistance without interruption between systole and diastole, e.g. patent ductus arteriosus–Gibson's murmur (heard in the left infraclavicular and left 2nd intercostal space), arterio venous fistula and coronary AV fistula.

MISCELLANEOUS AUSCULTATORY CARDIOVASCULAR EVENTS

Arterial Bruit

Systolic vascular sound heard over an artery either due to increased flow across a narrow artery or flow through an abnormal artery, e.g. bruit over the carotids in carotid atherosclerosis.

Venous Hum in the Neck

Can occur in healthy children:

- Pregnancy
- Thyrotoxicosis
- Severe anemia, etc.

Hum is heard due to increased venous flow

Genesis of Venous Hum in the Neck

Hum occurs due to the turbulence and disturbed laminar flow in the internal jugular vein.

Venous hum is better heard with rotation of the head.

Rotation of head causes angulation of jugular vein resulting in turbulence and disturbance in its laminar flow.

Method of Auscultation of Venous Hum in the Neck

- Patient is sitting upright.
- Bell of the stethoscope is applied to the medial aspect of the supraclavicular fossa lateral to the sternomastoid.
- Turn the patient's neck to the opposite side.
- Hum may be continuous, but louder during diastole.
- Hum is better heard on the right side and on deep inspiration (right internal jugular is larger than the left).
- Venous hum disappears by compression of the ipsilateral internal jugular vein above by fingers.

Mammary Souffle

Continuous arterial murmur.

Heard at second to sixth intercostal space during pregnancy and lactation.

PERICARDIAL DISORDERS

Pericardial Rub

Superficial coarse scratchy sound.

Characteristics

- Due to abnormal pericardial layers rubbing against each other.
- It has got 3 components—due to atrial systole, ventricular systole and rapid early diastolic filling of the ventricle.
- Pericardial rub may not disappear by the appearance of massive effusion (some portion of layers of the pericardium will be still in contact).
- It is a high-pitched leathery and scratchy sound.

Technique of Auscultation

- Patient is upright and leaning forward.
- Firm pressure of the stethoscope diaphragm to be applied over the precordium–lower left of the sternum.
- Better heard on expiration.

Pericardial Knock

- Occurs in patient with constrictive pericarditis.
- It is a low frequency diastolic sound.

Genesis of Pericardial Knock

Constrictive pericarditis results in sudden stoppage of ventricular filling during early diastolic phase causing vibration.

Dynamic Auscultation

By altering the circulatory dynamics, auscultatory events in the cardiovascular system can be made more prominent or less prominent. Circulatory dynamics can be altered by certain body manoeuvres and vasoactive substances.

Following manoeuvres or vasoactive substances are used for dynamic auscultation:

- *Manoeuvres:* Respiration, postural change, isometric exercise, valsalva manoeuvre.
- *Vasoactive amines:* Amyl nitrate, phenylephrine
- *Exercise:* Patient lying on a couch–sit up and lie down quickly (about 10 times).

- *Valsalva manoeuvre:* Patient is asked to take relatively deep inspiration followed by forced expiration (for about 10 to 12 seconds) against a closed glottis.

Variations of Murmurs during Dynamic Auscultation

Systolic Murmurs

- *Valvular AS:* ↑ with passive leg raising, sudden squatting, ↓ with valsalva release or amyl nitrate with hand grip and valsalva stain
- *HOCM:* Louder with valsalva strain, standing and amyl nitrate, decreases with squatting and hand grip.
- *PS:* ↑ on inspiration, amyl nitrate.
- *Rheumatic MR:* ↑ with squatting, hand grip and phenylephrine, ↓ with amyl nitrate.
- *MVP:*

Early click	standing
Early murmur	valsalva strain
Late click and	amyl nitrate
murmur	squatting
	recumbency

- *TR:* With inspiration and amyl nitrate

Diastolic Murmurs

- AR ↑ with squatting and hand grip or phenylephrine, ↓ with amyl nitrate
- PR ↑ on inspiration and with amyl nitrate
- MS ↑ with exercise, left lateral position, hand grip or amyl nitrate
- TS ↑ with inspiration and amyl nitrate.

Pattern of writing a diagnosis in cardiovascular disorders

- Aetiological diagnosis
- Existing cardiac lesion
- Presence of pulmonary hypertension
- Presence of cardiac failure
- Presence of infective endocarditis
- Associated cardiac rhythm abnormality
- Aetiological diagnosis:
  - Rheumatic heart disease
  - Congenital heart disease
  - Ischemic heart disease
  - Hypertensive heart disease
- Existing cardiac lesion with severity:
- For example, valvular heart disease. Mitral stenosis/mitral regurgitation/aortic stenosis/aortic regurgitation
- *Congenital heart disease:* ASD, VSD, PDA and Fallot's tetralogy
- Presence of pulmonary hypertension: If present–mild/severe
- *Presence of cardiac failure:* Right-sided/left-sided or biventricular failure
- *Presence of infective endocarditis:* Presence of fever, murmur along with splenomegaly.
- *Associated cardiac rhythm abnormality:* For example, normal sinus rhythm/multiple ectopics/atrial fibrillation.

Typical Example of a Case of Rheumatic Valvular Disease

History

20-year-old female presented with dyspnea, palpitation and PND of 6 months duration. Past history revealed history of polyarthritis and patient is on benzathine penicillin prophylaxis.

Peripheral Cardiac Examination Revealed

Irregularly irregular pulse with raised JVP, absence of a' wave in the JVP with pulse apex deficit of more than 10/minute. Precordial examination revealed:

- Tapping apical impulse and diastolic thrill at the apex
- Left parasternal heave and palpable P_2

Cardiac auscultation revealed

- Varying intensity of 1st heart sound
- Presence of an opening snap at the mitral area
- Prolonged rumbling mid-diastolic murmur at the mitral area without presystolic accentuation
- Tricuspid area auscultation revealed pansystolic murmur which is increasing on inspiration.

There is hepatomegaly with pedal edema. There is no history of fever and there is no evidence of splenomegaly.

The cardiovascular diagnosis of the above mentioned patient can be written as:

- Rheumatic heart disease
- Severe mitral stenosis with tricuspid regurgitation with congestive cardiac failure and severe pulmonary hypertension with atrial fibrillation without evidence of infective endocarditis.
- *Aetiological diagnosis:* Rheumatic heart disease
- *Evidence for rheumatic aetiology*: Past history of polyarthritis, benzathine penicillin prophylaxis.

Note: If there is no previous history of rheumatic fever multivalvular involvement or isolated mitral stenosis still favors the diagnosis of rheumatic etiology.

Existing Cardiac Lesion: Severe Mitral Stenosis

Evidence of mitral stenosis

- Tapping apex with diastolic thrill at the apex
- Opening snap at the apex
- Mid-diastolic murmur at the apex.

Severe mitral stenosis is suggested by

- Diastolic thrill at the apex
- Longer duration of mid-diastolic murmur
- Severe pulmonary hypertension

Evidence of CCF

Raised JVP, tender enlarged liver and pedal edema.

Evidence for pulmonary hypertension

- Left parasternal heave
- Palpable P_2
- Loud P_2

Severe pulmonary hypertension is suggested by presence of tricuspid regurgitation.

Evidence for tricuspid regurgitation: Pan systolic murmur in the tricuspid area increasing on inspiration.

Evidence for Atrial Fibrillation

- Irregularly irregular pulse
- Pulse apex deficit of >10/minute and absence of-a-wave in the JVP
- Varying intensity of 1st heart sound
- Absence of presystolic accentuation of the mid-diastolic murmur

Evidence not favoring infective endocarditis

No fever, no splenomegaly.

Abovesaid patient may be considered to have rheumatic activity if there is associated symptoms of fever and migratory polyarthritis.

IMPORTANT CARDIAC CONDITIONS WHICH ARE COMMONLY ENCOUNTERED IN CLINICAL PRACTICE

Mitral Stenosis

Normal mitral valve orifice area: 4 to 6 square cm.

- *Mild mitral stenosis:* Mitral valve orifice more than 2.5 square cm.
- *Moderate mitral stenosis:* Mitral valve orifice 1.5 to 2.5 square cm.
- *Severe mitral stenosis:* Mitral valve orifice less than 1 cm square.

Causes

- Rheumatic heart disease
- Calcified mitral valve
- Congenital mitral stenosis
- Mucopolysaccharidosis
- Collagen disease

Clinical Findings

- Tapping apical impulse
- Diastolic thrill at the apex
- Loud first heart sound
- Presence of an opening snap
- Mid-diastolic murmur at the apex.

Murmur of Mitral Stenosis

- Mid-diastolic murmur at the apex.
- Low-pitched rough and rumbling.
- Heard with the bell of the stethoscope and in the left lateral position associated with

presystolic accentuation. Breath held in expiration.

Pre-systolic Accentuation

Occurs due to:

1. At the last part of the diastole contraction of the left atrium causes increased flow across the mitral valve.
2. Due to the effect of onset of the ventricular contraction mitral valve starts to close causing turbulence.

(The 2nd mechanism contributes to the presence of presystolic murmur even in patients with atrial fibrillation).

Following features suggest severe mitral stenosis:

1. Longer duration of mid-diastolic murmur.
2. Decreased interval between the 2nd heart sound and opening snap.
3. Severe pulmonary hypertension.

Mitral Stenosis with Soft First Heart Sound

Causes

- Calcified mitral leaflets (opening snap also disappears).
- Associated significant mitral regurgitation.
- Severe mitral stenosis with extreme clockwise rotation of the heart.
- RV occupies the apex.

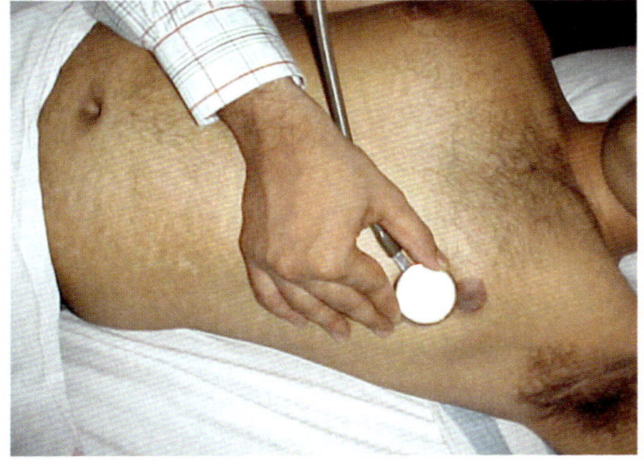

Fig. 2.10: Ascultation of cardiac apex–patient is in left lateral position (especially for the murmur of mitral stenosis)

Silent Mitral Stenosis

- Severe form of mitral stenosis.
- Marked pulmonary hypertension, RVH with decreased cardiac output.
- MDM murmur is not heard (or only heard in the axilla).

Causes of Mid-diastolic Murmur at the Apex apart from Organic Mitral Stenosis

a. Conditions which mimic—mitral stenosis:
   - Left atrial myxoma and left atrial ball-valve thrombosis.

b. Organic disease of the heart but mitral valve is not damaged:
   - Austin Flint and Carey-Coombs' murmur.

c. Mid-diastolic flow murmurs at the apex:
   - VSD and PDA.

Juvenile Mitral Stenosis

- Mitral stenosis can occur at early ages as a consequence of rheumatic fever (as early as 3–8 years).
- In South–East Asian region rheumatic fever assumes aggressive course due to lack of immunity, overcrowding and improper prophylaxis. This results in early valvular damage.
- Severe mitral stenosis with pin point size of the mitral valve.

Differences between Organic Mitral Stenosis and other Causes of MDM at the Apex

Organic Mitral Stenosis

- Diastolic thrill–present
- 1st heart sound–very loud
- Opening snap–present
- Murmur–rough and rumbling and of longer duration
- Presystolic accentuation–present

Other Causes of MDM at the Apex

- Diastolic thrill–absent
- 1st heart sound–normal or soft
- Opening snap–absent
- Murmur–soft and short
- Presystolic accentuation–absent

Complications of Mitral Stenosis

Due to raised pulmonary venous pressure

- Left atrial failure
- Hemoptysis

Due to raised pulmonary artery pressure:

- Pulmonary artery hypertension
- Right ventricular hypertrophy
- Right ventricular failure
- Hemoptysis

Due to enlarged left atrium

- Dysphagia: Due to compression of esophagus.
- Hoarseness of voice: Due to compression of recurrent laryngeal nerve (Ortner's syndrome).
- Due to left atrial clot formation: Embolism to the systemic, cerebral, visceral and peripheral circulation.
- Due to arrhythmias: Atrial and ventricular ectopics, atrial flutter and fibrillation.
- Due to infection : Bronchopulmonary infection, infective endocarditis (rare).

Mitral Regurgitation (MR)

Causes

1. Rheumatic
2. Mitral valve prolapse
3. Ischaemic damage to papillary muscle
4. Rupture of chordae tendinae (trauma, ischaemia and infective endocarditis)
5. LV dilatation with enlargement of mitral annulus.

Clinical Features

- High volume pulse
- Hyperdynamic apical impulse
- Systolic thrill at the apex
- Soft 1st heart sound
- Presence of left-sided 3rd heart sound
- Pansystolic murmur at the apex.

Murmur of MR

- *Pansystolic:* Soft blowing, high-pitched, heard better with diaphragm of the stethoscope and on expiration.

  Conducted to axilla if the anterior leaflet is involved (rheumatic).

  Conducted to the base of the heart (2nd left intercostal space) if the posterior leaflet is involved (MVP).
- *MR with loud first heart sound:* Consider associated dominant mitral stenosis.

  MR with normal first heart sound: Consider MVP, papillary muscle dysfunction.

Soft first heart sound in MR: Due to:

1. Defective closure of deformed valve leaflets.
2. Murmur starting with the first heart sound. Mitral regurgitation with late systolic murmur.

Causes

1. MVP
2. Ischaemic–papillary muscle dysfunction.

Severe MR

Presence of loud S_3, pansystolic murmur and mid-diastolic flow murmur across the mitral valve suggests severe MR.

Clinical signs of combined valvular lesion: Mitral stenosis with mitral regurgitation.

If mitral stenosis is the dominant lesion

- Pulse: Low volume

Differences between acute and chronic MR

	Acute MR	*Chronic MR*
Apex	• Not displaced	Displaced
Murmur	• Soft, low pitched and short	Harsh and pansystolic
Thrill	• Absent	Present
Location of murmur	• Base	Apex
Severe LVF	• Usually present	+/–

- *Apex:* Tapping apex
- *Thrill:* Diastolic thrill at the apex

Signs of pulmonary hypertension will be present. Left parasternal heave, palpable and loud P_2.

On auscultation

- Loud 1st heart sound
- Long mid-diastolic murmur with opening snap.
- Left-sided 3rd heart sound is absent
- Murmur of mitral regurgitation: Faint or absence of pansystolic murmur.

If mitral regurgitation is the dominant lesion

Pulse; normal or collapsing

- *Apex:* Hyperdynamic
- *Thrill:* Systolic thrill at the apex
- Signs of pulmonary hypertension and minimal

On auscultation

- Muffled 1st heart sound
- Left-sided 3rd heart sound is present
- Murmur of mitral regurgitation: Classical murmur present
- Signs of pulmonary hypertension minimal
- Short mid-diastolic murmur at the apex.

Heart sounds

- 1st heart sound muffled
- Presence of left-sided 3rd heart sound
- Absence of opening snap.

Murmur

- Classical pansystolic murmur of MR at the apex
- Short mid-diastolic murmur of mitral stenosis

Aortic Stenosis (AS)

Causes

1. Rheumatic
2. Congenital
3. Calcified aortic valve

Types of Aortic Stenosis

1. *Valvular:* Rheumatic heart disease
2. *Supravalvular:* Congenital along with hyper calcemia and elfin facies.
3. *Subvalvular:* Idiopathic hypertrophic subaortic stenosis.

Clinical Findings

- Low volume and slow raising pulse (pulsus parvus et tardus) and apicocarotid delay–severe aortic stenosis
- Heaving apical impulse
- Systolic thrill over the aortic area and over the carotids (in valvular stenosis)
- Ejection click (in valvular stenosis)
- 2nd heart sound—soft or single or paradoxically split
- Ejection systolic murmur at the aortic area.

Murmur of AS

Ejection systolic murmur with late peaking conducted to the carotids (in valvular stenosis).

Better heard on expiration with patient sitting up and stooping forward.

Sometimes the ejection systolic murmur of aortic stenosis can be heard at the apex with a different quality. This is called Gallavardin phenomenon.

Gallavardin Phenomenon

Harsh ejection systolic murmur of aortic stenosis is heard as musical quality murmur at the apex.

Occurs in elderly with aortic valve calcification and sclerosis.

Mechanism

Harsh aortic area murmur is due to high velocity of blood flow causing turbulence at the aortic root.

Musical component at the apex is due to high frequency vibration produced by the valve conducted to the apex.

Features of Severe Aortic Stenosis

- *Symptoms:* Symptoms of exertional syncope and angina.
- *Pulse:* Slow raising low volume pulse (pulses parvus and tardus, apicocarotid delay (carotid pulse is delayed).

- *Blood pressure:* Low systolic BP (systolic decapitation of blood pressure) systolic BP is usually less than 140–150 mm Hg.
- *Thrill:* Systolic thrill in the aortic area.
- Auscultation.
- *Heart sounds:* Presence of left-sided S_4, A_2 muffled or not heard, paradoxical splitting of 2nd heart sound.
- *Murmur:* Late peaking of ejection systolic murmur in the aortic area.

Complications of Aortic Stenosis

- Left ventricular failure
- Pulmonary artery hypertension
- Right ventricular failure
- Ventricular arrhythmias

Aortic stenosis can cause sudden death due to syncope, complete heart block and ventricular fibrillation.

Aortic Regurgitation (AR)

Murmur: Long early diastolic murmur with short ejection systolic murmur in the aortic area.

Causes

- *AS with AR:* Rheumatic fever and bicuspid aortic valve
- *Only AR:* AR due to syphilitic aortitis and Marfan's syndrome
- *Acute AR:* Infective endocarditis, dissecting aneurysm of aorta. Trauma to the chest.

Signs of AR

- Peripheral signs of AR
- Hyperdynamic or heaving apex (later stages)
- Diastolic thrill at the aortic area (severe AR)
- 2nd heart sound loud or musical
- *Murmur:* Early diastolic murmur of longer duration.

Decrescendo and high-pitched, on expiration heard with diaphragm of the stethoscope and on sitting up and stooping forward.

If the murmur of AR is better on right sternal border it signifies dilatation of the aortic root, e.g. syphilis, Marfan's syndrome.

If the murmur of AR is better heard on the left sternal border it signifies AR of valvular origin, e.g. rheumatic heart disease.

Musical murmur of AR (cooving dove): Due to either eversion or perforation of cusps.

Severe AR

- Dominant peripheral signs
- Diastolic thrill at the aortic area
- Long duration of early diastolic murmur
- Presence of austin flint murmur
- Presence of pulsus bisferiens.

Complications of AR

- LVF
- Pulmonary artery hypertension
- Right ventricular failure
- Infective endocarditis
- Cardiac conduction defect
- Arrhythmias

Clinical findings in a patient of combined aortic stenosis and aortic regurgitation. If aortic stenosis is the dominant lesion:

- *Pulse:* Low volume slow raising
- *Blood pressure:* Low systolic blood pressure.
- *Peripheral signs of aortic regurgitation:* Less prominent
- *Apex:* Heaving
- *Thrill:* Systolic thrill present in the aortic area.

Table 2.4: Differences between acute and chronic AR

	Acute AR	*Chronic AR*
• Peripheral signs	Absent	Present
• Apex	Not hyperdynamic and not displaced	Hyperdynamic and displaced
• AR murmur	Shorter	Longer

- Auscultation
- *Heart sounds:* Left-sided S_3 absent, left-sided S_4 present.

Murmur

- Prominent ejection systolic murmur in the aortic area
- Short early diastolic murmur in the aortic area.

If aortic regurgitation is the dominant lesion:

- *Pulse:* High volume collapsing and occasionally bisferience
- *Blood pressure:* High systolic and low diastolic blood pressure with wide pulse pressure
- Peripheral signs of AR marked
- *Apex beat:* Out and down and hyper dynamic
- *Thrill:* Diastolic thrill in the aortic area–rare
- Auscultation
- *Heart sounds:* Left-sided 3rd heart sound may be present
- *Ejection click:* Absent, instead ejection sound due to dilatation of aortic root may be present
- *Murmur:* Long early diastolic murmur with short ejection systolic murmur.

Cole Cecil Murmur

Murmur of AR radiates to axilla and apex.

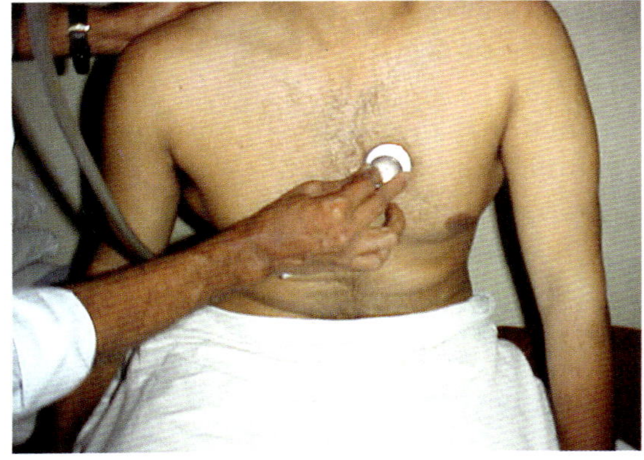

Fig. 2.11: Auscultation for aortic regurgitation murmur. Patient is sitting and leaning forward

Differences between Syphilitic AR and Rheumatic AR

Syphilitic AR	*Rheumatic AR*
Exposure to syphilis	H/o rheumatic fever
No associated mitral valve disease	Usually associated with mitral valve disease
Peripheral signs predominant	Peripheral signs less dominant
No associated AS	May be associated with AS

Aortic Aneurysm

Signs of Aneurysm of Ascending Aorta (Aneurysm of signs)

- Right parasternal pulsation and bulge
- Aortic regurgitation
- Loud A_2
- Compression of right main bronchus, phrenic nerve and cervical sympathetic chain.

Signs of Aneurysm of Arch of Aorta (Aneurysm of symptoms)

- Suprasternal pulsation
- Tracheal tug
- Pressure effect on left recurrent laryngeal nerve, cervical sympathetic and phrenic nerve.

Tricuspid Stenosis

Causes

- Rheumatic
- Tricuspid atresia
- Carcinoid syndrome

Signs: Opening snap:

Mid-diastolic murmur at the tricuspid area better heard on inspiration.

Tricuspid Regurgitation

Causes

Usually secondary to right ventricular dilatation causing stretching of the tricuspid annulus in patients with severe pulmonary hypertension.

Other causes

- Rheumatic
- Carcinoid syndrome
- Right-sided infective endocarditis
- Ebstein's anomaly

Signs

Prominent 'V' wave in the JVP and pulsatile liver.

Murmur

Pansystolic murmur, high-pitched, better heard on inspiration. (This is called Caravallo's sign.) This sign is absent in severe RV failure and hepatic outflow obstruction.

- Murmur is heard at the tricuspid area.
- Right-sided S_3 may be present.

Myxoma

- Tumour of the atrium raising from the interatrial septum.
- Commonly found in the left atrium.
- Can cause embolisation.
- Left atrial myxoma may obstruct the mitral valve and can produce mid-diastolic murmur at the apex.

Mid-diastolic Murmur of Left Atrial Myxoma

Characteristically appears on standing and may disappear on lying down. MDM may be associated with tumor plop sound rather than an opening snap.

Pulmonary Stenosis (Usually congenital)

Signs

- Right ventricular hypertrophy is usually present.
- Ejection click is heard in the pulmonary area which is better heard on expiration (valvular stenosis).
- 2nd heart sound pulmonary component may be soft and may be delayed.
- Ejection systolic murmur which is heard over the pulmonary area and better heard on inspiration.

Atrial Septal Defect (ASD)

Signs

- Left parasternal lift (due to right ventricular volume overload).
- Fixed and wide splitting of the 2nd heart sound.
- Ejection systolic murmur at pulmonary area (due to increased flow across the pulmonary valve).
- Mid-diastolic murmur at the tricuspid area due to increased flow across the tricuspid valve.
- ASD without fixed split: Sinus venosus type of ASD.
- ASD with thrill in the pulmonary area: Large ASD/ASD associated with valvular pulmonary stenosis.

Ventricular Septal Defect

Signs

1. Hyperdynamic apex.
2. Systolic thrill at the lower end of the left sternal border.
3. Pansystolic murmur at the left lower part of the sternum.
4. Murmur does not radiate to axilla.

Roger's malady: Small VSD with high velocity prominent pansystolic murmur.

Patent Ductus Arteriosus (PDA)

1. Continuous murmur and thrill at the pulmonary area—machinery murmur (accentuation of the murmur at the 2nd heart sound).
2. Functional mid-diastolic murmur at the mitral area.
3. Peripheral signs of wide pulse pressure.
4. With the onset of pulmonary hypertension, diastolic component of the murmur will be shortened.

Pulmonary Hypertension

Causes

- All causes of severe left heart disease, e.g. mitral valve disease.

- Ischaemic heart disease.
- Reversal of left to right shunt Eisenmenger's syndrome.
- Respiratory causes cor pulmonale, e.g. COPD and pulmonary embolism.
- Primary pulmonary hypertension.

Signs

- Prominent a wave in the JVP (due to stiff right ventricle)
- Left parasternal heave (due to RVH)
- P_2 palpable and loud
- Ejection systolic murmur at the pulmonary area
- Early diastolic murmur (Graham Steell's murmur) heard at the pulmonary area, better heard on inspiration due to dilatation of the pulmonary valve annulus and pulmonary regurgitation (PR).

Eisenmenger's Syndrome

- Occurs due to the development of pulmonary hypertension in an intracardiac shunt lesions.
- May cause left to right shunt to reverse and becomes right to left shunt.
- Occurs early in VSD (Eisenmenger's complex) and PDA and later in ASD.
- Patients with Eisenmenger's syndrome develop:
  - Clubbing
  - Central cyanosis
  - Prominent a wave in JVP
  - Signs of pulmonary artery hypertension. Murmurs of VSD, PDA and ASD become shorter and lesser in intensity.

Differences between Aortic (AR) and Pulmonary Regurgitation (PR)

AR	*PR*
Associated with peripheral signs	Signs of severe pulmonary hypertension
A_2 loud	P_2 loud
Murmur better heard in expiration	Murmur better heard on inspiration
Associated with LVH	Presence of RVH

Coarctation of Aorta

Signs

- Radio-femoral delay
- Left ventricular hypertrophy
- High blood pressure recorded in the upper limbs compared to lower limbs
- Ejection click at the aortic area
- ESM–at the aortic area due to bicuspid aortic valve
- Collaterals–around the scapulae.

Ebstein's Anomaly

Signs

- Central cyanosis
- Systolic thrill and murmur of TR
- Wide split of 1st and 2nd heart sounds with 3rd and 4th heart sounds.

Fallot's Tetralogy

Components

- Pulmonary stenosis (usually infundibular).
- Ventricular septal defect.
- Right ventricular hypertrophy.
- Overriding of the aorta (aorta arises from either ventricle).

Signs

- Central cyanosis
- Clubbing
- Relatively quiet precordium
- Ejection systolic murmur at the pulmonary area
- Single second heart sound (P_2 is absent)

Acyanotic Fallot (pink Fallot): Interventricular shunt with mild RV outflow obstruction.

Triology of Fallot: Pulmonary stenosis with reversed interatrial shunt.

Pentalogy of Fallot: Tetralogy with ASD.

Hypertrophic Obstructive Cardiomyopathy (HOCM)

Characterised by inappropriate hypertrophy of the left ventricle and septum.

Signs

- Jerky or sharp carotid pulse (due to abnormal pattern of blood flow from left ventricle).

- Double apical impulse.
- Stiff left ventricle produces loud S_4 at the apex.
- Obstruction to the LV outflow produces ejection systolic murmur at the left sternal border; murmur not conducted to the carotids.
- Papillary muscle abnormality in HOCM causes mitral regurgitant murmur.

Congestive Cardiac Failure

Signs

- Patient may be orthopneic (severe left heart failure).
- Pulse rate > 120/min
- Cheyne-Stokes breathing
- Due to prolonged circulation time to the medullary respiratory centre.

Left-sided Heart Failure

Signs

- Central cyanosis
- Low volume pulse
- Pulsus alternans
- Bilateral basal crepitations
- Left side 3rd heart sound.

Right-sided Heart Failure

Signs

- JVP increased.
- Congestive hepatomegaly (sometimes congestive splenomegaly).
- Ascites and pleural effusion may be present.
- Pedal oedema.
- Chronic congestive cardiac failure: Can cause severe weight loss (cardiac cachexia).

Atrial Fibrillation

Signs

- Irregularly irregular pulse.
- Pulse apex deficit (large).
- 'a' wave absent in the JVP.
- Varying intensity of the 1st heart sound.

Causes

Causes of atrial fibrillation can be remembered with the word **THRIL**

- **T**–Thyrotoxicosis
- **H**–Hypertensive heart disease
- **R**–Rheumatic heart disease
- **I**–Ischaemic heart disease
- **L**–Lone atrial fibrillation

Pericardial Effusion

Signs

- Apex not felt
- Cardiac dullness increased outside the apex
- Heart sounds muffled
- Pericardial rub may be audible

Ewart's sign: Dullness/bronchial breathing below angle of left scapula—due to compression of the left lung base by the effusion.

Pericardial Tamponade

- Pulsus paradoxus may be present
- Signs of pericardial effusion present.

Constrictive Pericarditis

- Kussmaul's sign present
- Pericardial knock present.

Acute Rheumatic Fever

Clinical signs of acute rheumatic carditis:

Rheumatic fever involves all layers of the heart. So it is pancarditis.

Signs of rheumatic carditis

- *Due to pericarditis*
  - Pericarditis with pericardial friction rub
  - Pericardial effusion
- *Due to myocarditis*
  - Related tachycardia (heart rate is disproportionately higher compared to the degree of fever)
  - Muffled heart sounds
  - Tic-Tac rhythm
  - Cardiomegaly
  - Cardiac failure
  - Conduction defects and rhythm disturbances.

- *Due to endocarditis*
  – Carey-Coombs' murmur
  – Systolic murmur due to acute mitral regurgitation.

EXAMINATION OF PERIPHERAL VASCULAR SYSTEM

VENOUS SYSTEM

Deep Vein Thrombosis

Features

- Sudden onset of pain in the limb with swelling
- Associated with mild degree of fever.

Signs

- Edema of limbs
- Tenderness in the muscles (calf tenderness in the DVT of leg)
- Homan's sign: Person feels pain in the calf when he dorsiflexes the foot.

Moses sign

Person feels pain on squeezing the calf muscles.

Risk Factors for DVT

- Long-term immobilisation
- Postoperative states
- Polycythemic states
- Protein C and S deficiency
- Oral contraceptive intake

Thrombophlebitis

- Reddish discoloration of the part affected
- Tenderness
- Cord-like feeling of veins

Varicose Veins

- Due to incompetence of venous valves
- Veins become tortuous and dilated.

Complications of Varicose Veins

- Venous stasis and ulcers
- Edema of limbs
- Thrombophlebitis

Predisposing Factors for Varicose Veins

- Occupations associated with long-term standing
- Congestive cardiac failure
- Extreme obesity
- Pregnancy
- Venous obstruction due to pelvic tumors.

Effect of Chronic Venous Stasis

- Varicose ulcers
- Varicose pigmentation
- Edema of limbs

  Usual sites of chronic venous stasis.

  Lower part of the lower limb on its medial aspect usually above the ankle.

LYMPHATIC SYSTEM

- Abnormalities–lymphedema
- Lymphangitis
- Lymphadenopathy
- For details *see* Chapter 1, general physical examination.

ARTERIAL SYSTEM

Pain due to ischaemia

- Pain may occur intermittently intermittent claudication.
- Pain may occur at rest and may be continuous.

Intermittent Claudication (Vascular)

- *Precipitating factors:* Walking for some distance
- Appearance of pain is directly related to the distance walked.
- *Sites of pain:* Usually calf
- Thigh/lumbar aspect with higher level of obstruction
- *Type of pain:* Aching/cramps-like pain
- *Relieving factors:* Stoppage of walking relieves pain.
- *Associated findings:* Peripheral pulse is feeble with evidence of ischaemia of limb.
- *Evidence of ischaemia:* Pallor, pain, pulse feeble, paraesthesia, cold limbs (poikilothermia).

Note: Differentiate vascular claudication from neurogenic claudication.

Features of Neurogenic Claudication

- *Precipitating factors:* Immediately upon standing or walking.
- *Site and type of pain:* Vague pain in the lower limb usually bilateral.
- Person may develop newer symptoms like parasthesia/weakness.
- *Relieving factors:* Forward bending/ stoppage of walking.
- *Associated findings:* Peripheral pulses are normal and no evidence of ischaemia.

Cause of Neurogenic Claudication

- Lumbar canal stenosis.
- Cauda equina/lumbar root compression.

Causes of Peripheral Vascular Disease

- *Inflammatory disorders (vasculitis)*
  - Collagen diseases, syphilis and endocarditis
- *Diseases associated with vascular obstruction*
  - Atherosclerosis and embolic obstruction
- *Functional disturbance of blood vessels*
  - Vasospasm, e.g. Raynaud's phenomenon
  - Hypertensive vascular disease.

Examples of congenital heart diseases and their associated malformations

Malformations	*Associated cardiac anomalies*
• **Holt Oram's syndrome**	
– Thumb with an extra phalanx	ASD
– Thumb lies in the same plane as other fingers	
– Radius and ulna may be deformed	
• **William's syndrome**	
– Microcephaly, elfin facies	Supravalvular AS
– Hypercalcemia, mental retardation	
• **Down's syndrome**	
– Mongoloid facies, hypertelorism	Endocardial cushion defect
– Mental retardation	ASD, VSD, tetralogy of Fallot
• **Turner's syndrome**	
– Short-statured female, broad chest	Coarctation of aorta
– Webbed neck, lymphedema, cubitus valgus	Bicuspid aortic valve
	Aortic dilatation
• **Noonan's syndrome**	
– Webbed neck, pectus excavatum	Pulmonary valve dysplasia
– Cryptorchidism	Cardiomyopathy
• **Rubella syndrome**	
– Deafness, cataract	PDA, ASD
– Microcephaly	Valvular pulmonary stenosis
• **Marfan's syndrome**	
– Arachnodactyly, iridodonesis	AR
– High-arched palate, Ht < arm span	Aortic dissection
– Upper segment < lower segment	
• **Foetal alcohol syndrome**	
– Cataract, deafness	VSD

Raynaud's Phenomenon

Causes

- Idiopathic–Raynaud's disease
- Secondary causes
  - Drug-induced (β-blockers, ergot derivatives)
  - *Collagen disease:* Systemic sclerosis, SLE and rheumatoid arthritis
  - *Hematological:* Cryoglobulinemia, Waldenström's macroglobulinemia
  - *Neurological:* Syringomyelia
  - *Traumatic:* Typing and vibration injury
- Precipitating factors
  - Exposure to cold results in spasm of terminal arteries

Features

Usually intermittent and mainly affects toes and fingers.

Sequence of Events in Raynand's Phenomenon

- *Initially pallor:* Due to vasospasm of arteries.
- *Cyanosis:* Due to dilatation of venules and capillaries containing deoxygenated blood.
- Redness appears last and is due to dilatation of capillaries and arteries.
- *Relieving factors:* Spontaneous/warming the part.

3 Respiratory System

CHECKLIST FOR GENERAL PHYSICAL EXAMINATION

- Symptoms and history of present illness
- Past history
- Family history
- Personal history
- Occupational and environmental exposure (exposure to organic and inorganic dusts)
- Treatment history
- General physical examination
- Examination of upper respiratory tract
- Examination of lower respiratory tract

SCHEME OF HISTORY TAKING

Symptoms and History of Present Illness

- Cough with expectoration
- Haemoptysis
- Dyspnoea
- Chest pain
- Fever
- Symptoms of upper respiratory illness
- Syncope
- Pedal edema and puffiness of face
- Bones and joint pain and muscle weakness
- Headache, altered mental status
- Personality changes and other neurological symptoms.
- Symptoms of other systemic illness.

Past History

- Tuberculosis
- Recurrent attacks of pleurisy and pneumonia since childhood
- Previous chest trauma and surgery
- History of altered consciousness and vomiting
- Previous history of allergy
- Risk factors for embolism

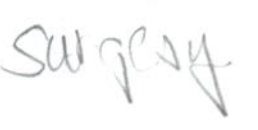

Family History

Tuberculosis, bronchial asthma, bronchiectasis, etc.

Personal History

- Loss of weight and appetite
- Smoking
- Alcoholism
- High-risk behavior

Occupational and environmental exposure (exposure to organic/inorganic dusts).

Treatment History

APPROACH TO A PATIENT OF RESPIRATORY DISEASE

COUGH

Definition

Sudden expulsion of irritant material and secretions from the lower respiratory tract through the glottis. Symptom of cough is analysed as follows:

1. Onset and duration
2. Type and nature
3. Dry or associated with expectoration
4. Aggravating factors

Onset and Duration

Causes of Sudden onset of Cough

- Acute pulmonary edema
- Pulmonary infarction
- Pneumothorax
- Aspiration into the lungs

Causes of Short Duration (2–3 Weeks) of Cough

- Infection of the upper respiratory tract
- Acute bronchitis
- Pneumonia
- Pneumothorax
- Pulmonary embolism
- Pulmonary edema

Causes of Longer duration of Cough (Weeks to months)

- Pulmonary tuberculosis
- Bronchogenic carcinoma
- Interstitial lung disease.

Causes of Cough (Months to years)

- COPD
- Bronchial asthma
- Bronchiectasis

Types and Nature of Cough

Brassy Cough

- Attacks of cough associated with production of metallic sound.
- Occasionally, harsh and barking type, e.g. tracheobronchitis, mediastinal mass, tumor or aortic aneurysm, compressing the trachea.

Bovine Cough

- Present in patients with vocal cord paralysis.
- Non-explosive cough associated with low-pitched sound.
- Usually accompanied by hoarseness of voice.
- Less effective in clearing secretions, e.g. vocal cord paralysis.

Whooping Cough

- Severe attack of prolonged cough.
- Characteristic sound (whoop) is produced due to inspired air entering through a narrow glottis. e.g. pertussis.

Aggravating Factors

Dust, pollen, and cold air can aggravate cough in patients with bronchial asthma.

Cough with expectoration: Cough may be dry or may be associated with expectoration (discussed below).

Analysis of Cough Depending on the other Associated Symptoms

Cough Associated with Chest Pain

Causes

- Pleuritis
- Diseases of the chest wall
- Tracheobronchitis
- Root pain due to dorsal spine disease.

Cough which is Predominantly Nocturnal and may also be Paroxysmal

- Left side cardiac failure
- Bronchial asthma
- Gastric contents aspirated into the lungs.

Cough Associated with Hoarseness of Voice

Causes

- *Infection:* Viral/bacterial laryngitis, TB larynx
- *Neoplastic:* Laryngeal tumors
- *Neurological:* Paralysis of larynx.

Note: Corticosteroid inhalation can also cause hoarseness of voice.

Cough with Diurnal Variation

Predominantly in the morning

- Bronchiectasis
- Chronic bronchitis
- Common in smokers

Predominantly in the evening

Day time exposure to irritants.

Occurrence of Cough during the Act of Eating and Swallowing

Due to:

- Aspiration into the lungs
- Defective swallowing mechanism
- Tracheoesophageal fistula.

Recent Change in the Nature of Cough

Recent change in the nature of cough in a chronic smoker may suggest the possibility of bronchial malignancy.

Complications of Severe Cough

- Vomiting
- Syncope
- *Cough fracture:* Elderly person with osteoporosis.

Causes of Recurrent Attacks of Cough since Childhood

- Childhood onset asthma
- Bronchiectasis (e.g. cystic fibrosis, ciliary abnormality)
- Cystic disease of the lung
- Congenital left to right shunts
- Hypogammaglobulinemia.

Cough with Expectoration

Most of the times cough is associated with expectoration except in the following situations wherein it may be dry.

Causes of Dry Cough

- Viral infection of the respiratory tract
- Interstitial lung disease
- Radiation injury to lungs
- Tumors in the lung
- Irritant gas inhalation

Occasionally, it may be difficult to differentiate sputum from saliva. Presence of alveolar macrophages on microscopy indicates the presence of sputum sample rather than saliva.

Clinical Evaluation of Expectoration

Quantity

Conditions associated with minimal sputum:

- Viral infection of the respiratory tract
- Bronchial asthma

Large quantity or sputum (>100 ml/day)

- Bronchiectasis
- Lung abscess
- Bronchopleural communication
- Bronchorrhea is the term used for expectoration of large (> 100 ml/day) quantity of watery sputum, e.g. bronchoalveolar carcinoma
- Chronic bronchitis.

Quality of sputum

Mucoid

- Gelatinous/sticky
- Colorless/white, e.g. chronic bronchitis and chronic bronchial asthma.

Serous

- Colorless and watery
- Occasionally frothy, e.g. left heart failure
- Bronchoalveolar carcinoma.

Purulent

- Yellow coloured
- Usually thick and viscous
- May be foul smelling
- Indicates pyogenic infection.

Note: Occasionally bronchial asthmatics can bring out casts of bronchial tree with mucus in the sputum.

Colour of sputum

- *Yellow*
  - Indicates infection with pus-forming organisms, e.g. streptococcal/staphylococcal infection
  - Occasionally, green color of the sputum may be due to the enzyme verdoperoxidase liberated by disintegrating cells.
- *Rusty colored*
  - Pneumococcal pneumonia
  - Rusty color is due to dispersion of blood evenly in the sputum.

Note: Patients of bronchial asthma may bring out green colored sputum even without infection due to the sputum containing excess eosinophils.

- Red currant jelly sputum (bright red and viscid), e.g. *Klebsiella pneumoniae*
- *Black coloured sputum (melanoptysis):* Found in coal miner patients and due to coal dust inhalation.

Note: Patients with infection due to Mycoplasma-like organisms will not have colored sputum.

Odour of sputum

Foul-smelling sputum is usually due to infection with anaerobic organisms, e.g. bronchiectasis and lung abscess.

Postural variation of sputum

Quantity of sputum expectorated is more in certain body postures.

Conditions associated with postural variation of sputum:

- Bronchiectasis
- Lung abscess
- Bronchopleural communication
- Gastroesophageal reflux and aspiration into the lungs
- Post-nasal drip

HAEMOPTYSIS

Coughing out of blood from the lower respiratory tract.

Clinical Evaluation and Approach to a Patient of Haemoptysis

True haemoptysis should be differentiated from:

1. *Spurious haemoptysis*: Bleeding from the upper respiratory tract trickling into the lower tract and coughed out.
2. *Pseudohaemoptysis*: Due to infection with organism like *Serratia marcescens* producing a red pigment.

Common Causes of Haemoptysis

Pulmonary causes

- Tuberculosis
- Necrotising pneumonia/lung abscess
- Bronchogenic carcinoma
- Acute bronchitis
- Bronchiectasis

Cardiac cause

Mitral stenosis

Haemoptysis should be differentiated from hemetemesis (Table 3.1)

Following are the differences between haemoptysis and hemetemesis:

Differential Diagnosis of Haemoptysis

- Enquire frequency, amount and duration of haemoptysis in all patients with haemoptysis.
- Massive haemoptysis without severe coughing can occur (> 600 ml/day) in patients with pulmonary cavity and tumors.
- Repeated expectoration of 2–3 ml of blood especially in a chronic smoker may suggest the possibility of bronchogenic carcinoma.
- Recent onset of cough, wheeze and purulent blood-streaked sputum is common in patients with acute bronchitis.
- Recurrent episodes of haemoptysis over many years with purulent sputum are usually found in patients with bronchiectasis.
- Patients with bronchiectasis may have massive haemoptysis (bright red) due to rupture of varicose bronchial vessels.
- High grade fever, chills, rigors and haemoptysis is a common manifestation of pneumonia.
- Mild to moderate fever, weight loss, cough and haemoptysis signifies pulmonary tuberculosis.
- Acute onset of dyspnoea with chest pain

Table 3.1: Differences between haemoptysis and hemetemesis

	Haemoptysis	*Hemetemesis*
1. History	Coughing	Nausea and vomiting
2. Food particles	Absent (contains sputum)	Present
3. Color	Bright red	Coffee ground
4. pH	Alkaline	Acidic
5. History of malena	Absent	Present

and haemoptysis may suggest pulmonary infarction especially with predisposing factors (acute heart failure may also have such a presentation).

- Consider Goodpasture's syndrome and collagen vascular disease in patients with haemoptysis associated with renal disease.

Rare Clinical Circumstances Associated with Haemoptysis

- Direct chest trauma causing lung damage can cause haemoptysis.
- Amoebic liver abscess: Rupture of amoebic abscess into the tracheobronchial tree can produce chocolate colored (anchovy sauce) sputum.
- Occasionally, anti-coagulant therapy may be a cause for haemoptysis.
- Patients with upper respiratory tract bleed may localise the site of bleed and describes it as spitting or hawking of blood rather than coughing.

Causes of Haemoptysis in a Patient of Tuberculosis

- Endobronchial lesion
- Cavitary lesion (rupture of Rasmussen's aneurysm—dilated vessel in a cavity)
- Secondary bacterial infection
- Post-tubercular bronchiectasis (bronchiectasis sicca)
- Erosion of a fully patent vessel located in the wall of a cavity.

DYSPNOEA

Respiratory Causes of Dyspnoea

Acute (Hours to days) (may be sudden onset)

- Bronchial asthma–acute attack pneumothorax
- Acute pneumonia
- Pulmonary embolism
- Laryngeal edema or foreign body
- ARDS

Subacute (Days to weeks)

- Pleural effusion
- Pneumonias
- Guillain-Barré syndrome
- Bronchial carcinoma

Chronic (Months to years)

- COPD
- Bronchial asthma
- Interstitial lung disease

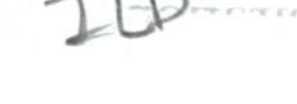

Approach to a Patient of Dyspnoea due Respiratory Disease and Wheeze

Exertional dyspnoea of respiratory origin may be due to:

- COPD
- Interstitial lung disease
- Bronchial asthma

Wheeze

When air passes through narrowed airways (bronchi) a musical sound is produced called wheeze.

Causes of Episodic Attacks of Respiratory Dyspnoea with Wheeze

- Bronchial asthma
- Pulmonary eosinophilia
- Bronchopulmonary aspergillosis.

Orthopnoea

Following respiratory disorders may be associated with orthopnoea

- Severe attack of asthma
- Massive pleural effusion
- Tension pneumothorax

Platypnea

Respiratory causes of platypnea

- Occasionally mass lesion in the upper airway
- Pulmonary AV fistula

Note: Patients with bronchial asthma can have an attack of dyspnoea after exposure to allergens.

Dyspnoea on returning to work after a day of rest, e.g. "Byssinosis" (monday morning chest tightness–due to exposure to cotton dust).

STRIDOR

Characteristics

- High-pitched inspiratory sound
- May be associated with cough and dyspnoea
- *Suggests:* Obstruction to the airflow during inspiration.

Site of Obstruction in Stridor

- Region of glottis (larynx or trachea–predominantly upper airway)
- May be due to narrowing, exudate or edema of upper airways.

Causes of Sudden onset of Stridor

- Laryngeal edema due to anaphylaxis
- Foreign body inhalation
- Inhalation of toxic gases

Causes of Stridor (may not be of sudden onset)

In children

- Foreign body in the upper respiratory tract
- Diphtheria
- Croup (acute laryngotracheobronchitis)

Adults

- Edema of larynx/laryngeal tumors
- Tracheal compression by lymph node
- Vocal cord paralysis–bilateral
- Tracheal malignancy.

APNEA

Suggests sudden stoppage of breathing

Definition: 10 secs pause of breathing.

Types

Obstructive: Due to oropharyngeal airway obstruction.

Causes

- Obesity, acromegaly and hypothyroidism
- Alcohol can aggravate obstructive apneas.

Central: Neuronal stimulation to the respiratory muscle is suddenly stopped.

Mixed: Obstructive with central component.

CHEST PAIN

Important symptom of respiratory disease.

Respiratory Causes of Chest Pain

Pleuritic pain: Pleural involvement due to:

- Pneumonia
- Tuberculosis
- Malignancy
- Pulmonary infarction

Pain due to chest wall disease

- Intercostal myalgia
- Costochondritis
- Rib fracture
- Herpes zoster–spinal root involvement
- Tumor invasion of the chest wall

Pain predominantly central

- Tracheobronchitis
- Inflammatory and neoplastic disease of mediastinum

Chest Pain of Respiratory Disease is Analyzed

Chest wall disorder and musculoskeletal pain

- Chest pain increases with respiratory movement and chest movement.
- Intensity is less compared to pleuritic pain.
- Associated with local tenderness.
- Pain in the distribution of C_8,T_1 root is common in patients with Pancoast's tumor. There will be local tenderness over the 1st and 2nd ribs associated with atrophy of hand muscles.

Pulmonary and Pleural Causes of Chest Pain

Tracheitis and Tracheobronchitis

- Retrosternal or central chest pain
- Increases after coughing.

Pulmonary Hypertension

- Retrosternal pain
- Exercise and stress precipitates pain.

- Pain is not present at rest.
- Dyspnoea may be associated with the pain.

Pulmonary Mass Lesion

- Pain may be localised to an area of chest or may be diffuse.
- Present continuously.
- Dull aching/sharp pain.
- Pain is due to tumour invading the parietal pleura/chest wall.

Pleuritic Pain

Characteristics of Pleuritic Pain

- Severe catching type of pain
- Increases on coughing and inspiration.
- Pain is due to stretch of inflamed parietal pleura.
- Visceral pleura is insensitive to pain.
- Pain originates in the parietal pleura.
- On inspiration parietal pleura gets stretched giving rise to pain.
- Inflammation of diaphragmatic pleura gives rise to the pain which may be referred to the tip of the shoulder and hypochondrium.

FEVER

Fever is a common manifestation of respiratory infection. Occasionally, fever may also be due to bronchogenic malignancy.

Significance of Fever in a Respiratory Disorder

- *Moderate fever:* URTI and tracheobronchitis.
- *Fever with chills, rigors:* Pneumonia, lung abscess and empyema thoracis.
- *Fever associated with night sweats:* Soaking of bedclothes at night, e.g. pulmonary tuberculosis.
- Fever in a patient of bronchogenic carcinoma may be due to necrosis of tumour or secondary infection.
- Mesothelioma of pleura may present with febrile illness.

Fever is not a Dominant Symptom in the Respiratory Disorders

- Pneumoconiosis
- Idiopathic pulmonary fibrosis
- Sarcoidosis—unless extensive
- Multiple pulmonary secondaries.

Symptoms of Upper Respiratory Illness (Table 3.2)

Disorders of Nose and Nasopharynx

- Discharge from the nose
- Nasal obstruction
- Epistaxis
- Repeated sneezing, e.g. allergic rhinitis
- Headache due to recurrent sinusitis.

Miscellaneous Symptoms of Respiratory Disease

Syncope

Respiratory causes

- Severe and prolonged coughing
- Severe pulmonary hypertension
- Massive pulmonary embolism.

Edema and Puffiness of Face

Puffiness of face: Pancoast's tumour with superior vena caval obstruction can produce puffiness of face.

Pedal edema: Common in patients with cor pulmonale and CCF.

Note: Occasionally, long-standing bronchiectasis can result in amyloid deposition in the kidney causing nephrotic syndrome and edema.

Bone and Joint Pain and Muscle Weakness

- Bony pain can be due to hypertrophic pulmonary osteoarthropathy or hypercalcemia associated with bronchogenic carcinoma.
- Bony pain in the region of 1st and 2nd rib may be due to tumour invasion (Pancoast's tumor).
- Myasthenic type of muscle weakness may be associated with paraneoplastic manifestation of bronchogenic carcinoma.

Table 3.2: Symptoms of laryngeal disease and associated disorders

Symptom	Associated disorder
Hoarseness of voice throat pain	Due to laryngeal infection or growth
Harsh, barking and dry cough	Laryngitis
Bovine cough	Laryngeal paralysis
Stridor	Laryngeal obstruction

Symptoms of tracheal disease
- Tracheitis–retrosternal chest pain more on coughing
- Tracheal obstruction–dyspnoea and stridor

Neurological Symptoms

Headache, personality changes and mental state alteration.

Hypoxia and hypercapnea associated with respiratory failure can manifest with headache, altered mentation and personality changes.

Convulsions and focal neurological deficits may be due to tuberculosis and cerebral abscess which may be associated with pulmonary tuberculosis and lung abscess or bronchiectasis respectively.

Bronchogenic carcinoma can cause neurological disturbances either due to metastasis or due to non-metastatic manifestation.

Systemic Symptoms

Primary disorder of liver, cardiovascular system, gastrointestinal or musculoskeletal system can involve the respiratory system. A detailed enquiry about the symptoms of systemic illness is essential in patients with respiratory disease.

Past History

- Importance of previous history of pulmonary tuberculosis:
  - Childhood tuberculosis can become reactivated in the adult.
  - Prior pulmonary tuberculosis may cause bronchiectasis later.
  - Extensive pulmonary fibrosis due to tuberculosis can result in significant alteration in the lung function and hypoxia.
  - Details of prior treatment of tuberculosis, duration, drug therapy, etc. should be elicited in detail as it will be useful in deciding the effectiveness of therapy.
- Haemoptysis may occur due to formation of aspergilloma in a TB cavity.
- Recurrent attacks of pleurisy and pneumonia (may be since childhood) are common in patients with:
  - Cystic fibrosis
  - Bronchiectasis
  - Hypogammaglobulinemia.
- Childhood measles and whooping cough may be responsible for adult bronchiectasis.
- *Previous chest trauma and surgery:* Haemothorax caused by previous chest trauma can cause pleural thickening with diminished chest expansion. Previous chest surgery can cause chest deformity.
- Recent history of altered consciousness, general anesthesia, vomiting or oropharynges surgery may suggest aspiration of septic material from URT and development of lung abscess.
- Previous history of eczema, urticaria and exacerbation of symptoms after exposure to pollens and dusts–common with atopic asthma.
- Long-standing history of cough with sputum, wheeze and breathlessness with recurrent exacerbations–common in patients of COPD, bronchial asthma and bronchiectasis.
- Recent surgery, severe illness or prolonged bedridden states are important risk factors for pulmonary embolism.

It is beneficial to obtain the previous chest radiographs with dates for comparison of the present radiological status and also for previous evidence of respiratory disease.

Family History

Respiratory disorders with familial occurrence

- Bronchial asthma
- Cystic fibrosis (bronchiectasis)
- Ciliary dyskinesia
- Alpha I-antitrypsin deficiency (emphysema).

Pulmonary tuberculosis can manifest in several members of a family as it can get transmitted due to close contact and overcrowding.

Personal History

Loss of weight and appetite: Most of the acute and chronic respiratory disorders can manifest with loss of appetite.

Significant weight loss occurs with pulmonary tuberculosis, malignant disorders of lung, emphysema and chronic suppurative lung diseases.

Infection with human immunodeficiency virus should always be considered in all patients with extreme weight loss and respiratory symptoms.

Extreme obesity: Predisposes for hypoventilation and obstructive sleep apnea syndrome.

They are more likely to develop hypoxic pulmonary hypertension.

Smoking

- Smoking 20 cigarettes per day for 1 year constitutes a pack year and number of pack years smoked should be enquired. This has got direct relationship with disorders like COPD and bronchogenic carcinoma. Smokers are more predisposed for the development of pulmonary tuberculosis.
- Chronic smokers have 8 to 20 times more chance of developing bronchogenic carcinoma.

Chronic exposure to smoking (passive smoking) increases the risk of developing bronchogenic carcinoma by 1.5 times.

Alcoholism: Aspiration pneumonia is common in alcoholics specially with altered sensorium.

Alcoholics have decreased immunity predisposing them for respiratory infection.

High-risk behaviour: Intravenous drug abusers and persons having multiple sexual partners can contract HIV infection and associated respiratory diseases. Occupational and environmental exposure.

1. Prolonged exposure to inorganic dusts results in the development of pneumoconiosis and can also exacerbate asthma.
2. Chronic exposure to asbestos can cause asbestos–related lung disease and mesothelioma of pleura.
3. Exposure to organic substances like moulds, animal products may cause extrinsic allergic alveolitis or precipitate an attack of asthma.
4. Contact with pet animals may be responsible for conditions like ornithosis. Hanta virus pneumonia can occur secondary to exposure to mouse droppings.

Persons from coastal areas of India have more chance of developing tropical pulmonary eosinophilia.

Treatment History

- Details of prior treatment with ATT–duration, combination of the drugs used and their dosage should be enquired. This is important in the treatment of reactivation or resistant pulmonary tuberculosis.
- All patients with recent onset of cough–enquire about ACE inhibitor therapy.
- Antihypertensive like beta-blockers can precipitate an attack of asthma.
- Treatment with methotrexate, bleomycin can cause pulmonary fibrosis.
- Chronic nitrofurantoin therapy can rarely result in interstitial pulmonary fibrosis.

EXAMINATION OF THE RESPIRATORY SYSTEM

General Physical Examination

Build and nourishment.

Vital signs

- Pulse
- BP
- Temperature
- Respiratory rate
  - Pallor
  - Jaundice
  - Cyanosis
  - Lymphadenopathy
  - Clubbing
  - Pedal edema

Examination

- Eyes
- Oral cavity
- Neck
- Skin

Examination of the Upper Respiratory Tract

Nose and paranasal sinuses

- Nostril
- Nasal septum
- Sinus tenderness
- Pharynx
- Tonsil

Examination of the Lower Respiratory Tract

Inspection

- Shape and symmetry of chest
- Position of trachea and apical impulse
- Respiratory movement
- Visible pulsations
- Visible veins and scar mark
- Spine

Palpation

- Position of trachea and apical impulse
- Respiratory movements and measurements
- Vocal fremitus
- Intercostal and rib tenderness
- Palpable respiratory sounds (fremitus)
- Rib crowding

Percussion

- Normal lung resonance, abnormal percussion notes
- Liver dullness and cardiac dullness
- Percussion in specific circumstances:
- Shifting dullness
- Tidal percussion
- Traube's area

Auscultation

- Breath sound intensity
- Type of breathing and alteration of inspiration and expiration
- Added sounds
- Vocal resonance

Examination of other systems

- CVS
- GIT
- CNS
- Other related systems

Build and Nourishment

Respiratory causes of severe emaciation and weight loss

- Pulmonary tuberculosis
- Bronchogenic malignancy
- Emphysema
- Suppurative lung disease
- Respiratory disorders associated with HIV infection.

Recording of Weight is Important

- It is required for calculating the dose of medication.
- For monitoring the benefit of therapy.
- Extreme degree of obesity may be associated with hypoxia and pulmonary hypertension, e.g. Pickwickian syndrome.

Vital Signs

Pulse: Record the rate, rhythm, volume and character of the pulse.

Important Pulse Abnormalities Related to Respiratory Disorders

Tachycardia (rate > 120/min):
- Severe form of pneumonia
- Severe airflow obstruction

High volume bounding pulse: CO_2 retention (type 2 respiratory failure).

Pulsus paradoxus: Severe airflow obstruction (acute severe asthma).

Respiration

- Rate: Normal rate 16–20/min.
- Normal ratio of pulse to respiration—4:1
- *Tachypnoea:* Respiratory rate > 20/min.

Causes of Tachypnoea

- *Physiological:* Anxiety neurosis (hysterical hyperventilation) exertion.
- *Pathological:* Diseases of the chest wall and lungs
- Hypoxic conditions
- Metabolic acidosis

Bradypnea

Respiratory rate < 12/min

Causes

- Narcotic overdosage
- Head trauma
- Hypothermia

Counting the respiratory rate: Observe and count the chest or abdominal movement while counting the radial pulse rate (to divert the patient's attention).

Normal Breathing Pattern and Muscles of Respiration

Muscles of Inspiration

Main group of muscles: External intercostals, diaphragm.

Accessory muscles: Strap muscles of neck, muscles of pharynx and face.

Muscles of Expiration

Main group of muscles: Abdominals

Accessory muscles: Internal intercostals

Breathing Pattern in Males

Predominantly abdominothoracic

Abdomen moves outward during inspiration.

In females: More of chest wall movement than diaphragm (thoracoabdominal).

Causes of Purely Thoracic Breathing

- Peritonitis
- Pregnancy
- Ascites, ovarian cyst

Causes of Purely Abdominal Breathing

- Paralysis of intercostal muscles
- Pleuritic pain
- Defective chest expansion due to ankylosing spondylitis.

Abnormal Patterns and Rhythm of Respiration

1. Increased depth of breathing (hyperapnoea), e.g. Kussmaul breathing (metabolic acidosis).
2. *Stertorous breathing:* Due to vibrations of soft tissues of the nasopharynx, larynx and cheeks resulting from loss of muscle tone. *Causes:* Coma from any cause, during snoring.
3. *Abnormal rhythm of respiration: See* under examination of an unconscious patient.
4. *Prolonged inspiration:* Obstruction to the upper airways. Patient will have stridor.
5. *Prolonged expiration:* Obstruction to the intrathoracic airways.

Abdominal paradox: Due to fatigue of the diaphragm.

Characteristics

During inspiration: Abdomen moves inwards (opposite to normal), e.g. severe COPD.

Blood pressure: Recording of blood pressure is important in monitoring of the patient for noting hypotension and recording of pulsus paradoxus.

Temperature: For making out febrile disorders.

Pallor

Significant pallor may be found in patients with pulmonary tuberculosis, bronchogenic carcinoma and chronic suppurative lung disease.

Patients with chronic hypoxic states like COPD, bronchial asthma can have suffused conjunctiva due to polycythemia.

Icterus

Following respiratory conditions may be associated with icterus:

- Hepatitis due to anti-tuberculous drugs
- Disseminated tuberculosis
- Bronchogenic carcinoma with secondaries in the liver
- Pneumonia with toxic hepatitis
- Pulmonary infarction

Cyanosis

Respiratory disorders which cause type II respiratory failure (acute or chronic) cause central cyanosis, e.g.

Acute: Foreign body inhalation, acute severe asthma, respiratory muscle paralysis

Chronic: COPD, ankylosing spondylitis and kyphoscoliosis

Clubbing

Causes of respiratory disorders associated with clubbing:

- *Suppurative lung diseases:* Lung abscess and bronchiectasis
- Pleural diseases like empyema thoracis and mesothelioma of pleura
- *Malignant disease:* Bronchogenic carcinoma
- Secondaries in the lung
- Interstitial lung disease

Bronchogenic carcinoma and bronchiectasis may also be associated with hypertrophic pulmonary osteoarthropathy (*see* Chapter 1, general physical examination.)

Edema

Edema of feet can occur in following respiratory conditions

- Cor pulmonale with CCF
- Bronchiectasis with nephrotic syndrome due to amyloidosis.
- Hypoproteinemia associated with respiratory diseases.
- Puffiness of face can occur in patients with bronchogenic carcinoma due to SVC obstruction.

Lymphadenopathy

Respiratory disorders may be associated with localised lymphadenopathy like cervical or axillary lymphadenopathy.

Respiratory diseases associated with cervical lymphadenopathy.

1. Bronchogenic carcinoma with secondaries in the neck.
2. Hodgkin's lymphoma with cervical and mediastinal lymphadenopathy.

Lungs can also be involved in conditions like sarcoidosis, tuberculosis, etc. which may cause generalised lymphadenopathy (right supraclavicular lymph node is involved in malignancies of right lung and left lower lobe. Left upper lobe malignancy may involve the left supraclavicular node).

Pathology in the chest wall may cause enlargement of the axillary node.

Scalene node significance: See Chapter 1, general physical examination.

Examination of Eyes, Neck and Skin in Relation to Respiratory Disorders: Examination of Eye (Table 3.3)

Neck

Neck should be examined for the following abnormalities:

- Cervical lymphadenopathy—see above
- Previous lymph node biopsy scar—tuberculosis/malignancy
- Excessive contraction of neck muscles—dyspnoeic patient.

Note: Distended neck veins: Cor pulmonale with CCF and SVC obstruction.

Severe emphysema: Neck vein distend during expiration and collapse during inspiration.

Table 3.3: Examination of skin, neck and eyes in relation to respiratory disorders

Abnormalities	*Conditions associated*
Eye: Eye should be examined for the following abnormalities:	
• Papilledema	SVC obstruction CO_2 retention
• Conjunctival suffusion	CO_2 retention/polycythemia
• Scleritis	TB, sarcoidosis with lung involvement
• Uveitis	Due to collagen disease
• Choroid tubercles phlycten	Pulmonary TB
• Ptosis (Horner's syndrome)	Pancoast's tumor

Thyroid enlargement—may cause tracheal shift.

Tracheal descent with respiration—severe airflow obstruction.

SYSTEMIC EXAMINATION OF THE RESPIRATORY SYSTEM

Upper Respiratory Tract (URT)

Upper respiratory tract extends from external nostril to the junction of larynx and trachea (glottis).

Examination of the Different Parts of the URT with Related Abnormalities

Nose and nasopharynx	
Abnormalities	*Conditions*
• Nasal discharge • Post-nasal drip	Rhinitis
• Deviated nasal septum	produces nasal obstruction
• Hypertrophied turbinates • Nasal polyps	Allergic rhinitis

Paranasal Sinuses and Ear

Paranasal sinus tenderness—suggestive of acute/chronic sinusitis.

Recurrent sinusitis and otitis media are associated with ciliary dyskinesia syndrome and bronchiectasis.

Necrotising granuloma of nasal passage: Rule out Wegener's granulomatosis.

Tonsils and pharynx: Look for tonsillar infection.

Posterior pharyngeal wall congestion: Suggests pharyngitis.

Oral cavity: Check for gingival suppuration–aspiration may lead onto acquired lung abscess.

Examination of the Lower Respiratory Tract

Important Anatomical Landmarks

- Sternal angle or angle of Louis-Bony ridge corresponds to the junction of 2nd rib with the sternum.
- Tracheal bifurcation
  - Anteriorly at the level of angle of Louis
  - Posteriorly at the lower border of T_4 vertebra
- Midclavicular line—line drawn from the mid-point of the left and right clavicles.
- Hilum or root of the lung: Corresponds to 4th, 5th, 6th thoracic spines.
- Apices of upper lobe: Lie 2 to 3 cm above the clavicles.
- Spine of the scapula corresponds to the level of 2nd thoracic vertebra.
- Angle of the scapula corresponds to the T_7 vertebra.

Major Interlobar Fissure (Oblique fissure)

Draw a line from T_2 spine along the scapular border through the 5th rib in the mid-axillary line so as to meet the 6th rib anteriorly in the midclavicular line.

Minor Fissure (Horizontal fissure)

Draw a horizontal line on the right side from the 4th rib at the sternal border to meet the major fissure at 5th rib in the mid-axillary line.

Examination of skin reveals several abnormalities in patients with respiratory disease as mentioned below	
Abnormalities	*Disorder associated*
• Butterfly rash of SLE	SLE with pleural and pulmonary involvement
• Herpes labialis	Pneumonia
• Herpes zoster	Can cause unilateral chest pain
• Metastatic tumour nodules	Secondary from Bronchogenic carcinoma
• Erythema nodosum	TB/collagen disease/sarcoidosis

Lung Borders

Normally

- On the right side (lower border)
- Midclavicular line at 6th rib
- Mid-axillary line at 8th rib
- Scapular line at 10th rib
- Paravertebral line at the spine of 10th vertebra.

Left side: Almost like the right side.

Bronchopulmonary Segments (Fig. 3.1)

Part of the lung tissue correspondingly supplied by a single bronchus, corresponding artery and vein.

Distributions of Bronchopulmonary Segments

Right lung	*Left lung*
Right upper lobe	*Left upper lobe*
• Apical (1)	Apicoposterior (1) and (2)
• Posterior (2)	Anterior (3)
• Anterior (3)	
Right middle lobe	*Lingula*
• Lateral (4)	Superior (4)
• Medial (5)	Inferior (5)
Right lower lobe	*Left lower lobe*
• Apical (6)	Apical (6)
• Medial basal (7)	Anteromedial basal (7) and (8)
• Anterior basal (8)	Lateral basal (9)
• Lateral basal (9)	Posterior basal (10)
• Posterior basal (10)	

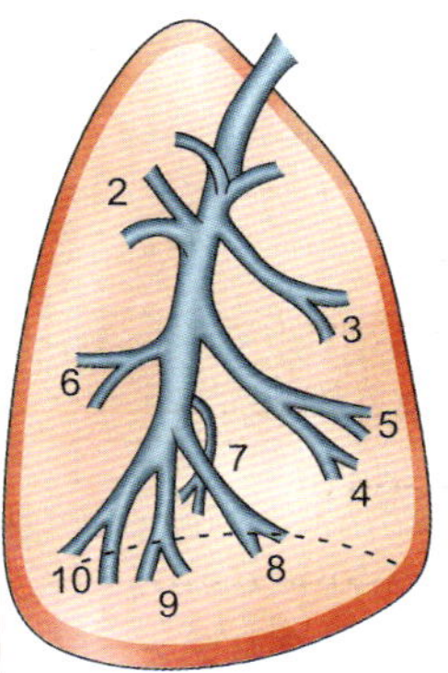

Bronchial tree on the right side (lateral view)

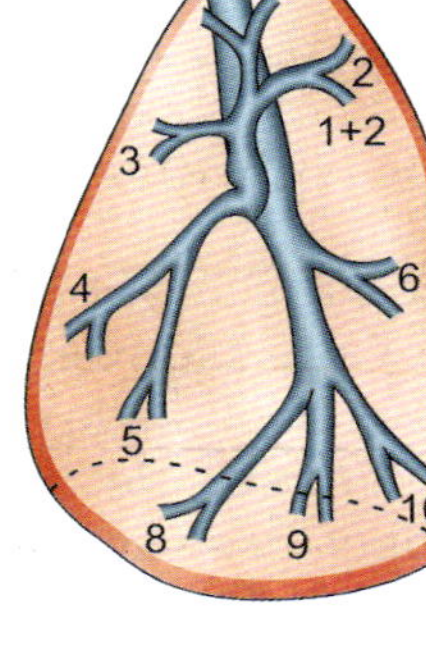

Bronchial tree on the left side (lateral view)

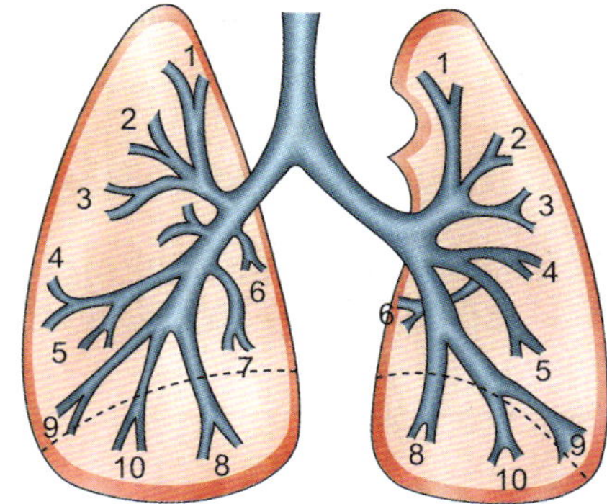

Fig. 3.1: Anterior view of bronchial bifurcations

Respiratory disorders like consolidation or atelectasis usually correspond to bronchopulmonary segments.

INSPECTIONS OF THE CHEST

Position of the patient

For anterior and posterior aspect: Patient sitting upright

Note: Semi-reclining position may also be used for inspection of the respiratory system. In case of bedridden patients, inspection can be carried out from the foot end of the bed.

Normal Chest in Healthy Adults

- Elliptical in cross-section
- Bilaterally symmetrical
- Transverse diameter is more than antero-posterior diameter in the ratio of 7:5.
- Subcostal angle is 90° or less than 90°.

Abnormalities of Shape of the Chest

Barrel-shaped Chest

Characteristic features

- Ribs are more horizontal with flaring upwards of lower ribs.
- Prominent angle of Louis.
- Anteroposterior diameter has increased.
- Upper thoracic spine is kyphotic.
- Subcostal angle becomes obtuse (> 90°).

Causes: Long-standing airflow obstruction, e.g. emphysema.

Pectus Excavatum

- Lower or all parts of the sternum are depressed.
- Costal cartilages attached to sternum may also be depressed.
- Severe pectus excavatum can cause shift of cardiac apex and restriction of lung expansion.

Conditions associated

- Congenital
- Rickets

Pectus Carinatum

Prominent anterior protrusion of sternum and costal cartilages attached to it, e.g. rickets and chronic respiratory disease since childhood (e.g. childhood asthma).

Harrison's Sulcus

- Sulci or depressions on either side of the xiphisternum and the groove corresponds to the diaphragmatic attachment to the ribs.
- It is due to the pulling in of the softened ribs at their attachments by the diaphragm, e.g. rickets.

Lesions of the Chest Wall (Table 3.4)

Symmetry of the chest

Normal chest is bilaterally symmetrical.

Asymmetry of the chest may be due to

Previous thoracic surgery, kyphoscoliosis, chest trauma, lung/pleural disease.

Pathological causes of chest asymmetry

Unilateral flattening and shoulder droop suggest volume loss on the same side, e.g. pulmonary collapse and fibrosis, pleural fibrosis. Unilateral fullness of the chest may be due to:

- Pleural effusion and empyema
- Occasionally pneumothorax.

Localised bulging of the chest: Can occur due to:

- Empyema necessities (empyema pointing through chest wall)
- Aortic aneurysm
- Malignancy of the lung and chest wall

Table 3.4: Lesions of the chest wall

Lesions of the chest wall	
Superficial skin lesions and their significance	
Bleeding spots over the chest wall	• Bleeding disorder with haemoptysis
Vesicles over the chest wall	• Herpes zoster with root pain
Scar over the chest wall	• May be suggestive of previous surgery
Deeper skin lesions–look for	• Axillary lymphadenopathy • Metastatic deposits • Neurofibromas/lipomas

Subcutaneous Emphysema

Feel for the cracking sensation (produced by the air) when the subcutaneous tissues are palpated.

Causes

Severe asthma with air leaking into the mediastinum.

Leaking of air from intercostal tube drainage for pneumothorax/empyema.

Local Tenderness

Causes

Intercostal tenderness—Empyema/pleuritis.

Bony tenderness—Fracture/secondaries/tumour invasion of the chest wall.

Venous engorgement: Due to prominent chest wall veins in SVC obstruction (*see* SVC obstruction).

Arterial Lesions Over the Chest Wall

Causes

- Spider naevi in cirrhotics
- Collaterals around scapulae in coarctation of aorta
- Breast lesions: Look for breast lesions in female patient (*see* examination of breast).

Trachea: Normally 4–5 cm of trachea above the suprasternal notch is palpable.

Trail's sign (sternomastoid sign): Tracheal shift to one side results in sternomastoid on that side to become prominent called Trail's sign.

Apex Beat

Note the position of apical impulse. Shift of the apex may be indicative of mediastinal shift.

Apical impulse may be difficult to visualize–in patients with:

- Thick chest wall, pleural effusion
- Emphysema, pericardial effusion.

Respiratory Movement

Observe the movements of the different parts of the chest.

Different Areas of Chest

- Supraclavicular
- Clavicular
- Infraclavicular (up to 3rd rib)
- Mammary (3rd to 6th rib)
- Axillary (up to 6th rib)
- Infra-axillary (below 6th rib)
- Suprascapular
- Interscapular
- Infrascapular (up to 11th rib)

Localised decrease of movements or decrease of movement on one side localises the site of the disease to that side.

Flail Chest

Occurs due to multiple rib fractures:

Characteristics of Flail chest: On inspiration: Affected area moves inwards.

On expiration: Affected area moves outwards.

Abnormal Respiratory Movements

Excessive contraction of sternomastoid and scalene muscles.

Causes

- Advanced COPD
- Acute severe asthma
- Laryngeal and tracheal obstruction.

Indrawing of intercostal spaces, suprasternal space and supraclavicular fossae occurs in conditions like:

- COPD
- Bronchial asthma
- Severe upper airway obstruction.

Breathing Pattern in Patients with Advanced Emphysema

Person is breathless.

Person tries to increase the effort of expiration by sitting upright and catching the edge of the bed or chair.

Above maneuver fixes the shoulder girdle and allows latissimus dorsi to help in expiration.

Pursed Lip Breathing

Observed in patients with advanced emphysema.

Expiration is carried through the mouth with pursing of lips.

In persons with advanced airflow obstruction high intra-alveolar pressure (due to air trapping) tends to collapse the intrathoracic airways. Purse lip breathing prevents the airway collapse by keeping intra-airway pressure above the intra-alveolar pressure.

Litten's Sign

Sign for observing the movement of diaphragm.

Elicitation of Litten's sign

- Patient lies down supine with lower part of the chest wall exposed to light.
- Examiner sits on the side of the patient.
- Movement of diaphragm is made out as a waveform (phrenic wave) moving up and down in the lower part of the chest with each respiration.
- Persons who are obese or with shallow breathing it may be difficult to make out abnormal movement.

Significance: Unilateral absence of movement suggests defective movement of diaphragm on that side.

Note: Bilateral diaphragm paralysis will be associated with thoracoabdominal discordination of respiratory movement.

Hoover's Sign

- Found in patients with advanced COPD.
- There will be indrawing of intercostals during inspiration.

Spine

- It is preferable to ask the patient to stand while examining the spine.
- Kyphosis suggests posterior bending of the spine.

Scoliosis: Lateral bending of the spine (convexity determines the side of scoliosis).

Kyphoscoliosis can cause change in the position of the mediastinum.

Scar Mark

Look for:

- Previous surgery scar (lobectomy/pneumonectomy)
- Mark of pleural aspiration/biopsy.

PALPATION

Schematic Approach to the Palpation of the Chest

Trachea

- Normal length of the trachea above the suprasternal notch is 4–5 cm.
- Thyroid enlargement may occasionally be responsible for tracheal shift.

Technique of palpation for position of trachea (Fig. 3.2)

- Introduce the tip of the index finger into the suprasternal notch in the midline and note the relationship of the trachea and sternomastoid.
- Observe the resistance offered on each side of the trachea by introducing the finger in between the trachea and sternal insertion of sternomastoid.
- Deviation of trachea to one side will offer more resistance to palpation on that side. Normally trachea is central or minimally deviated to right side.

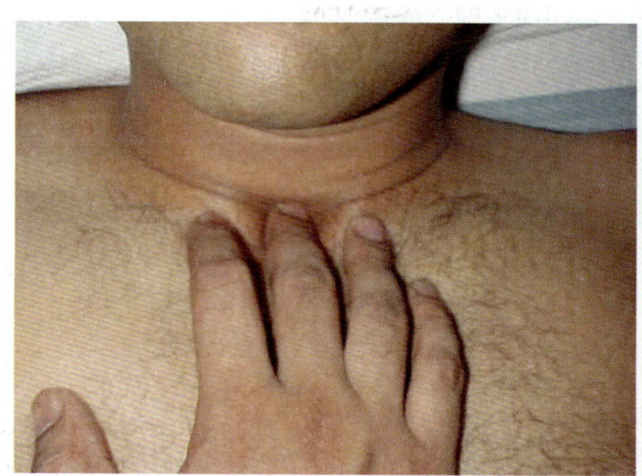

Fig. 3.2: Palpation of trachea

Position of the Apical Impulse

Palpate for the position of the apical impulse and observe for any shift.

Diseases of the lung and pleura may cause shift of the mediastinum.

Only shift of trachea can occur with pathology of the upper lobe and pathology involving only the lower lobe can cause only shift of cardiac apex.

Respiratory Disorders causing Shift of Trachea and Apex (Mediastinum)

- Shift of mediastinum to the same side of pathology:
  - Pulmonary fibrosis
  - Pulmonary collapse
- Shift of mediastinum to the opposite side of pathology:
  - Pleural effusion
  - Empyema thoracis
  - Pneumothorax
  - Upper lobe pulmonary mass
- Respiratory disorders usually without mediastinal shift:
  - COPD
  - Bronchial asthma
  - Bronchiectasis
  - Interstitial lung disease
- Non respiratory causes of shift of cardiac apex:
  - Scoliosis
  - Cardiomegaly
  - Pectus excavatum

Respiratory Movements

Movement of different areas of chest

1. Infraclavicular area movement:

   Technique of palpation

   - Patient is either sitting up or in supine position.
   - Look tangentially at the infraclavicular area on both sides of chest.
   - While patient is breathing steadily, observe for any difference in movement.
   - Movement can also be made out by the movement of two hands, which are kept in the infraclavicular area on either side.

2. Movement of mammary and lower part of the chest (Fig. 3.3):

   Technique of palpation

   - Sides of the chest are grasped with fingers so as to approximate the tips of outstretched thumbs in the region of:
     1. Mammary area.
     2. Xiphoid process (for lower part of chest).
   - A loose fold of skin in between the two thumbs is produced by the adjustment of the hands and with each chest expansion hands move apart.
   - Degree of movement on the two sides of the chest can be estimated by the relative movements of two thumbs with each respiration.

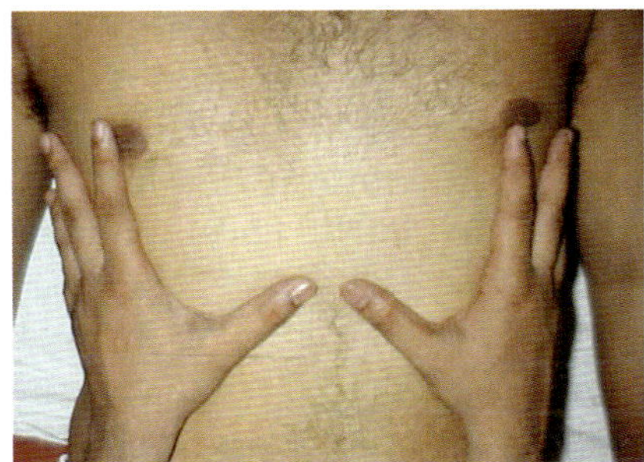

Fig. 3.3: Demonstration of respiratory movement—anterior lower part of chest

3. Posterior movement (Fig. 3.4): Chest is grasped from behind as mentioned above in the region of the lower thoracic spine (10th). Degree of movement of two thumbs on either side is noted.

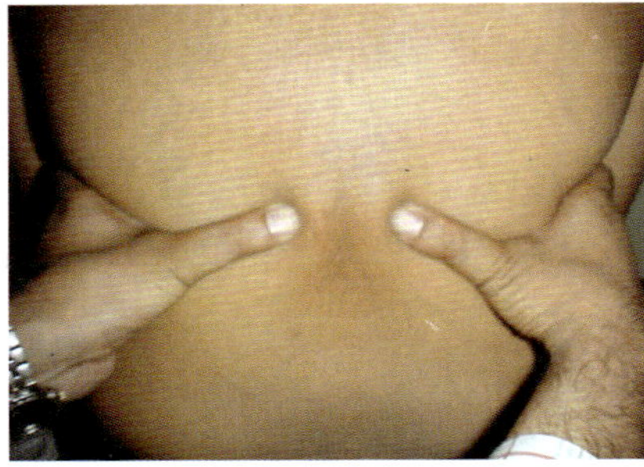

Fig. 3.4: Demonstration of posterior movement

Localised Impairment of Respiratory Movement

Unilateral Decrease of Chest Movement

Causes

1. Empyema and pleural effusion
2. Consolidation
3. Pulmonary collapse
4. Pneumothorax
5. Pleural and pulmonary fibrosis.

Bilateral Decrease of Chest Movement

Causes

1. Airflow obstruction (COPD, bronchial asthma).
2. Diffuse pulmonary fibrosis.

Chest Expansion

Place a measuring tape around the chest at the lower part of the chest (xiphoid process/ T_8 vertebra).

Record the maximum inspiratory/expiratory difference in the chest circumference which indicates chest expansion.

Normal chest expansion: 3–5 cm and above. Expansion of less than 2 cm is suggestive of diminished expansion.

Causes of Diminished Chest Expansion

Unilateral diseases of lungs, pleura and chest wall decrease the chest expansion on the affected side.

Causes of bilateral diminution of chest expansion

- Severe bronchial asthma
- Emphysema
- Interstitial lung disease
- Ankylosing spondylitis

Tests for Integrity of Diaphragm

Ask the patient to sniff—patients with paralysis of diaphragm will have difficulty in sniffing.

Vocal Fremitus (VF)

Definition: Tactile perception of vibrations produced in the larynx communicated to the chest wall through the lungs and tracheobronchial tree.

Technique of Palpation for VF

Keep the ulnar border of the palpating hand on identical areas of both sides of the chest while the patient is repeating 'one-one'. Compare the 2 sides of the chest for the intensity of vibrations felt by the palpating hand.

Normally, VF is equally felt on both sides of the chest.

Unilateral Increase of Vocal Fremitus

- Pneumonic consolidation
- Pulmonary cavity

Unilateral Decrease of VF

- Fibrosis, pleural effusion
- Collapse, pneumothorax

Measurement of Anteroposterior (AP) and Transverse (Tr) Diameter

AP diameter: Measure the distance between the sternum and thoracic spine at the mammary level.

Transverse diameter: Measure the distance between the 2 sides of the chest at the mammary level.

Normal transverse: AP diameter is 7:5. In emphysema ratio becomes almost equal.

Other palpable sounds over the chest (tactile fremitus)

- Crepitations
- Rhonchi
- Pleural rub

Tenderness Over the Chest Wall

- Intercostal tenderness—acute pleurisy, empyema
- Rib tenderness—fracture rib, malignant deposit.

Examination of the Spine

- Evidence of kyphoscoliosis can be made out with palpation of spine.

- Extreme degree of kyphoscoliosis may cause hypoxia and pulmonary hypertension.

PERCUSSION

Rules of Percussion

- Middle finger (pleximeter finger) of the left hand is placed firmly on the part to be percussed.
- Strike the middle phalanx of the left middle finger with the tip of middle finger of the right hand (percussing finger).
- Movement should be at the wrist joint.
- Striking should be perpendicular and repeated heavy striking should be avoided.
- Sound and feel of percussion should be felt.
- Percuss directly over the bones and percuss from resonance to dull area.
- It is ideal to percuss only 2 to 3 times over each area of percussion.

Position of patient for percussion of respiratory system

- Ideal position: Patient is sitting up.
- Percussion of anterior chest: Patient upright and is asked to keep the hands over his head/or in resting position.
- Percussion of posterior chest wall: Patient is sitting up with the head slightly bent forwards and arms folded across the chest anteriorly.
- Axillary percussion: Patient is asked to keep the hands over his head.

Areas of Percussion (Fig. 3.5)

Anteriorly	Supraclavicular area Clavicles Infraclavicular region up to 5th intercostal space.
Laterally	Apex of axilla up to 7th intercostal space.
Posteriorly	Chest wall–above the scapula (above the spine of scapula) Interscapular region (in between scapulae) Infrascapular up to 10th intercostal space (below the angle of scapula up to the 11th rib)

Key Points

- Percussion over the normal lung should be learnt by practice.
- It is ideal to percuss identical areas of chest for comparison.
- Percuss the normal side first.
- Use light percussion while percussing clavicles and anterior chest (with less depth of tissues).
- Use heavy percussion while percussing the posterior chest (greater depth of tissues).

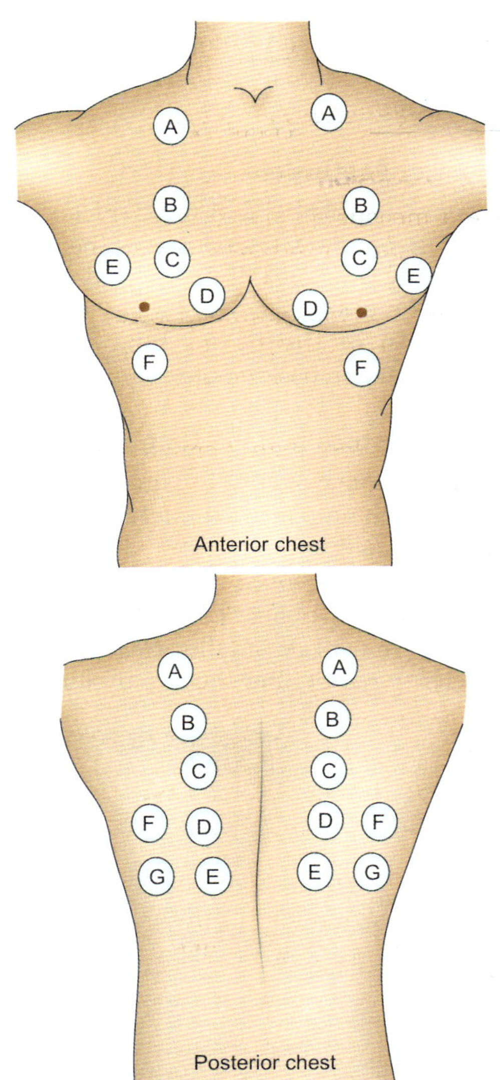

Fig. 3.5: Areas of percussion and auscultation of chest

Percussion of Lung Apex (Fig. 3.6)

Corresponds roughly to the supraclavicular area.

Keep the middle finger of the left hand over the trapezius from behind and percuss with downward movement. Main causes of dullness over the apex:

- Upper lobe pneumonia
- Tuberculosis
- Pancoast's tumour

Cardiac Dullness

Percuss the cardiac borders. Obliteration or diminished cardiac dullness—indicates emphysema.

Clavicular Percussion

Percuss the medial 1/3 of the clavicle.

- Percussion of the lateral part of the clavicle normally produces dull note due to lateral muscle mass.
- A lesion of the upper lobe produces abnormal percussion note over the clavicle.

Normal Percussion of the Lung

Normal lung is resonant to percuss.

Percussion note is moderately low in pitch and heard easily.

Anterior aspect of the chest is more resonant than the back. Lesions 5 cm deeper to the chest wall or smaller than 2–3 cm in diameter may not alter the percussion note.

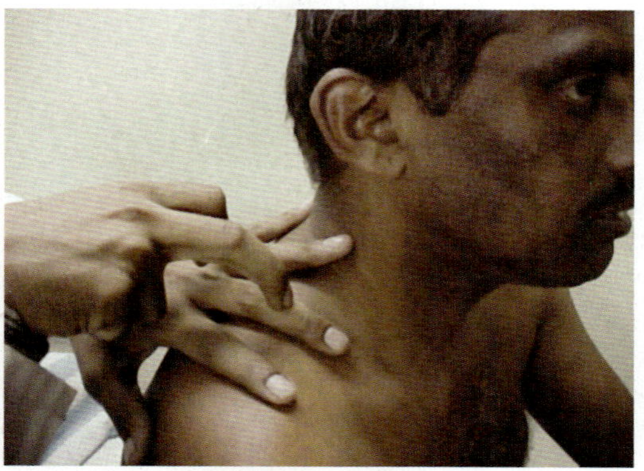

Fig. 3.6: Percussion of the apex of the lung

Genesis of Normal Percussion Note

- Vibrations of the pleximeter fingers, chest wall and underlying tissues together produce composite notes, which is felt or heard when the chest is percussed. Selective resonating action of the thorax reinforces the percussion note.
- Density of the medium through which the sounds travel determines the quality of the percussion note. Quieter notes are produced by denser medium.
- If vibrations are undampened and continue for a longer time percussion note will be resonant.

Abnormal Percussion Notes

Hyperresonant Note

Unilateral hyper resonance, e.g. pneumothorax, compensatory emphysema, large thin-walled cavity.

Hyperresonance over localised area of chest, e.g. obstructive emphysema.

Bilateral hyperresonance, e.g. emphysema of the lung.

Tympanitic note: Abnormally low-pitched (loudest note), e.g. drum-like note, heard over the hollow viscus.

Hyperresonance and tympanitic notes are due to the vibrations produced by percussion which are undampened, continue for significant time due to large acoustic mismatch of the conducting media, e.g. tissues overlying the air—filled space.

Decrease or Absence of Resonance

Impaired note: Decrease of resonance due to airless lung. Percussion note is short in duration with low intensity, e.g. consolidation, pulmonary collapse, pulmonary fibrosis.

Dull/note: Significant or total decrease of resonance, e.g. consolidation, pulmonary collapse/fibrosis, pleural thickening.

Stony dull note: Absolute decrease of resonance (quietest note) with resistance felt by the percussing finger (as though percussion over muscles), e.g. pleural effusion.

Mechanism of impaired or dull note

- Due to rapid decrease of vibrations
- Underlying tissue is similar to the surface tissues and vibrations decay quickly.

Traube's Area

A Semilunar Area

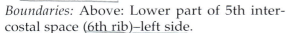

Boundaries: Above: Lower part of 5th intercostal space (6th rib)–left side.

Below: Costal margin on the left side.

Lateral: Mid-axillary line on the left side.

Significance

- Normally resonant to percuss due to the fundus of the stomach.
- Becomes dull in cases of left-sided pleural effusion and massive splenomegaly.

Skodiac Resonance

Resonant percussion note heard above the level of pleural effusion (when the underlying lung is compressed by the fluid).

Shifting Dullness Over the Chest

Significance: Indicates the presence of air and fluid in the pleural space (hydropneumothorax).

If the pleural cavity contains fluid and air, upper border of the dullness will be horizontal.

Percussion can detect change in the level of fluid if the patient's position is changed.

Elicitation of shifting dull note: Keep the patient upright:

- Percuss the chest from above downwards and detect the upper border of dull note (upper part will be hyperresonant due to associated pneumothorax).
- Change the position of the patient—patient is asked to lie down and, while keeping the pleximeter finger in the same area of previous dull note.
- Observe for resonant note while percussing the previously dull area after changing the patient's position.
- Note the degree of shift of fluid by percussing downwards in the newer position of the patient.

Key Points

- Ideal position for auscultation is either the patient sitting up/standing.
- Corresponding areas on either side of the chest should be auscultated and compared.
- Avoid deep breathing as it may produce dizziness and tetany (occasionally).

Myotatic Irritability

Percussion of the anterior part of the chest near to the sternum may produce transient flickering of the neighbouring muscle, e.g. in case of extreme emaciation in diseases like pulmonary tuberculosis.

Percussion for Movement of Diaphragm (Tidal percussion)

Significance: To make out the lower border of lung resonance and lung expansion.

Technique of Tidal Percussion

- Percuss the upper border of the liver dullness—normally in the right 5th intercostal space.
- Ask the patient to take deep inspiration.
- Percuss for the liver dullness at the height of inspiration.
- Normally liver dullness moves down by 1–2 intercostal spaces.

Decreased Movement of Lower Border of Lung Resonance (Tidal percussion negative)

For example: Pulmonary fibrosis, pleural effusion.

Conditions associated with decreased movement of diaphragm.

Note: In patients with emphysema on tidal percussion there is no change in the lower border of the lung resonance as the lung is already fully expanded.

In patients with pushed up diaphragm due to infradiaphragmatic causes upper border of dullness moves down on deep inspiration.

Tidal percussion can also be carried out posteriorly by noting the change in the level of lower border of lung resonance on inspiration and expiration.

AUSCULTATION

Auscultate the following areas of chest

- Anteriorly from supraclavicular area up to the liver dullness (5th intercostal space).
- Lateral sides apex of axilla to the 8th rib.
- Posteriorly from suprascapular area to the 11th rib.
- Avoid auscultation within 2–3 cm of midline.
- Auscultation after coughing is helpful in detection of crepitations and post-tussive suction (avoid coughing in patient with severe pleuritic pain).
- Auscultation of upper lobe—supra- and infraclavicular areas.
- Auscultation of lower lobe—infrascapular area.
- Right mid lobe and lingula—anteriorly on either side of lower 1/3rd of sternum.
- All lobes—auscultatory events of all lobes can be heard in the axilla.

Schematic Auscultation of the Respiratory System

Check for

1. Intensity of breath sounds
2. Type of breathing
3. Comparison of inspiratory and expiratory components of breathing
4. Added sounds
   - Crackles
   - Rhonchi
   - Pleural rub
5. Voice sounds
   - Vocal resonance
   - Bronchophony
   - Aegophony
   - Whispering pectoriloquey

Breath Sounds

Genesis of normal breath sounds: Normal breathing pattern is vesicular which resembles rustling of trees.

Predominantly produced in the major airways (200–2000 Hz) and is heard at the chest wall with low frequency (200–400 Hz) due to filtering of high frequency sounds by the lung and chest wall.

Inspiration is of longer duration (3 times) than expiration.

Inspiratory sound is due to the gas turbulence in the major airways.

Expiratory sound is due to elastic recoil of the lung and produced by central airways and at their bifurcations due to convergence of airflow, maximal at the onset of expiration.

Expiration contains predominantly low frequency sounds and ear is less sensitive to low frequency sounds (falls below the threshold of audibility early in expiration).

Characteristics of Vesicular Breathing (Fig. 3.7)

Normally heard over the chest except over the larynx, trachea, upper part of sternum, lower cervical vertebra and 3rd and 4th dorsal vertebra.

- Rustling in quality
- Inspiration is longer than expiration
- There is no gap between inspiration and expiration.

Intensity (Loudness) of Breath Sounds

Normal intensity depends on the acoustic density of the conducting medium of the sound.

Normally, breath sounds are of equal intensity on both sides of the chest (normally inflated lung).

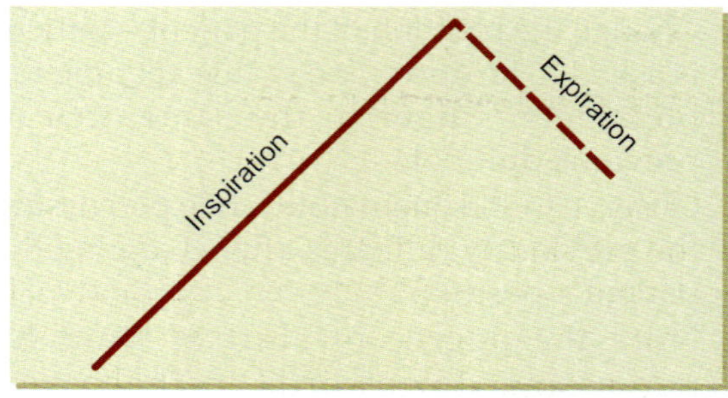

Fig. 3.7: Vesicular breathing

Diminished Intensity of Breath Sounds

Impedance and resistance to transmission of sound can occur as the sound waves pass through tissues of different acoustic density resulting in sound reflection resulting in decreased intensity of sound.

The sound reflection can occur at boundaries between gas-liquid (alveoli), lung-pleura and pleura-chest wall with different acoustic properties due to the underlying pathology.

Conditions Associated with Diminished Breath Sounds

Bilaterally diminished breath sounds—hyperinflated chest, e.g. emphysema, attack of bronchial asthma.

Chest wall and hyperinflated lung will have different acoustic property resulting in reflection of sound at the pleural surface causing decreased intensity of breath sound.

Bilaterally breath sounds can also be decreased due to respiratory muscle paralysis.

Unilateral Decrease of Breath Sounds

- *Pleural effusion:* Decreased intensity of breath sound is due to sounds getting reflected at the pleural surface because of the different acoustic density of the conducting media
- Pneumothorax
- Pleural thickening
- Pulmonary collapse (breath sounds absent)

Causes of prolonged inspiration, e.g. upper airway obstruction produces stridor.

Causes of prolonged expiration—smaller airway obstruction, e.g. bronchial asthma, COPD.

Bronchial Breathing (Fig. 3.8)

Characteristics

- Greater in intensity
- Harsh blowing in quality
- There is a pause in between inspiration and expiration.
- Expiratory sound is of equal duration and louder as that of inspiration.

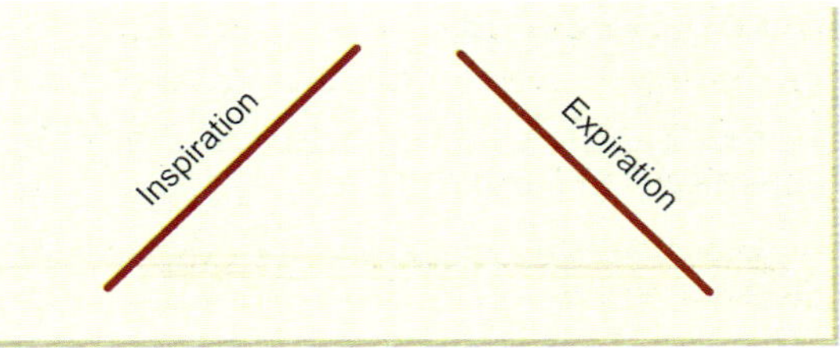

Fig. 3.8: Bronchial breathing

Different Types and Causes of Bronchial Breathing

1. *Tubular breathing:* Resembles tracheal breathing (high-pitched), e.g. pneumonic consolidation.

   Occasionally, upper lobe fibrosis with tracheal shift.

   Sometimes direct transmission of the sound from the trachea can occur as mediastinal surface of right upper lobe is in direct contact with the trachea (irrespective of patency of right upper lobe bronchus).

   Pulled trachea syndrome: In patients with right upper lobe fibrosis tracheal shift to right side can cause bronchial breathing in the infraclavicular area (not heard in the axilla).
2. Cavernous breathing, e.g. cavity.

   Cavity acts as a resonating chamber producing a hollow quality (low-pitched) cavernous breathing.
3. Amphoric breathing: High-pitched metallic quality bronchial breathing as though blowing through top of a bottle, e.g. large cavity, tension pneumothorax (with bronchopleural communication).

Bronchovesicular Breathing

Type of breathing which is intermediate between bronchial and vesicular in its character.

Inspiration and expiration are almost of equal duration and character.

There is no gap between inspiration and expiration.

Normally heard over upper interscapular and suprascapular areas.

Adventitious Sounds

Classification

- Continuous sounds, wheeze (rhonchi)/stridor
- Discontinuous sounds—crackles (crepitations)

Even though rhonchi are relatively lower pitched than wheeze (high-pitched), two terms can be used interchangeably.

Rhonchi

Continuous musical sounds produced due to the narrowing of the medium sized airways.

Characteristics of rhonchi/wheeze

- Musical sounds lasting longer than 250 millisecs.
- Due to the vibrations of an airway at the point of closure.
- Expiration is prolonged.

Genesis of Rhonchi

Produced in the medium-sized airways.

Acceleration of airflow through a narrowing airway will decrease the pressure in that airway (Bernoulli effect) and then tends to close it. This, in turn, decreases flow and airway opens producing rapid vibrations of airways generating wheeze/rhonchi. Narrowing of airways may be due to:

- Mucosal edema
- Spasm of bronchial musculature
- Partial obstruction.

Different Types of Rhonchi

1. *Monophonic:* Single musical note

   Generated from single airway with partial obstruction, e.g. tumor, foreign body, rarely stricture.

   Fixed monophonic wheeze: Localised wheeze which does not change on coughing.

   Suggests fixed partial obstruction to single bronchus. Evidence of associated obstructive emphysema may be present.
2. *Polyphonic wheeze:* Multiple varieties of musical notes.

   Suggests—widespread narrowing of airways (multiple or diffuse).

   Always associated with airway disease with prolonged expiration, e.g. COPD, bronchial asthma, acute bronchitis.

Causes of Rhonchi

- Inspiratory and expiratory—bronchial asthma (predominantly expiratory)
- COPD (both inspiratory and expiratory)
- Pulmonary eosinophilia
- Bronchopulmonary aspergillosis
- Pulmonary edema.

Significance of absence of wheeze in an asthmatic

Severe attack of asthma—flow rate decreases below the critical level necessary to generate oscillations of airways.

It will be associated with severe airflow obstruction.

Stridor

Inspiratory sound can be heard to a distance, best heard over the neck.

Suggests upper airway obstruction (larynx/trachea), e.g. foreign body, carcinoma, hypocalcemia, anaphylaxis.

Crepitations (Crackles)

Fine crepitations

- Non-musical discontinuous sounds
- Higher in pitch and less louder than coarse crepitations.

Genesis of fine crepitations: Occurs due to sudden reopening of closed airways during inspiration, which were closed during previous expiration.

When two areas of lung contain gas at widely different pressures, if the pressure becomes suddenly equalized, airways reopen and gas is set into oscillations producing crepitations.

Examples of crepitations: Early inspiratory: Produced at proximal bronchi, e.g. chronic bronchitis, bronchial asthma, late inspiratory (fine crepitations).

Generated at the distal airways and alveolar level, e.g. pulmonary edema, fibrosing alveolitis, early pneumonia.

Coarse Crepitations

Non-musical discontinuous sounds.

Low-pitched and of longer duration.

Bubbling sounds—produced due to air passing through liquids/secretions.

May be palpable over the chest wall.

May be heard in both inspiration and expiration.

Crepitations can decrease after coughing, e.g. bronchiectasis, pulmonary cavity, resolving pneumonia.

Post-tussive Crepitations

Crepitations appear after coughing.

Characteristically found in patients with early pulmonary tuberculosis in the apical region.

Leathery Crepitations

Coarse crepitations–characteristic of bronchiectasis.

Velcro Crepitations

End inspiratory crepitations—sound resembles that produced when adhered two strips of velcro tapes are separated apart.

Found in patients with interstitial lung disease.

Voice Sounds

Voice Resonance (VR)

Sounds auscultated over the various parts of the chest during phonation.

Technique of auscultation for vocal resonance: Patient is asked to repeat words like one-one-one.

Auscultate symmetrical areas on either side of chest and compare the intensity of sounds.

Normal regional variations of VR: Suprasternal and interscapular areas have increased intensity of VR.

Pathological Variations of VR

Increased VR

- Consolidation
- Cavity

Decreased VR

Unilateral

- Pleural effusion
- Pneumothorax
- Pulmonary collapse
- Pulmonary fibrosis

Bilateral

- Emphysema
- Diffuse airflow obstruction

Bronchophony

Voice sounds which are spoken are heard with greater clarity (e.g. one-one-one) (distinction between individual syllable is not possible).

Bronchophony is due to the better transmission of higher frequency sounds, e.g. consolidation, cavity.

Aegophony

Voice sounds: Heard by the stethoscope over the chest with nasal quality (bleating of a goat), e.g. consolidation, cavity, above the level of pleural effusion.

Aegophony may be an extreme degree of bronchophony. It is due to better transmission of amplified higher frequency sound.

Whispering Pectoriloquy (WP)

Characterized by better appreciation of whispered voice sounds by the stethoscope.

Technique of Auscultation of WP

Patient is asked to repeat with whispered voice sounds (one-one-one).

Auscultate symmetrical areas of chest.

Whispered voice sounds are better heard with clarity and each syllable can be distinguished, e.g. cavity and consolidation.

These higher frequency sounds are better transmitted through airless lung (consolidation and cavity).

Whispered voice sounds are not transmitted by normal lung as it transmits predominantly low frequency sounds.

Whispering pectoriloquey is a confirmatory sign of consolidation.

Pleural Rub

Sound generated by the movement of inflamed layers of pleura.

Characteristics

1. Superficial coarse scratching sound.
2. Present on both phases of respiration.
3. Sound does not alter by coughing.
4. Associated with pleural pain.
5. Intensified by pressure of diaphragm of the stethoscope.

Pleural rub is usually heard at infrascapular and infraaxillary area (due to maximum movement of pleural layers).

Causes

- Pleuritis due to: Viral infection
- Tuberculosis
- Pneumonias
- Malignant disorder
- Collagen disease

Distinguishing Features between Coarse Crepitations and Pleural Rub

Crepitations	*Pleural rub*
Present only on one phase of respiration	Both phases of respiration
Altered by coughing on	Does not change coughing
Not associated with pleuritic pain	Associated with pleuritic pain

Succussion Splash (Hippocratic splash)

Apply the stethoscope over the area of chest at the level of fluid and air and shake the patient—a splashing sound is heard—classically heard in a patient of hydropneumothorax.

Causes of succussion splash heard over the chest

- Hydro/pyopneumothorax
- Large cavity with fluid
- Herniation of stomach into the thorax

Coin Test

Tap a coin, which is held flat against the chest wall with another coin.

Auscultate the opposite chest wall—for a metallic sound.

Heard in patients with pneumothorax.

Post-tussive Suction

Ask the patient to cough and take a deep inspiration.

Auscultate for the suction sound while the patient is taking deep inspiration.

Suggests

- Thin-walled collapsible cavity communicating with the bronchus.
- Sucking sound is heard due to entry of air into an empty cavity during inspiration.

D'Espine's Sign

Whispered voice sounds, which are heard below the T_3 vertebra in adults.

Suggests: Posterior mediastinal mass.

Note: Normally whispered voice sounds are heard only up to T_2 vertebra.

Pneumothorax Click (Hamman's sign)

Rhythmical sound which is heard synchronous with each cardiac systole.

Suggests: Pneumomediastinum.

Note: In suspected cases of exercise-induced asthma person may become breathless and can have rhonchi after exercise.

COMMON RESPIRATORY CONDITIONS IN CLINICAL PRACTICE

Pleurisy

Suggests: Inflammation of the pleura—also called dry pleurisy (there is no accumulation of fluid in the pleural cavity).

Signs

- Audible pleural rub
- Intercostal tenderness

Important causes

- Viral infection
- Bacterial pneumonia
- Tuberculosis

Pleural Effusion

Suggests: Presence of fluid in the pleural cavity.

Signs

- Mediastinal shift to opposite side.
- Decreased chest movement and expansion on the affected side.
- Stony dull note on percussion.
- Decreased or absent breath sound.

Causes

Transudates	*Exudates*
• Cirrhosis of liver	Tuberculosis
• Nephrotic syndrome	Malignant effusion
• CCF	Pneumonia

Causes of Hemorrhagic Pleural Effusion

- Malignancy of pleura—primary, secondary
- Tuberculosis
- Trauma to the chest
- Bleeding diathesis
- Pulmonary infarction
- Anticoagulant therapy

Causes of Predominant Right-sided Pleural Effusion

- Congestive cardiac failure
- Cirrhosis of liver (hepatic hydrothorax)
- Rupture of amoebic liver abscess into the pleural cavity
- Subphrenic abscess on the right side
- Meig's syndrome

Causes of Predominant Left-sided Pleural Effusion

- Acute pancreatitis
- Rupture of esophagus
- Post myocardial infarction (Dressler's syndrome).

Empyema Thoracis

(Presence of pus in the pleural cavity)

Features

- Rigors
- Clubbing
- Tachycardia
- Inter costal fullness and tenderness
- Skin over is red and edematous
- Signs of pleural effusion

Empyema Necessities

Bulge over the chest wall due to subcutaneous collection of pus communicating with the empyema cavity.

Causes of Pleural Effusion with Position of Trachea in the Centre

- Minimal pleural effusion
- Encysted pleural effusion
- Bilateral pleural effusion
- Fixed mediastinum due to growth and mediastinal fibrosis.
- Mesothelioma of pleura

Causes of pleural effusion with shifting of trachea to the same side of effusion

Endobronchial growth/compression of bronchus: obstructing the bronchus on the side of pleural effusion. Causing collapse of the lung with shift of trachea towards the side of pleural effusion.

Pneumothorax

Suggests: Presence of air in the pleural cavity.

Signs

- Mediastinal shift to opposite side.
- Decreased chest expansion and movement on the affected side.
- Hyperresonant note on percussion.
- Absence of breath sounds.

Causes

- Tuberculosis
- Rupture of emphysematous bulla
- Rupture of pulmonary cavity

Types of pneumothorax

- Open type
- Closed type
- Tension type

Hydropneumothorax

Suggests: Presence of air and fluid in the pleural cavity.

Causes

- Tuberculosis
- After aspiration of pleural fluid
- Trauma to the chest
- Rupture of lung abscess cavity into pleural space.

Signs

- Hyperresonant note above and stony dull note below with—horizontal level of dullness in between.
- Shifting dullness
- Succussion splash
- Mediastinum shifted to opposite

Pneumonic Consolidation

Signs

- Mediastinum not shifted
- Movement is decreased on the affected side (due to associated pleuritis)
- Dull percussion note
- Tubular bronchial breathing
- Presence of crepitations (early stage–fine crepitations
- Late stage—coarse crepitations

Classification of pneumonia

Depending on the host condition

- Primary
- Secondary

Depending on the etiology

- Bacterial
- Fungal
- Viral
- Chemical

Depending on the anatomical site involved

- Lobar
- Segmental
- Bronchopneumonia

Lung Abscess

Causes

- Community acquired
- Septic embolisation into the lungs
- Aspiration of septic material from the URT/oral cavity

Signs

- Toxemia
- Clubbing
- Signs of consolidation/cavity

Bronchial Asthma

Signs during an acute attack

- Dyspnoeic patient
- Diminished chest expansion
- Hyperresonant percussion note
- Diminished intensity of breath sounds
- Rhonchi and prolonged expiration

Signs of acute severe asthma

- Dyspnoeic patient
- Presence of central cyanosis
- Tachycardia and pulsus paradoxus
- Hyperresonant chest percussion
- Silent chest on auscultation

Pulmonary Fibrosis

Signs

- Signs of volume loss on the affected side.
- Mediastinum is shifted to same side of pathology.

- Movements and expansion are decreased on the affected side.
- Impaired percussion note.
- Breath sound is diminished with presence of crepitations.

Causes

- Pulmonary TB
- Lung abscess
- Interstitial lung disease
- Pneumoconiosis

Note: Upper lobe fibrosis can result in tracheal breathing in the infraclavicular area on the affected side due to tracheal shift.

Cavity in the Lung

Signs

- Cavernous type of bronchial breathing.
- Presence of crepitations.
- Presence of post-tussive suction in a thin-walled collapsible cavity.

Causes

- Pulmonary tuberculosis
- Lung abscess
- Malignancy undergoing cavitation

Pulmonary Collapse

Signs

- Decreased movement and expansion on the affected side.
- Signs of volume loss on the affected side.
- Mediastinum shifted to the same side of pathology.
- Impaired or dull percussion note.
- Absence of breath sounds.

Causes

Bronchial obstruction due to:

- Foreign body
- Intrabronchial growth
- Extrinsic compression of the bronchus.

Bronchiectasis

Signs

- Halitosis
- Clubbing
- Coarse leathery crepitations

Causes

- Congenital: Ciliary abnormality
- Cystic fibrosis
- Acquired: Necrotising pneumonia
- Pulmonary tuberculosis
- Obstruction to the bronchus

Bronchiectasis sicca

- Secondary to pulmonary tuberculosis
- Patient will have haemoptysis
- Affects the upper lobe

Central/proximal: Bronchitis

Causes: Aspergillosis

COPD (Chronic bronchitis and emphysema)

Signs

Only chronic bronchitis—presence of rhonchi and crepitations.

Signs of airflow obstructions—rhonchi, prolonged expiration.

Signs of emphysema

- Barrel-shaped chest
- Decreased chest expansion
- Hyperresonant percussion note
- Cardiac dullness obliterated
- Liver dullness pushed down
- Decreased breath sounds

Causes of chronic bronchitis

- Chronic smoking
- Atmospheric pollution
- Occupational exposure to dust and minerals
- Repeated respiratory infection

Causes of emphysema

- Chronic bronchitis
- Pneumoconiosis
- Alpha 1-antitrypsin deficiency

Different types of emphysema

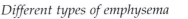

- Pulmonary emphysema (secondary to COPD)
- Obstructive emphysema
- Surgical emphysema
- Compensatory emphysema
- Mediastinal emphysema

Pink Puffer

- Occurs in patient with predominant emphysema
- Patient is severely breathless but not cyanosed
- They are able to maintain the near normal PO_2 and PCO_2.

Blue Bloater

- Occurs in patient with predominant chronic bronchitis
- Patients are cyanosed and edematous
- Due to severe hypoxia in patient with predominant chronic bronchitis—patient develops severe pulmonary hypertension , right-sided cardiac failure (bloated) and hypercapnia (cyanosed-blue).

Obstructive Emphysema

Causes

- Fixed partial intrabronchial obstruction
- Foreign body/tumour
- Signs
- Fixed monophonic wheeze
- Localised hyperresonance

Bronchial Carcinoma

May present with

- Pleural effusion
- SVC obstruction
- Mass lesion
- Mediastinal mass
- Pulmonary collapse

Mass Lesion in the Lung

Signs

- Dull note
- Diminished breath sounds

Note: Occasionally, mass lesion can result in bronchial breathing due to better conduction of breath sounds.

Upper Lobe Bronchial Carcinoma (Pancoast's tumour)

Signs

- Wasting of small muscles of hand
- 1st and 2nd rib tenderness
- Horner's syndrome
- Signs of mass in the upper lobe.

Evidences of Mediastinal Mass

- SVC obstruction
- Horner's syndrome
- Hoarseness of voice
- Diaphragm paralysis
- Dullness on percussion over the sternum/ either side of the sternum
- D'Espine's sign

Differential Diagnosis of Dullness at Right Lung Base

Due to conditions above the diaphragm

- Pulmonary causes: Lower lobe consolidation, collapse and fibrosis
- Pleural causes: Pleural effusion, pleural fibrosis

Table 3.5: Differences between compensatory emphysema and emphysema secondary to COPD

Emphysema (secondary to COPD)	*Compensatory emphysema*
Bilateral	Unilateral
Cardiac dullness obliterated	Cardiac dullness is not obliterated
Breath sounds decreased	Breath sound intensity normal or harsh vesicular
Expiration is prolonged	Expiration is not prolonged
	Evidence of significant lung disease with volume loss on the opposite side

Due to conditions below the diaphragm

- Elevated diaphragm due to massive ascites
- Upward enlargement of liver
- Subdiaphragmatic abscess.

Features of SVC Obstruction

Above the joining of azygos

- Chest wall veins are not prominent
- Main collaterals: Superior intercostal veins.

SVC obstruction involving azygos

Collaterals:

- Veins inside and outside the chest carrying the blood to inferior vena cava.
- There will be prominent veins over the chest.

Patients with SVC obstruction will also have facial puffiness, non-pulsatile and engorged veins over the neck and edema of upper limbs.

Causes of SVC obstruction

- Carcinoma bronchus
- Lymphoma
- Mediastinal secondaries (e.g. testicular tumor, carcinoma breast)
- Retrosternal goiter
- Aortic aneurysm
- Fibrosing mediastinitis.

4 Gastrointestinal and Hepatobiliary System

CHECKLIST FOR GENERAL PHYSICAL EXAMINATION

- Symptoms and history of present illness
- Past history
- Family history
- Personal history
- Occupational history
- General physical examination
- Signs of liver cell failure
- Examination of oral cavity
- Examination of abdomen
- Per rectal examination

HISTORY AND APPROACH TO A PATIENT OF GASTROINTESTINAL DISEASE

Symptoms and History of Present Illness

- Abdomen pain
- Nausea and vomiting
- Heart burn, flatulence and waterbrash
- Hemetemesis and malena
- Distension of abdomen
- Dysphagia
- Constipation and diarrhoea
- Altered bowel habit
- Jaundice, itching and high coloured urine
- Fever
- Weight loss

Miscellaneous symptoms

- Pain in the oral cavity
- Dry mouth and altered taste
- Halitosis
- Hiccups

SPECIFIC SYMPTOMS OF LIVER DISEASE

Past History

- Jaundice
- Pain abdomen and dyspepsia
- Transfusions, vaccinations and injections
- Abdominal surgery
- Drug intake
- High-risk behavior

Family History

History suggestive of gastrointestinal/liver disease in the family.

Personal History

- Loss of appetite
- Loss/gain in weight
- Smoking
- Alcoholism
- Sleep disturbance
- Urine and stool
- High-risk behavior

Occupational History

Menstrual History

SYMPTOM ANALYSIS OF GASTROINTESTINAL AND HEPATOBILIARY DISORDERS

Abdomen Pain

- Significant symptom of gastrointestinal disease.
- Pain abdomen is invariably organic in origin.

Different Mechanisms Contributing for Pain Abdomen

1. *Visceral pain:* Pain may be due to distension, inflammation or perforation of viscera.

   Pain is conducted by sympathetic supply from T_5 to L_2 segments.

   Unpaired intra-abdominal organs can cause midline pain.
2. *Parietal peritoneal pain:* Due to irritation or inflammation of parietal peritoneum.

   Pain is felt in the distribution of somatic supply of the peritoneum.
3. Excessive smooth muscle contraction: Specific pain and usually colicky in nature and well localised, e.g. biliary or intestinal colic.

Check list in a patient of abdominal pain

- Onset
- Site
- Type of pain
- Aggravating factors
- Relieving factors
- Referred/radiation of pain
- Other associated symptoms

Onset and Duration of Pain (Table 4.1)

Causes of acute onset of pain abdomen

- Biliary, ureteric or intestinal colic
- Torsion of testis, ovary, caecum or sigmoid colon.

Aggravating Factors

1. *Food aggravating pain*
   - Gastric ulcer
   - Biliary colic
   - Occasionally pancreatitis
   - Allergy to food
2. *Pain on physical activity and jolting*
   Biliary/ureteric calculus
3. *Pain on reclining forwards*
   Hiatus hernia
4. *Pain after roughage intake*
   Inflammatory bowel disease
5. *Pain increases during menstruation*
   - Spasmodic dysmenorrhea
   - Endometriosis
   - Pelvic inflammatory disease
6. *Hunger pain (may be nocturnal)*
   Duodenal ulcer.
7. *Drug-induced pain (NSAIDs, corticosteroids)*
   Peptic ulcer disease.
8. Abdominal pain, which increases after passing stool, may suggest local colonic disease.

Posture and Abdominal Pain

- Abdominal pain predominantly on reclining may be due to hiatus hernia.
- Abdominal pain occurring on jolting may suggest biliary or ureteric colic.
- Patients of acute peritonitis are usually immobile in the bed.
- Pain of chronic pancreatitis decreases on knee elbow position.

Table 4.1: Characteristics of different types of pain abdomen depending on the onset

Hollow viscous perforation Aortic aneurysm rupture Occlusion of mesenteric artery	Person was asymptomatic before Acute/sudden onset of severe pain Pain progresses rapidly and becomes diffuse allover the abdomen
Acute appendicitis Acute cholecystitis/ Acute diverticulitis	Pain progress is slow and in a steady manner Pain persists for hours to days
Chronic pancreatitis Peptic ulcer	Pain will be persisting for few months to years There will be recurrent exacerbation of pain

Note: Suspect massive GI bleed, acute pancreatitis. Aortic aneurysm rupture or rupture of ectopic pregnancy (in a female) in all patients with abdominal pain and shock.

Different causes of abdomen pain depending on the site of pain	
Epigastric pain	Peptic ulcer
Umbilical	Small intestinal disease
Right hypochondrium	Diseases of the liver and gall bladder, hepatic flexure of colon
Left hypochondrium	Diseases of the spleen, pancreas and splenic flexure of colon
Right iliac pain	Disease of the appendix, caecum, terminal ileum, mesentery, right urinary tract and right uterine adnexa
Left iliac fossa	Diseases of the sigmoid colon, diverticulitis, left urinary tract and left uterine adnexa
Hypogastric region	Usually urinary bladder in origin
Types of abdomen pain with corresponding disorders	
Burning type of pain	Peptic ulcer disease
Colicky type of pain	Intermittent, spasmodic pain–pain of hollow viscous, e.g. ureteric colic, biliary colic
Diffuse abdominal pain	Peritonitis, intestinal obstruction, and gaseous distension of abdomen
Dull aching pain	Enlargement of solid viscera like liver and spleen (rapid stretch of liver capsule (Glisson's) and splenic capsule causes pain)
Nocturnal pain	Usually organic, e.g. pain of duodenal ulcer

Relieving Factors

- Food relieves pain in a patient of duodenal ulcer.
- Pain responding only to antispasmodics suggests colicky pain.
- Sitting up and stooping forward relieves pain in a patient of pancreatitis.
- Abdominal pain, which is relieved by passing flatus and stool, may be seen in patients with irritable bowel syndrome.

Referred Pain

Pain is felt in the area of somatic supply (cutaneous area) which converges on the same segment of the spinal cord to which the visceral pain is conveyed, e.g. pain from the liver abscess, tumor invading the diaphragm and subdiaphragmatic abscess may be referred to shoulders.

Radiation of Pain

Pain radiates from the original site of pain to a distant site.

Examples of pain radiation

Pain of penetrating peptic ulcer—from epigastrium to back

Pain of pancreatic disease—from centre of the abdomen to back.

Pain of rectum and sigmoid colon—radiates posteriorly to the sacral area.

Importance of Associated Symptoms with Abdominal Pain

- Onset of abdominal pain in a patient with previous history of constipation may suggest the possibility of carcinoma colon or diverticular disease.
- Suspect aortic aneurysm rupture in a patient of severe hypertension with abdominal pain and shock.
- Suspect mesenteric ischaemia in a patient of abdominal pain with CCF, atrial fibrillation and peripheral vascular disease.
- Preceding history of dyspepsia (belching, bloating, nausea, anorexia and vomiting) with sudden onset of abdominal pain may suggest peptic ulcer perforation.
- Follicular rupture usually causes pain abdomen in the middle of menstrual cycles.

Metabolic Causes of Pain Abdomen

- Hypercalcemia
- Porphyria

- Diabetic ketoacidosis
- Haemochromatosis

Non-gastrointestinal Causes of Abdominal Pain

- Diaphragmatic pleurisy
- Sickle cell disease
- Myocardial infarction
- Dissecting aneurysm
- Herpes zoster
- Collagen vascular disease

Characteristic Features of Common Types of Abdominal Pain

Peptic ulcer

- Episodic attacks of pain.
- Nocturnal or hunger pain relieved with food/antacids.
- Pain may be severe–burning/colicky type.
- May radiate posteriorly to the back.

Biliary colic

- Severe spasmodic pain associated with vomiting.
- Pain is felt in the right hypochondrium/epigastrium.
- Pain may be of longer duration for hours. Pain refers to right scapula/shoulder tip.

Ureteric colic

- Pain starts in the loin, spreads to groin and genitalia, constant, severe and may be up to 24 hours. Restlessness, vomiting, haematuria and dysuria may be associated with pain.

Appendicitis

- Colicky/severe pain
- Associated with fever and vomiting
- Initial visceral pain—vague pain around the umbilicus
- Involvement of parietal peritoneum—pain will be felt in the right iliac fossa
- Rupture of appendix—generalised abdominal pain due to peritonitis.
- "Consider appendicitis in all cases of acute right iliac pain."

Pancreatitis

- Acute onset severe pain epigastrium/hypochondrium.
- Pain may increase after food/alcohol.
- Pain decreases with sitting up and stooping forward.
- Pain may persist for hours, associated with vomiting, jaundice and shock.

Nausea and Vomiting

Nausea

Feeling or discomfort that occurs before vomiting. Nausea may be associated with symptoms like sweating, faintness and salivation.

Vomiting

Forceful expulsion of contents of gastro-intestinal tract through the oral cavity.

Regurgitation

- Contents of stomach enter the oral cavity through reflux.
- Not associated with forceful act of vomiting.

Approach to a Patient of Nausea and Vomiting

All acute abdominal conditions are associated with vomiting, e.g. acute gastritis, pancreatitis, cholecystitis and acute hepatitis.

Vomiting associated with pain abdomen, e.g. peptic ulcer disease:

- Carcinoma stomach
- Ureteric colic
- Pancreatitis
- Intestinal obstruction
- Biliary obstruction and cholecystitis.

Vomiting without pain abdomen, e.g. pregnancy:

- Alcoholism
- Pyloric obstruction
- Psychogenic
- Renal failure

Projectile vomiting

- There is no preceding nausea before vomiting.

- Raised intracranial tension is a common cause of projectile vomiting.

> *Note:* Oesophageal and gastric obstruction and achalasia cardia may not have nausea before vomiting.

Self induced vomiting

- Patients themselves may induce vomiting for pain relief in peptic ulcer disease.
- In conditions like bulimia nervosa also person himself may induce vomiting.

Causes of severe vomiting

- Duodenal ulcer
- Food hypersensitivity
- Meniere's disease
- Migrainous headaches

Conditions associated with early morning vomiting

- Chronic alcoholism
- Incipient uremia
- Psychogenic vomiting
- Pregnancy

Relationship between the time of onset of vomiting and consumption of food

- Peptic ulcer disease and psychogenic vomiting: May vomit immediately after food.
- Pyloric/duodenal obstruction:
  - Vomiting may occur later in the day
  - Recurrent vomiting few hours after food
  - Vomitus may contain food eaten on the previous day.

> *Note:*
> - Patients with carcinoma stomach can have foul-smelling vomitus.
> - Pyloric obstruction will not have bile-stained vomitus.
> - Rarely vomitus may contain pus (swallowed) or parasites like round worms.

Non-gastrointestinal Causes of Vomiting

Vomiting is invariably the manifestation of gastrointestinal tract.

But following conditions are the examples of non-gastrointestinal causes of vomiting:

Metabolic: Hypercalcaemia, hypoadrenalism, diabetic ketoacidosis and renal failure.

Neurological: Increased intracranial tension, labyrinthine disease, migraine, severe pain and febrile states.

Drug-induced: NSAIDs, digoxin, morphine and alcohol.

Psychogenic: Bulimia and anorexia nervosa.

Psychogenic Vomiting

- Symptoms of depression are usually associated with psychogenic vomiting.
- Vomiting is usually in the early morning and late evening hours.
- No organic cause can be found out.

HEARTBURN, INDIGESTION AND FLATULENCE

Heartburn (Pyrosis)

- Person feels burning type of sensation behind the sternum.
- Food intake, lying down immediately after food and forward bending increases the retrosternal burning.
- Antacids and H_2-blockers relieve heartburn.
- Reflux of acid, pepsin or bile into the oesophagus causes heartburn.

> *Note*:
> - Heartburn can also be a manifestation of duodenal ulcer.
> - Occasionally cardiac pain may present like heartburn.

Causes of Heartburn

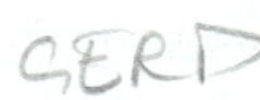

- Reflux oesophagitis
- Hiatus hernia
- Reflux of acid can occur due to relaxation of lower oesophageal sphincter or increased intra abdominal pressure.

Waterbrash

Condition associated with reflux increase of salivation and mouth fills with excess saliva. Waterbrash is usually associated with reflux oesophagitis and duodenal ulcer.

Dyspepsia

Benign disorder.

Characteristics

- Symptoms of peptic ulcer disease.
- Endoscopy fails to detect an ulcer.

Different types of dyspeptic disorders

- Reflux type of symptoms, e.g. retrosternal burning.
- Peptic ulcer-like symptoms: Pain and vomiting. Food or antacids relieve pain.
- Symptoms of disturbed motility: Early fullness, recurrent belching.
- Peptic ulcer disease and occasionally IHD can cause symptoms of dyspepsia.

Flatulence

- Condition associated with increased belching and passing excess flatus through the rectum.
- Flatulence may be associated with audible bowel sounds (Borborygmi) due to movement of fluid and gas due to altered intestinal motility.
- Excess flatus production can occur due to:
  - Aerophagia (swallowing of air)
  - Malabsorption
  - Lactase deficiency
- Intestinal obstruction can result in total absence of passing flatus.

Note: Normally flatus is produced by fermentation of carbohydrates by colonic bacteria due to poor absorption.

Hemetemesis

Indicates presence of blood in the vomitus.

Common causes of hemetemesis

- Oesophageal variceal bleed
- Erosive gastritis
- Mallory–Weiss syndrome
- Peptic ulcer disease
- Stomach/oesophageal malignancy.

Approach to a Patient of Upper GI Bleed

- Vomiting of bright red vomitus indicates bleeding at the pharyngeal or oesophageal level.
- *Coffee-ground vomitus:* Suggests bleeding into the stomach. Color of the vomitus is characteristically brownish and may contain coffee-ground sediment.

  Color is due to the conversion of haemoglobin to acid hematin by gastric acid.
- Previous history of chronic pain abdomen and dyspepsia with upper GI bleed is common with peptic ulcer disease.
- History of retching and violent vomiting especially after alcohol indicates Mallory–Weiss tear.
- Consumption of NSAIDs and steroids prior to hemetemesis is common with erosive gastritis.
- Presence of chronic liver disease with hemetemesis is usually indicative of variceal bleed.
- Elderly person with weight loss and hemetemesis may be suggestive of upper gastrointestinal malignancy.

Lower Gastrointestinal Bleed

Causes

- Acute bacterial or amoebic dysentery
- Lower gastrointestinal malignancy (>40 years of age, recent change of bowel habit).
- *Diverticulosis*

  Characteristics: Abdominal discomfort, constipation and altered bowel habit
- Ulcerative colitis and Crohn's disease and ischemic colitis.

  Characteristics
  - Lower abdominal pain
  - Diarrhoea
  - Rectal bleeding
- *Acute mesenteric infarction*

  Characteristics: Abdominal rigidity, altered bowel habit, lower GI bleed.

Malena

- Term is given to the passing of black tarry stools.
- Suggests upper gastrointestinal bleed above the attachment of ligament of Treitz.

- Minimal of 60 ml of bleeding is required for the appearance of malena.
- Tarry color is due to the action of lower bowel secretions on the blood.
- Malena stool is usually sticky (intake of iron and bismuth salts will produce tarry stool but will not be sticky).
- Stool color may remain black for several days even after the stoppage of bleed.

Hematochezia

Indicates passing frank blood per rectum.

Common causes

- Colitis
- Bleeding piles
- Fissure in ano
- Malignancy rectal/colon
- Inflammatory bowel disease

Rare causes

- Diverticulosis
- Polyposis of colon
- Ischaemia of bowel
- Massive upper GI bleed with rapid intestinal transit

Bleeding from the Anal Canal and Rectum

Characteristics

Bleeding piles:

- Massive bleeding with splashing of blood.
- Bleeding continues even after passing the stool.

Anal canal bleed: Can only soil the toilet paper. Usually bright red and separate from the faecal matter.

Anal fissure bleed: Severe pain is associated with bleeding while passing the stool.

Infection/inflammation of colon: Loose stools associated with blood and mucus and tenesmus.

Abdominal Distension

Five common causes of abdominal distension:

- **F**—fluid accumulation
- **F**—fat accumulation
- **F**—faecal matter (e.g. intestinal obstruction, chronic constipation)
- **F**—flatus (e.g. intestinal obstruction)
- **F**—fetus

Check list for abdominal distension

- Onset and duration
- Pain abdomen
- Vomiting
- Constipation
- Puffiness of face
- Pedal edema
- Urine output

Note:

- Acute and rapid distension of abdomen along with pain may be due to peritonitis.
- Distension of abdomen associated with vomiting, abdominal pain and absolute constipation suggests presence of intestinal obstruction.
- Gradually progressive distension may also be due to accumulation of fluid.
- Combination of puffiness of face, swelling of feet and abdominal distension occurs in conditions like cirrhosis of liver, nephrotic syndrome and congestive cardiac failure.
- In cirrhotic patients—abdominal distension is predominant compared to pedal edema due to the combined effect of hypoalbuminemia and portal hypertension.

Key Points

- Constipation, distension of abdomen and the child not soiling the clothes with faecal matter may suggest Hirschsprung's disease.
- Acute development of tense ascites is usually due to intra-abdominal malignancy, infectious peritonitis, hepatic or portal vein obstruction.
- Painless abdominal distension in women may be indicative of pregnancy or ovarian cyst.
- Abdominal distension in an elderly may occasionally be due to pseudo obstruction as a result of autonomic neuropathy or use of anticholinergics.
- Massive enlargement of liver/spleen or any abdominal viscera can cause non-uniform distension of abdomen.

Dysphagia

Term indicates difficulty in swallowing.

Felt as a sensation of food sticking in the throat or chest while swallowing.

Causes of Dysphagia

1. Painful lesions of mouth, throat and oesophagus, e.g. ulcers, peritonsillar abscess
2. *Mechanical causes*
   - Neoplasm of oral cavity, pharynx and oesophagus
   - Extrinsic compression of oesophagus
   - Stricture of oesophagus
   - Oesophageal webs, e.g. post-cricoid web in iron deficiency anemia.
3. *Neuromuscular disorders*
   - Bulbar and pseudobulbar palsy
   - Myasthenia gravis
   - Achalasia cardia
4. Miscellaneous: Globus hystericus.

Approach to a Patient of Dysphagia

Following details are important in a patient of dysphagia:

- Duration of dysphagia
- Level at which dysphagia occurs (sensation of food sticking)
- Intermittent/progressive
- Associated with pain or without pain
- Type of dysphagia (for solids/liquids)
- Associated symptoms of reflux.

Types of Dysphagia

- Symptoms of dysphagia occurring immediately (1–2 secs) after food usually suggests: pathology in the oral cavity or pharynx.

  Patients with difficulty in swallowing initially for liquids than solids associated with coughing suggests—neurological cause for dysphagia.
- Dysphagia initially for solids and later both for solids and liquids suggests—mechanical cause for dysphagia.
- In patients with long—standing oesophageal obstruction food may be regurgitated long after it was taken.
- Achalasia cardia may cause initially intermittent dysphagia.

Level of Dysphagia

1. Dysphagia occurring at the level of cricoid cartilage may be due to growth, narrowing of oesophagus or even pharyngeal pouch.
2. Obstruction anywhere along the course of oesophagus may cause sensation of dysphagia at suprasternal notch.
3. Dysphagia occurring at the lower part of the oesophagus usually due to disease of the lower oesophagus like growth, achalasia cardia or oesophagitis due to reflux disease.

Pain and Dysphagia

Severe pain can be felt at the site of narrowing due to food impaction.

Regurgitation of food or passing of food downwards can relieve the pain.

Causes of painful dysphagia e.g. infective/inflammatory disorders of oral cavity, reflux oesophagitis.

Note: Oesophageal pain may be due to muscle contraction above the level of obstruction to the oesophagus.

- Oesophageal pain may be retrosternal and may radiate to the neck and interscapular area.
- Lower oesophageal burning type of pain may be due to reflux oesophagitis.
- Occasionally, painless dysphagia can be due to tumor invasion causing denervation.

Globus Hystericus

- Not a true form of dysphagia.
- Person feels as though there is a foreign body or lump sticking in the throat.
- Person has no difficulty in swallowing or eating.

- There will be associated history of suppressed emotional feeling.
- Crying or emotional outbursts can relieve dysphagia.

Diarrhoea

Definition: Frequent passage of unformed stools with stool quantity more than 200 gm/day.

Causes

Acute (less than 2 weeks):

- Infective—viral, bacterial, amoebic dysentery.
- Drug allergy.

Causes of chronic diarrhoea (more than 4 weeks)

- Tuberculosis of intestine
- Colonic neoplasm
- Malabsorption syndrome
- Parasitic infestation
- Inflammatory bowel disease
- Endocrinal—thyrotoxicosis, Addison's disease
- Irritable bowel syndrome Zollinger-Ellison syndrome.

Constipation

The term is used if the stool frequency is less than 3 times/week (term is highly individualised and depends on the bowel habit of each individual).

Causes of Constipation

- Lesions causing pain on defecation, e.g. proctitis, fissure in ano.
- Endocrine disorders—hypercalcemia, hypothyroidism
- Intestinal obstruction—carcinoma, stricture
- Hirschsprung's disease
- Lesions involving sacral nerve roots–cauda equina syndrome
- Drugs—aluminium hydroxide, opiates, decreased fibre intake
- Lack of physical activity, psychogenic factors like depression.

Dyschezia

Difficulty in emptying rectum with requirement of excess straining at stool.

A form of rectal constipation.

Due to the loss of tone of rectal musculature—requiring greater amount of stool collection to initiate the act.

Altered Bowel Habit

Irritable bowel syndrome is a common cause of alternate diarrhoea and constipation (especially below the age of 50 years).

Recent changes in the bowel habit in an elderly person—consider and rule out malignant disease of the bowel.

Tenesmus

A sensation of incomplete rectal emptying or frequent desire to pass stool.

Common causes of tenesmus

- Colonic infection
- Irritable bowel syndrome

Approach to a patient of diarrhoea

Diarrhoea associated with fever and abdominal pain	Infective or inflammatory disease of the intestine
Diarrhoea associated with arthritis, skin rash and ocular symptoms	Inflammatory bowel disease
Presence of pale bulky greasy stool (steatorrhea) Foul smelling stools, excessive flatulence, difficult to flush the pan Presence of abdominal bloating with flatulence and diarrhea Blood and mucus with stool	} Ulcerative lesion in the colon
Diarrhoea alternating with constipation with large quantities of mucus History of diarrhoea in several members of close community	} Irritable bowel syndrome Food poisoning

Key Points

- Diarrhoea associated with weight loss and diarrhoea that is nocturnal is usually organic.
- Enquire the history of consumption of laxatives, antacids and long-term antibiotics as they themselves can cause diarrhoea.
- Diarrhoea after consumption of milk or milk products suggests either primary or secondary lactase deficiency.
- Constipation and rectal impaction can cause overflow resulting in spurious diarrhoea.
- Small intestinal diarrhoea is usually characterised by large volume with less frequency.
- Large bowel diarrhoea is characterised by small volume with more frequency.
- Presence of tenesmus suggests rectal pathology and presence of blood mixed with stool suggests ulcerative lesion in the colon.
- Consider tuberculosis, HIV infection and thyrotoxicosis in a patient with diarrhoea associated with significant weight loss.

- Carcinoma rectum
- Prolapse of the rectum.

Jaundice

Yellowish discoloration of skin, sclera and mucosa due to excess of circulating bilirubin.

Check list for jaundice

- Duration
- Colour of urine
- Fever
- Obstructive symptoms
- Pain abdomen
- Appetite and weight loss
- Altered bowel habits
- Bleeding tendencies
- Abdominal pain.

Duration

Acute causes of jaundice:

- Acute hepatitis
- Acute cholecystitis
- Acute hemolysis

Gradually progressive jaundice

- Chronic parenchymal liver disease
- Chronic hepatitis.

Causes of progressive jaundice due to obstruction to the bile flow

- Gallstones
- Carcinoma head of pancreas
- Carcinoma ampulla of Vater.

Colour of urine

Deep yellow (high coloured) urine with jaundice: Due to the presence of conjugated bilirubin in the urine, e.g. parenchymal liver disease, extrahepatic biliary obstruction.

Presence of jaundice with normal urine colour

Due to increase of unconjugated bilirubin in circulation which cannot be excreted in the urine (acholuric jaundice), e.g. hemolytic jaundice.

Symptoms of obstructive jaundice: High colored urine, itching and clay coloured stool.

Colour of stool: Clay coloured stool in a patient of jaundice suggests obstruction to the biliary flow (due to the absence of stercobilinogen in the stool).

Itching: Suggests obstructive jaundice with increased level of bile salts.

Fever: Jaundice associated with fever, e.g. acute hepatitis of any cause

- Acute cholecystitis
- Sepsis syndrome
- Acute malaria

Jaundice with bony pain and bleeding tendencies

- Defective absorption of vitamin D and vitamin K occurs in patients with obstructive jaundice.
- Defective vitamin D metabolism causes bony pain and defective vitamin K metabolism causes bleeding tendencies.

Note: All causes of hepatocellular jaundice and primary biliary cirrhosis can cause intrahepatic cholestasis and obstructive jaundice.

Jaundice with abdominal pain

- Dull aching abdominal pain is associated with hepatomegaly and parenchymal liver disease.

Key Points

- Painless progressive jaundice may be due to carcinoma head of pancreas.
- Fluctuating jaundice may be due to gall stone disease.
- Recurrent attack of jaundice since childhood may be due to hemolytic disease or familial hyperbilirubinemias

- Colicky pain in the right hypochondrium suggests obstructive biliary tract disease.
- Epigastric pain radiating to the back suggests pancreatic disease.

Fever

Gastrointestinal disorders associated with fever (all infective and inflammatory disorders of gastrointestinal tract), e.g. acute peritonitis

- Pyelonephritis
- Tuberculosis abdomen
- Inflammatory bowel disease
- Malignancies like abdominal lymphoma, pancreatic carcinoma and renal cell carcinoma. RCC

MISCELLANEOUS SYMPTOMS OF GASTROINTESTINAL DISEASE

Symptoms of Oral Disease

Dryness of Mouth

Causes

- Mouth breathing
- Mumps
- Sjögren's syndrome
- Salivary calculi
- Conditions associated with excessive thirst. dehydration

Excessive Salivation

Causes

- Stomatitis
- Irritation of buccal mucosa
- Parkinsonism
- Defective swallowing
- Oesophageal obstruction.

Bad Breath (Halitosis)

Bad breath is usually due to putrefaction of food in the oral cavity.

Putrefaction of food occurs as a result of overgrowth of organisms in the oral cavity, gum or tonsil.

Conditions associated with bad breath

- Disease of the oral cavity
- Bronchiectasis/lung abscess
- Diabetic ketoacidosis—acetone odour
- Hepatic encephalopathy—musty odour
- Carcinoma stomach
- Intestinal obstruction
- Uraemia—ammoniacal odour

Hiccups

Occurs as a result of diaphragm and intercostal muscle contraction resulting in sudden inspiration which is terminated by closure of glottis.

Some of the causes of hiccups

- Dilatation of stomach
- Oesophageal irritation
- Diaphragmatic irritation
- Ischaemic heart disease IHD
- Hyponatremia
- Alcoholism

Cough

Cough may rarely be a manifestation of alimentary disease like gastroesophageal reflux disease and hiatus hernia.

SPECIFIC SYMPTOMATOLOGY OF LIVER DISEASE

Fatigability, anorexia and weight loss occurring in all forms of acute and chronic liver disease.

1. Patients with cirrhosis can have weight gain due to fluid retention.
2. *Disordered taste and smell:* Jaundiced persons (usually with viral hepatitis) cannot tolerate cigarette smell.
3. *Nausea and vomiting:* Occurs in parenchymal and obstructive liver disease.

Pain in the oral cavity

Causes	
Nutritional deficiency	Glossitis due to B complex and iron deficiency
Mechanical causes	Ill-fitting denture
	Carcinoma
Infections	Oral thrush
	Herpes simplex infection
	Vincent's angina
Dermatological	Ulcers due to lichen planus and due to pemphigus
Drug therapy	Ulcers due to drug allergy
	Stevens-Johnson syndrome
Collagen disease	Mouth ulcers
Idiopathic	Aphthous ulcers

4. *Abdominal distension and pain:* Abdominal pain—parenchymal and biliary tract disease (*see* abdominal pain).
   Abdominal distension and pedal edema - occurs in (*see* abdominal distension) cirrhosis with ascites. Abdominal distension can also occur due to enlarged liver and spleen.
5. *Jaundice: See* Jaundice.
6. *Bowel function and stool:*
   Constipation precipitates encephalopathy in cirrhosis.
   Clay-coloured stool suggests cholestasis.
   Steatorrhoea occurs in chronic biliary obstruction.
   Black tarry stool can occur as a result of upper GI bleeding due to oesophageal varices.
7. *Oliguria and nocturia:* Oliguria can occur in cirrhotics and hepatic outflow obstruction. Nocturia occurs due to increased renal blood flow in recumbent position (may be in cirrhotics).

Pruritus of Hepatobiliary Disease

- Common in patients with cholestasis.
- Pruritus may be mild to severe, more on hands and feet.
- Increases after hot bath and troublesome at night.
- Alcoholic liver disease is a rarer cause of pruritus.
- Pruritus is supposed to be due to increasing concentration of circulating bile salts, irritating the nerve endings.

Fever with Rigors and Skin Eruption

- Viral hepatitis especially hepatitis B is associated with fever and rash.
- Fever with rigors occurs in conditions like cholecystitis, liver abscess and cholangitis.

Hepatic Encephalopathy Symptoms

- Inverse sleep rhythm: Somnolence during the day with lack of sleep at night.
- Change in mental functions with neuropsychiatric manifestations.
- Altered consciousness.
- Memory impairment and decreased intelligence.

Impotence and Sexual Dysfunction

- Common in patients with chronic parenchymal disease like cirrhosis.
- Impotence is more common in alcoholic cirrhotics than non-alcoholics.
- Sexual desire significantly decreases in cirrhotics.
- Menstrual irregularities occur in female patients with liver disease.

Bleeding Tendency, Night Blindness and Bony Pain

Defective absorption of fat soluble vitamins like vitamins K, A and D in patients with hepatobiliary disease result in bleeding tendency, night blindness and bony pain, respectively. Bleeding tendency may also be

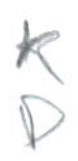

due to defective prothrombin synthesis in parenchymal liver disease.

Symptoms of Systemic Disease

Enquire always symptoms of other systemic diseases, which can secondarily involve the liver.

Past History

- Previous history of fever with jaundice may be present in patients of chronic liver disease due to hepatitis B and C.
- Recurrent history of jaundice occurs in patients with chronic hepatitis, gallstone disease and hepatic decompensation.
- Previous history of pain abdomen, dyspeptic symptoms are common in patients with peptic ulcer complications like perforation and hemorrhage.
- Previous history of transfusions, vaccinations, injections and needle sharing is significant in patients with acute hepatitis B and C and in chronic liver disease of viral etiology.
- High-risk behaviors like intravenous drug abuse and multiple sexual partners is important in patients with parenchymal liver diseases like hepatitis B and C and HIV infection.
- Previous history of abdominal surgery is significant in patients with biliary stricture, retained gallstones and damage to portal vein.
- History of staying in endemic areas of schistosomiasis should be enquired in patients with portal hypertension.

History of Taking Drugs

Drugs Causing Corresponding Hepatic Abnormalities

- INH, rifampicin, pyrazinamide, methyldopa–hepatitis
- Sex hormones—cholestatic jaundice, adenomatous changes in the liver
- Anabolic steroids—hepatocellular carcinoma
- Paracetamol > 10 gm (single dose) can cause hepatic necrosis
- Long duration of methotrexate therapy can cause cirrhotic changes in the liver.

Family History

GIT disorders with familial tendency

- Peptic ulcer
- Gluten sensitive enteropathy
- Inflammatory bowel disease
- Familial polyposis coli
- GI malignancy

Liver disorders with familial tendency

- Wilson's disease
- Congenital hyperbilirubinemia
- Alpha 1-antitrypsin deficiency

History of parental consanguinity is important in patients with Wilson's disease, galactosemia and hereditary fructose intolerance.

Several family members can be affected with viral hepatitis and it is ideal to vaccinate other partners of hepatitis B patients.

Personal History

Loss of appetite

Appetite loss occurs in all disorders of hepatobiliary and gastrointestinal tract.

Loss of weight

- Occurs in acute and chronic liver disease.
- Chronic disorders of gastrointestinal tract like malignancy, malabsorption, tuberculosis, HIV-induced gastrointestinal disorders are associated with significant weight loss.
- Patients of chronic duodenal ulcer can gain weight due to excessive eating to relieve hunger pain.
- Weight gain can also occur due to fluid retention in cirrhotics.

Smoking

Details of amount and duration of smoking should be enquired.

- Smoking can contribute to the development of peptic ulcer disease and reflux esophagitis.
- Smoking can also delay the healing of peptic ulcer.
- Patients with acute viral hepatitis may not tolerate the smell of cigarette smoke.

Alcohol

Amount and duration of alcohol consumed is important in causing liver disease.

Consumption of 60–80 gm of alcohol/day for about 10 years may be necessary in males for the development of cirrhosis of liver (females tolerate alcohol less than males—about 30 gm/day for 10 years is adequate to develop cirrhosis).

Hepatic abnormalities caused by alcohol are as follows:

- Fatty liver
- Acute hepatitis
- Chronic hepatitis
- Cirrhosis of liver
- Hepatocellular carcinoma

Gastrointestinal disorders caused by alcohol

- Pancreatitis
- Peptic ulcer disease
- Reflux oesophagitis

Sleep

- Reversal of sleep rhythm occurs in patients with early hepatic encephalopathy.
- Hunger pain disturbing sleep can occur in patients with chronic duodenal ulcer.
- Urine and stool—*see* history of present illness.
- High-risk behavior—*see* past history

Occupational History

- Occupations related to alcohol are more predisposed for the development of alcoholic liver disease.
- Laborers coming in contact with contaminated water can develop leptospirosis.
- Medical and paramedical personnel have additional risk of contacting hepatitis B and 'C'.
- History of travel to endemic areas of viral hepatitis should be enquired in patients with jaundice.
- Occupations associated with stress and irregular eating pattern are more likely to be associated with peptic ulcer disease.

Menstrual History

Patients with chronic parenchymal liver disease will have decreased menstrual flow or amenorrhea.

EXAMINATION OF THE GASTROINTESTINAL TRACT

SCHEME OF EXAMINATION

General Physical Examination

- Build
- Nourishment
- Vital signs:
  - Pulse
  - Blood pressure
  - Respiratory rate
  - Temperature
- Pallor, clubbing, edema, icterus, cyanosis, lymphadenopathy
- Examination of eyes and face in relation to gastrointestinal tract
- Signs of liver cell failure

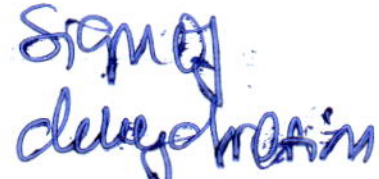

Examination of Oral Cavity

Examination of the Abdomen

Inspection

- Shape of the abdomen
- Pulsations over the abdomen
- Flanks
- Visible veins
- Umbilicus
- Peristalsis
- Movement of different parts of the abdomen
- Visible mass
- Scar mark
- Hernial orifices
- Genitalia

Palpation

- *Superficial palpation:* Tenderness, temperature, guarding/rigidity
- *Deep palpation:* Liver, spleen, kidney or any other mass.

Percussion

Liver and splenic dullness, free fluid.

Auscultation

Bowel sounds, bruit, venous hum.

Examination of other Systems

Examination of the Gastrointestinal Tract

Build and Nourishment

Loss of muscle bulk and subcutaneous fat occurs with chronic liver disease and chronic gastrointestinal disorders.

Rarely anabolic steroid abuse can cause unduly large muscles.

Pallor

Significant anemia develops in following gastrointestinal disorders:

- Gastrointestinal bleeding
- Malabsorption syndrome

Chronic liver disease can result in anemia due to the following reasons

- Bleeding due to oesophageal varices
- Portal hypertension with splenomegaly causing hypersplenism
- Bleeding tendencies due to defective prothrombin synthesis
- Anemia of chronic disease.

Icterus

Icterus appears when serum bilirubin level reaches above 3 mg/dl.

Icterus appears early in the sclera than in any other parts of the body.

Causes

See Chapter 1, general physical examination

Clubbing

Gastrointestinal and hepatic causes of clubbing:

- Cirrhosis especially in biliary cirrhosis
- Hepatocellular carcinoma
- Ulcerative colitis and Crohn's disease
- Malabsorption syndrome.

Cyanosis

Portal hypertension can cause pulmonary AV shunting, O_2 desaturation and hypoxia and central cyanosis.

Lymphadenopathy

Causes of significant lymphadenopathy associated with gastrointestinal disease:

Left supraclavicular node—Virchow's node (Troisier's sign):

Node enlarges due to metastasis from gastrointestinal and testicular malignancy spreading through the thoracic duct.

Viral infections, lymphoma and leukemias associated with generalised lymphadenopathy can also involve gastrointestinal tract and para-aortic nodes.

Pedal Oedema

- Cirrhosis of liver is associated with swelling of feet.
- Patients of hepatic outflow and inferior vena caval obstruction can also have pedal edema.

Examination of Face and Eyes in Relation to Gastrointestinal Tract

- *Exophthalmos:* Thyrotoxicosis can be associated with diarrhea and weight loss.
- *Jaundice:* Suggestive of hepatobiliary disease.
- *Subconjunctival hemorrhage:* Leptospirosis is associated with subconjunctival hemorrhage and liver involvement.
- *Kayser-Fleischer ring:* Brownish green ring appears due to deposition of copper on the Descemet's membrane of the cornea—found in patients with Wilson's disease.
- *Xanthelasma:* Yellowish deposit near the eyelids, associated with chronic cholestasis.

Nails: Nails become white (leuconychia), e.g. cirrhosis of liver.

Skin

- Needle tracks may be visible with IV drug abusers.
- Skin excoriations are seen in patients with severe itching due to primary biliary cirrhosis and sclerosing cholangitis. Skin pigmentation may be a feature of haemochromatosis, primary biliary cirrhosis or chronic cholestasis.

Note: Vitiligo can be associated with autoimmune hepatitis/primary biliary cirrhosis. Chronic cholestasis, primary biliary cirrhosis and liver disease associated with haemochromatosis can he associated with skin pigmentation.

SIGNS OF LIVER CELL FAILURE

Icterus

Parenchymal and obstructive hepatobiliary diseases are associated with icterus.

Parotid Swelling

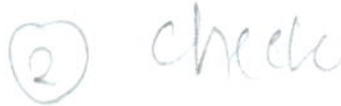

- Parotid swellings are commonly associated with alcoholic liver disease.
- Parotid enlargements are usually not painful.
- Parotid swelling may be related to alcohol itself or due to malnutrition.

Spider Naevi

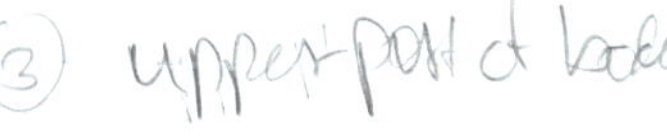

Characteristics: Central arteriole with radiating small vessels resembling spider legs which blanch on pressure.

- Pinhead to 10 mm size.
- Giant spiders seen to pulsate and may bleed.

Distribution of spider naevi: Upper part of the body in the territory of superior vena cava.

Causes of spider naevi

- Cirrhosis of liver
- Thyrotoxicosis
- Pregnancy
- Rheumatoid arthritis
- Alcoholic hepatitis
- Estrogen therapy

Note: Occasionally normal persons can have spiders (usually less than 5 in number).

Increase in the size of previous spider or appearance of new spider is abnormal.

Skin of upper part of the body may be more vulnerable to skin damage making it prone to develop spiders whenever appropriate endocrine abnormalities occur. Differential diagnosis of spider naevi:

- Campbell de Morgan spots
- Hereditary telangiectasia

Palmar Erythema

- Redness of thenar and hypothenar eminences.
- Sole of feet, pulp of fingers can also become erythematous.
- Hands are usually warm, bright red, blanches on pressure with rapid return of colour.

Causes of palmar erythema

- Cirrhosis of liver
- Pregnancy
- Thyrotoxicosis
- Chronic rheumatoid arthritis

Gynaecomastia

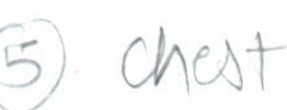

Palpable enlargement of glandular tissue beneath the areola. Areola may become enlarged and pigmented.

Gynaecomastia may be tender. (For further details *see* endocrinology.)

Common causes of gynaecomastia

1. Cirrhosis of liver
2. Spironolactone therapy
3. Testicular disease

Testicular Atrophy

- Testis becomes soft and small.
- Normal testicular size in adult males is around 4–6 cm (15–20 ml/vol) measured by Prader orchidometer.

- Testicular size less than 3 cm usually suggests testicular atrophy. Testicular atrophy is more commonly related to alcoholic liver disease and alcohol-induced pituitary abnormality.

Dupuytren's Contracture

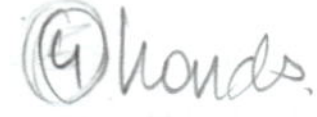

Common in patients with alcoholic liver disease.

Characterised by flexion deformities of fingers due to thickening and shortening of palmar fascia.

Occurs as a result of free radical damage to the connective tissues caused by alcohol. Mainly related to alcohol rather than cirrhosis itself.

Breast Atrophy in Females

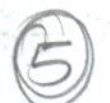

Female patients with cirrhosis develop atrophy of gonads and ovulatory failure. They may develop breast atrophy and infertility. Menstrual cycles become altered with oligomenorrhea or amenorrhea.

All these are closely related to alcoholic liver disease.

Loss of Axillary and Pubic Hair

Cirrhotic men will shave less and will have loss of axillary and pubic hairs.

Bleeding Tendencies

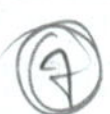

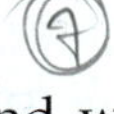

Petechiae and ecchymoses can occur due to: Hypoprothrombinaemia due to liver disease and also due to decrease in platelets as a result of hypersplenism due to portal hypertension.

Pedal Edema

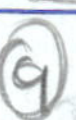

Patients of cirrhosis of liver will have pedal edema due to decrease of albumin synthesis.

Hepatic Encephalopathy

Characteristic features

- Altered conscious level
- Personality changes–loss of family concern and irritability.
- Handwriting becomes impaired.
- Intellectual deterioration–deterioration of intellectual function
- Constructional apraxia–inability to reproduce simple diagrams with blocks or matches.
- Flapping tremors
- Other features–hypothermia, fetor hepaticus.

Flapping Tremors (Asterixis)

Failure to actively maintain posture results in flapping tremors.

Significance of flapping tremor

- Indicates hepatic encephalopathy in a patient of liver disease.
- Flapping tremors are due to difficulty in maintaining posture. These are not seen on voluntary movement and are absent at rest.
- Sustained posture is more likely to result in flapping tremor and is usually bilateral.

Elicitation of flapping termor

Ask the patient to outstretch the arms and keep the wrist hyperextended while supporting the forearm and maintain this position for about 15 secs.

Observe for

- Lateral movement of fingers.
- Flexion and extension movement of wrist and metacarpophalangeal joints.

Pathogenesis of asterixis

- Defective posture maintenance is due to defective relay of joint sense and other informations to brain stem reticular formation concerned with posture maintenance.
- Other causes of flapping tremor are CCF, uraemia, CO_2 narcosis.

Mechanisms behind Spider Naevi and Palmar Erythema

Due to oestrogen-induced vasodilatation and altered ratio of oestrogen/free testosterone.

Pathogenesis of Endocrine Abnormalities in Cirrhosis

- Alcohol-induced liver damage.
- Decompensated liver disease with abnormal hormone metabolism.
- Alcohol-induced pituitary dysfunction.
- Spironolactone-induced anti-androgen effect.

EXAMINATION OF THE ORAL CAVITY

Buccal Mucosa

Observe for mouth ulcers.

Causes of mouth ulcers

- Aphthous ulcers
- Malignancy
- Collagen vascular disease
- Herpes simplex stomatitis
- Herpes zoster
- Inflammatory bowel disease
- See also under causes of pain in the oral cavity

Characteristics of Lesions in the Oral Cavity

Infective Disorders

Oral thrush (moniliasis).

Caused by Candida albicans: Lesions will have sheets of curdy white patches difficult to remove and leave behind a raw surface after removal.

Conditions associated with oral thrush

- Immunosuppressive and corticosteroids therapy
- Long-term antibiotic therapy
- Diabetes mellitus
- Acquired immune deficiency syndrome.

Causes of White Lesions in the Oral Cavity apart from Oral Thrush

- Lichen planus
- Leukoplakia
- Ulcers of other causes

Streptococcal tonsillitis: Exudates appear as yellow punctate lesions over the tonsil.

Infectious mononucleosis

- Redness of pharynx
- Fauces and palate are edematous
- Tonsils are enlarged and covered with white exudate.

Diphtheria

- Characterised by white or greenish coloured membrane formation.
- Membrane spreads from tonsil to pharynx.

Herpes zoster: Vesicles over the oral mucosa.

Measles: Characterised by the presence of Koplik's spots.

Koplik's spots

- Bluish white spots surrounded by an area of redness.
- Usually seen opposite the molar teeth.

Chickenpox: Vesicles can appear in the oral mucosa.

Pigmentation of the Oral Cavity

Causes

- Congenital
- Addison's disease
- Malabsorption syndrome
- Haemochromatosis
- Peutz-Jeghers syndrome (associated with multiple polyposis of intestine).

Miscellaneous lesions in the oral cavity

- Cleft palate
- Telangiectasia
- Haemorrhages
- Pallor, cyanosis and jaundice
- Abnormal palate and uvula movement in 10th nerve palsy.

Gross oral sepsis can lead to endocarditis, lung **abscess** and can aggravate dyspepsia and gastritis.

Examination of the Teeth

Teeth Abnormalities

Check for:

- Number and condition of the teeth
- Discolouration

- Decaying (caries)
- Abnormal configuration and artificial denture.

Causes of discolouration of teeth

- Staining due to tobacco
- Fluorosis causes pitted, mottled yellow teeth
- Tetracycline therapy in children yellow teeth

Hutchinson's teeth

- Incisors are notched (may be peg-shaped)
- Found in patients with congenital syphilis.

Hypoplastic teeth (poorly developed)

- Occurs in patients with hypoparathyroidism.
- Delayed teeth eruption occurs due to hypocalcaemia in infancy.

Gums

Gingivitis: Deep red congestion of gums, which bleed easily on touch.

Pyorrhea

- Teeth are loose, covered with a greenish-yellow exudate
- Pus can be squeezed from the gum margins.

Acute herpetic gingivostomatitis: Caused by herpes simplex virus associated with greenish-gray slough with halitosis.

Vincent's angina

- Ulceration and sloughing of gingiva.
- Caused by infection due to spirochetes and fusiform bacilli.

Lead poisoning: Blue line at gum may be due to deposition of lead sulfide in gum tissues.

Scurvy: Gums are soft, spongy, swollen and bleed easily.

Hypertrophy of Gums

Causes

- Pregnancy
- Long-term phenytoin treatment
- Scurvy
- Acute myeloid leukemia (gums are hypertrophied and bleed easily).

Tongue

Check for following abnormalities

- Atrophy of papillae
- Tremors
- Ulcers and white lesions
- Atrophy of musculature
- Enlargement of tongue

Atrophy of papillae

- Pale and bald tongue—iron deficiency
- Pink and bald—B complex deficiency
- Magenta coloured—riboflavin deficiency
- Beefy red—niacin deficiency

Tremors of tongue

- Thyrotoxicosis
- Parkinsonism
- Anxiety states

Ulcers of tongue: All causes of ulcers in the oral cavity.

Atrophy of musculature: LMN type of 12th nerve palsy.

Enlargement of Tongue

Causes

- Acromegaly
- Myxedema
- Amyloidosis
- Down's syndrome (may be fissured).

Miscellaneous lesion in the tongue: Curdy white patches over the tongue: suggests oral candidiasis.

Hairy leukoplakia

- White lesions, usually on the lateral surface of the tongue.
- Hairy surface is due to keratin projections.
- Caused by Epstein-Barr virus and may progress to squamous cell carcinoma.

Central cyanosis

- Bluish discoloration of the tip of the tongue.
- *Ventral surface of the tongue:* Hemorrhages, neoplastic ulcers, leukoplakia and jaundice can be made out.

EXAMINATION OF THE ABDOMEN

GENERAL PRINCIPLES

- Proper positioning of the patient is essential for examination of the abdomen. Patient should be completely resting supine with the arms on sides.
- Examiner stands on the right side of the patient.
- Expose the abdomen preferably from xiphisternum to inguinal region. Cover the genitalia except during the examination of that part.
- For the purpose of description abdomen is divided into 9 different regions as shown in Fig. 4.1.

Vertical line 1 and 2: Line drawn upwards from midinguinal region to midclavicular region.

Horizontal line I: Connects the lowest part of 10th costal cartilage on both sides.

Horizontal line II: Connects the highest points of iliac crest on both sides.

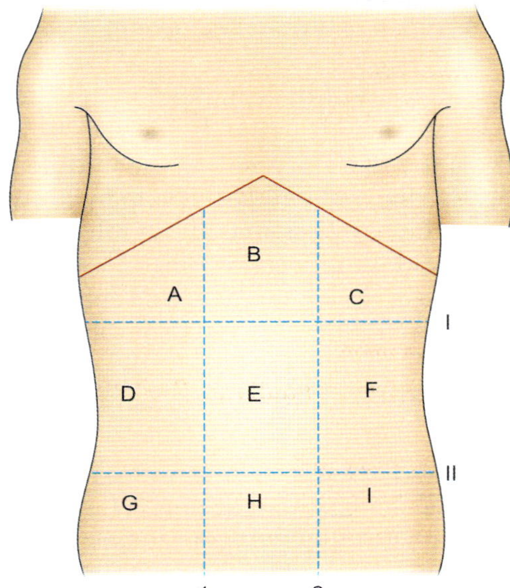

A and C: Rt and Lt hypochondrium; B–epigastrium
A and F: Rt and Lt lumbar; E–umbilical
G and I: Rt and Lt fossae; H–suprapubic/hypogastrium

Fig. 4.1: Different parts of the abdomen

INSPECTION OF THE ABDOMEN

Distension of Abdomen

Uniform distension caused by 5 Fs (discussed above).

Ascites is the most important cause of uniform distension of abdomen.

Flanks become full in patients with uniform distension of abdomen.

Localised distension: Caused by massive enlargement of intra-abdominal viscera.

Epigastric fullness: Occurs in patients with distension of stomach due to pyloric obstruction.

Fullness of suprapubic region

- Occurs due to uterine enlargement
- Distended urinary bladder
- Ovarian tumors

Scaphoid abdomen

- Causes: Severe starvation
- Disorders like TB/malignancy

Umbilicus

Normal position of the umbilicus is at the centre of the abdomen. It may be inverted and retracted.

Bulging of the umbilicus—occurs due to umbilical hernia which can be confirmed by impulse on coughing.

Umbilicus is transversely stretched in patients with massive ascites.

Discharge from the umbilicus

- Serous and seropurulent discharge occurs due to infection of the umbilicus and patent urachus.
- Displacement of umbilicus can occur in upper and lower abdominal mass lesions.

Skin Striae

White, colourless lines over the abdomen occur in patients with gross distension of the abdomen.

Enormous stretching of the skin causes rupture of elastic fibers causing white striae, e.g. pregnancy, massive ascites, excessive weight gain

Purple striae: Occurs in patients with Cushing's syndrome.

Campbell de Morgan spots: Small angiomas occur in elderly patients.

Scars

Previous surgery or laparoscopy (immediately below the umbilicus) can cause multiple scars over the abdomen.

Discolouration of Skin

Cullen's sign: Bluish discolouration around the umbilicus suggests bleeding into the peritoneal cavity, e.g. rupture of ectopic pregnancy, acute pancreatitis.

Turner's sign: Bluish discolouration (ecchymosis) of flanks—due to hemoglobin undergoing tissue catabolism, e.g. acute pancreatitis.

Sister Mary Joseph nodule

- Metastatic nodule in the umbilical area
- Indicates intraperitoneal tumor with metastasis
- Branding marks of different size and shape indicate pain and distress in that part of the abdomen.

Movement of the Different Parts of the Abdomen

- Normally all parts of the abdomen move equally with respiration.
- In males abdomen moves outwards during inspiration.
- Localised or generalised peritonitis or intra-abdominal disease causes decreased movement of that region of the abdomen.
- Tense ascites can also cause decreased movement of the abdomen.

Visible Pulsations

Visible epigastric pulsation may be due to

- Abdominal aorta in thin individuals
- Right ventricular hypertrophy

Pulsatile liver causes predominantly right hypochondrial pulsation.

Aortic aneurysm produces expansile pulsation. Mass overlying the aorta can have transmitted pulsations through the mass. (Pulsation will decrease on knee elbow position as the mass falls away from the aorta.)

Divarication of Rectus Abdominis

Persons with chronic intra-abdominal pressure increase will have wide separation of recti muscles in the midline (may be due to weakness of muscles).

When the person is asked to sit upright from supine position without support, linea alba bulges between the two recti, e.g. common in multiparous individuals. Can also occur in patients with long-standing massive ascites.

Visible Veins

Normally, there may be thin small veins below the costal margin.

Dilated tortuous veins are more of pathological significance.

Visibility of veins is made out better in standing position.

Demonstration of direction of flow in a collateral vein

- Select a part of the collateral vein of about 3–4 cm which is free of branches.
- Press the two fingers over the middle part of this vein and empty the vein by drawing apart the two fingers without releasing the finger pressure being applied.
- Lift one of the fingers at a time and note the direction of filling up of the emptied vein.

Caput Medusa (Fig. 4.2)

Characteristics

- Veins radiating away from the umbilicus.
- Flow is away from the umbilicus.
- Caput medusa suggests—intrahepatic portal hypertension.
- Portal vein drains through collateral vessels along the falciform ligament.
- In extrahepatic portal hypertension, umbilical veins are not prominent.

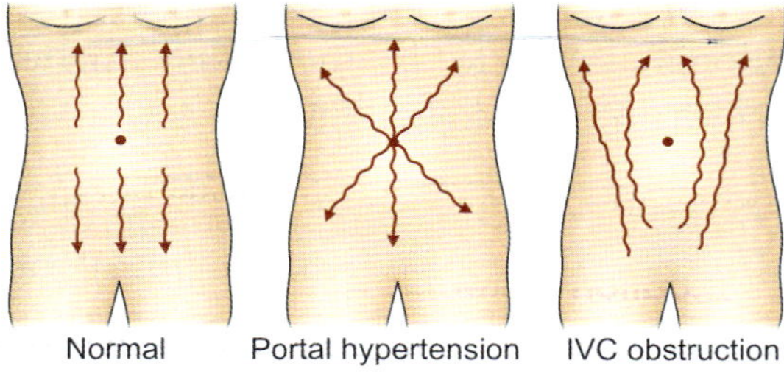

Fig. 4.2: Abdominal venous flow patterns in different disorders

Inferior Vena Caval Obstruction

Dilated anastamotic channels predominantly seen over the flanks and back.

Blood flow is from below upwards.

Anastamoses occur between superficial epigastric and superficial circumflex iliac veins below and lateral thoracic veins above.

Hepatic Outflow Obstruction

Patient may have prominent back veins draining from below upwards.

Visible Mass

Visible mass appears as an area of localised fullness of the abdomen.

Massively enlarged liver and spleen can produce visible mass in the hypochondrium.

Visible Peristalsis

Visible peristalsis may be a normal feature in a very thin elderly person with lax abdominal muscles.

Vigorous tapping or flickering the skin of the abdomen can augment peristalsis.

Pyloric Obstruction

Massively enlarged stomach can cause epigastric fullness.

Ask the patient to drink water and observe for peristaltic waves moving from left to right hypochondrium.

Small Intestinal Obstruction

Abdomen is usually distended. Peristalsis appears as writhing movement in the centre of the abdomen or may appear as a ladder pattern.

Colonic Obstruction

In transverse colonic obstruction, waveform appears moving from right to left in the upper abdomen.

In ascending and descending colonic obstruction—waveform appears to be moving up and down or appears as an alternatively appearing or disappearing mass.

Hernial Orifices

Hernial orifices should be carefully inspected especially on standing and on coughing for cough impulse.

Umbilical hernia: Appears as a bulge through the umbilicus.

Epigastric hernia: Extraperitoneal fat bulging through the defect in the linea alba producing a small epigastric swelling.

Incisional hernia: Herniation occurs due to defective healing of the incision wound after the surgery.

Femoral and inguinal hernia

- Herniation through the femoral and inguinal hernial orifices.
- Inspect the groin in a male for any abnormality of penis, scrotum, position of the testis and testicular swelling.

PALPATION OF THE ABDOMEN

Methods of Palpation

Different methods of abdominal palpation

- Superficial palpation
- Deep palpation
- Bimanual palpation
- Ballottement
- Dipping method.

Superficial Palpation

Gentle and light palpation is required predominantly with the flat of the hand and observe for tenderness, guarding and rigidity.

Key Points

- Patient's position: Patient is lying down comfortably on his back.
  Head is raised slightly and arms are kept to the side.
  Knees are semiflexed (for relaxing the abdomen).
  Cover the genital region except during its examination.
- Examiner sits by the side of the patient and keeps the palpating hand parallel to the abdomen.
- Patient should breath more deeply than normal with mouth open.
- Use flat of the hand and mould it to the abdominal wall and exert pressure by the fingertips and avoid sudden poking of the abdomen.
- Avoid palpating the tender area unles required.

Area of tenderness

- Indicative of inflammatory lesions of underlying viscera and surrounding peritoneum.
- Generalised tenderness over the abdomen occurs in patients with generalised peritonitis.

Rebound Tenderness

- Initial routine palpation does not result in pain.
- Slow and deep palpation over the abdomen and then sudden release of pressure by withdrawing the hand—patient experiences pain. This indicates peritoneal inflammation.
- Pain on release of hand is due to sudden movement of intra-abdominal inflamed structure or viscera.

Note:
- Pressure in the left iliac fossa may cause pain in the right iliac fossa in cases of appendicitis.
- Gaseous distension of intestinal coils may give rise to temporary abdominal tenderness.

Guarding and Rigidity

Indicate resistance of the muscle for palpation.

Guarding: State of voluntary contraction of the abdominal muscles by the patient (patient expects a painful palpation).

Rigidity

- State of reflex involuntary spasm of the muscles of the whole of the abdominal wall.
- Rigidity is indicative of generalised peritonitis and abdominal wall does not move with respiration.
- Whole abdominal wall becomes hard and board-like (board-like rigidity).

Edema of the Abdominal Wall

Abdominal wall edema is demonstrated by applying finger pressure or pinching a fold of skin over the abdominal wall producing a depression (pitting). Abdominal wall edema occurs in patients with anasarca.

Deep Palpation

Each area of the abdomen should be palpated starting from remote area of tenderness and observe for palpability of underlying mass or viscera.

Structures which may be felt normally on palpation

- Lower border of the liver on deep respiration.
- Lower pole of right kidney: Felt in thin and lax abdominal wall on deep inspiration.
- Abdominal aorta: Palpable in thin individuals.

In thin individuals with lax abdominal wall occasionally pelvic colon, caecum and transverse colon may become palpable.

An intra-abdominal mass may become less prominent if the person is asked to raise the head from supine position without support, whereas mass arising from the abdominal wall becomes more prominent.

PALPATION OF LIVER

Palpation in the Right Hypochondrium (Fig. 4.3)

- Examiner sits on the side of the patient.
- Flat of one hand or both hands are kept

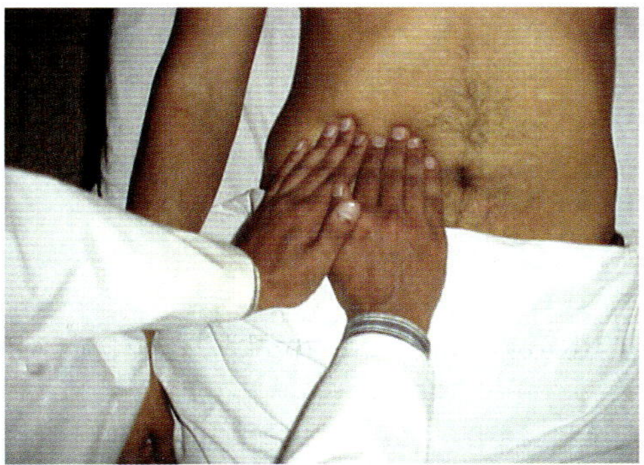

Fig. 4.3: Palpation of liver—right hypochondrium

side-by-side lateral to the rectus abdominus below the costal margin and the patient is asked to take deep breath.

- It is preferable to move the hand upwards from much below the costal margin to avoid missing a greatly enlarged liver.
- Firm upward and inward pressure is given with the hand with the fingers directed towards the costal margin.
- Border of the liver is felt by the tips of the fingers.
- Define the border of the liver from the right hypochondrium to the epigastrium.
- Liver normally moves about 1–3 cm downwards on inspiration.

Palpation from the Right Iliac Fossa (Fig. 4.4)

- Keep the right hand in the right iliac fossa with its border parallel to the costal margin.

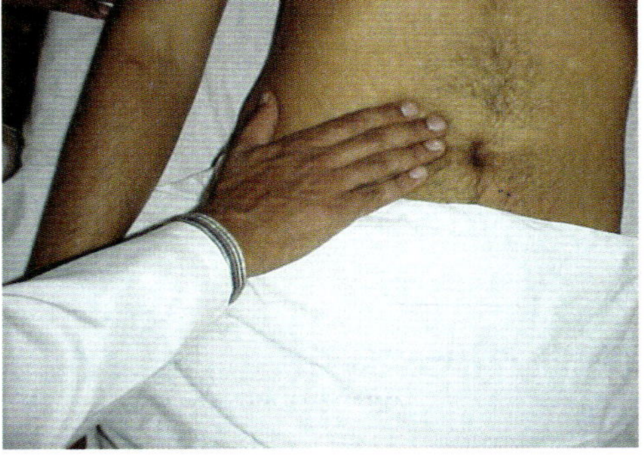

Fig. 4.4: Palpation of liver—right iliac fossa

- Move the hand upwards until the edge of the liver is felt by the border of the hand.

Note the following features whenever the liver is palpable

1. Extent of enlargement from the costal margin in the midclavicular and midsternal line
2. Edge or border
3. Surface
4. Consistency
5. Tenderness
6. Movement with inspiration
7. Pulsation

Features Favoring a Hepatic Mass

- Presence in the right hypochondrium.
- Movement with respiration.
- Getting above the mass is not possible.
- Finger cannot be insinuated between the costal margin and the mass.

Left Lobe of Liver

- Left lobe of the liver may be palpable in the epigastrium between the xiphoid process and umbilicus.
- Left lobe is continuous with the right lobe in the hypochondrium.

Reidel's Lobe

Part of the liver, which is felt superficially in the midclavicular line, occasionally may also become palpable at the level of the umbilicus.

Reidel's lobe moves freely with respiration, and may be mistaken for a mobile kidney or a gall bladder.

Significance of Caudate Lobe of the Liver

Caudate lobe

- Present on the right lobe of the liver on the posterior superior surface
- Does not get affected in hepatic outflow obstruction.

Due to its own anastamoses and separate venous supply with inferior vena cava its blood supply is not affected in hepatic outflow obstruction and it may undergo hypertrophy inpatients with hepatic outflow obstruction.

Features of Normal Liver

Sharp and regular border, soft in consistency, smooth surface, moves with respiration.

Hepatomegaly

Indicates enlargement of liver with increase in the liver span.

In conditions like pleural effusion and emphysema liver may be pushed down, becoming palpable without enlargement (normal liver span).

Causes of Hepatomegaly

Acute

- Viral hepatitis
- Enteric fever
- Acute malaria

Chronic

- Cirrhosis of liver
- Fatty liver
- Lymphoma and leukemias

Tender and Enlarged Liver

Causes

- Congestive cardiac failure
- Amoebic liver abscess (may cause predominant upward enlargement)
- Viral hepatitis
- Pyogenic liver abscess

Abnormalities of Palpable Liver

Round border liver, e.g. congestive cardiac failure.

Firm liver: All causes of chronic liver disease, e.g. cirrhosis.

Nodular liver

1. Macronodular cirrhosis, e.g. post-necrotic cirrhosis
2. Malignancy of liver
3. Hepar lobatum—congenital syphilis

Hard liver

1. Primary hepatocellular carcinoma
2. Secondaries in the liver

Differences between hepatocellular carcinoma and secondaries in the liver

Hepatocellular carcinoma

- Hard enlarged liver
- Bruit over the liver

Secondaries in the liver

- Hard single or multiple nodules
- Umbilication over the nodule (central softening due to degeneration of cells)
- Bruit is absent

Pulsatile Liver

Causes: Tricuspid stenosis, tricuspid regurgitation and aortic regurgitation.

Palpation of pulsatile liver: Place two fingers over the surface of the liver well separated. Observe for further separation of two fingers with each pulsation suggesting pulsatile liver.

Causes of Massive Liver Enlargement

(> 10 cm below the costal margin)

Common causes

- Tricuspid regurgitation and CCF
- Malignancy of liver
- Hepatic amoebiasis
- Hepatic outflow obstruction (caudate lobe is not involved due to separate venous supply).

Rare causes

- Myelofibrosis
- Chronic myeloid leukemia
- Lymphoma

Causes of Painless Hepatomegaly (Firm enlarged liver)

- Cirrhosis of liver
- Fatty liver
- Chronic malaria
- Infiltrative and storage disorders
- Hematological disorders (leukemia, lymphoma, etc.)
- Biliary obstruction
- Amyloidosis

GALL BLADDER

- Normally not palpable.
- Enlarged gall bladder is felt as a round smooth swelling.
- Gall bladder swelling usually moves with respiration.
- Enlarged gall bladder is felt at the angle formed by the lateral border of the rectus abdominus and the right costal margin.

Enlarged gall bladder without jaundice: Cystic duct obstruction can cause enlarged gall bladder due to mucocele or empyema without causing jaundice.

Causes of palpable gall bladder

- Carcinoma of head of pancreas—patient is deeply jaundiced
- Mucocele of gall bladder—patient is not jaundiced
- Carcinoma of gall bladder—felt as a hard irregular swelling.

Murphy's Sign

- In patients with acute cholecystitis (usually secondary to gallstone) tenderness is felt below the right costal margin, midway between the xiphisternum and the flank.
- In patients of acute cholecystitis, if the fingers are kept over the above said area and the patient is asked to take deep breath–Inspiration suddenly gets arrested due to sudden occurrence of pain (Murphy's sign).

Palpation of Spleen (Fig. 4.5)

Palpation

- Normally spleen is not palpable.
- Spleen should enlarge by 2–3 times to become palpable.
- Direction of enlargement of spleen is in the long axis of spleen towards the right iliac fossa.

Method of Palpation of Spleen

- Examiner sits or stands on the right side of the patient.
- Flat of the right hand is placed in the right iliac fossa with the fingers pointing towards the left costal margin.

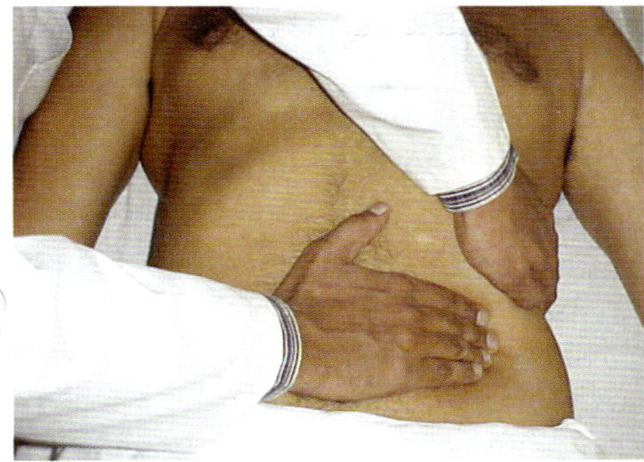

Fig. 4.5: Palpation of spleen

- Flat of the left hand is placed over the lower left rib cage posterolaterally and continuous pressure is applied medially and downwards.
- Right hand is moved upwards after each inspiration until spleen is felt. (Pressing the finger upwards and inwards may be helpful.)
- Entire left costal margin is to be palpated starting from lateral to medial aspect.
- Spleen is felt as a round border swelling with direction of enlargement towards the right iliac fossa.

Method of Palpation for Just Palpable Spleen (Fig. 4.6)

- Turn and keep the patient on the right lateral position.
- Apply inward pressure from the left hand, which is applied over the posterolateral aspect of left lower rib cage.

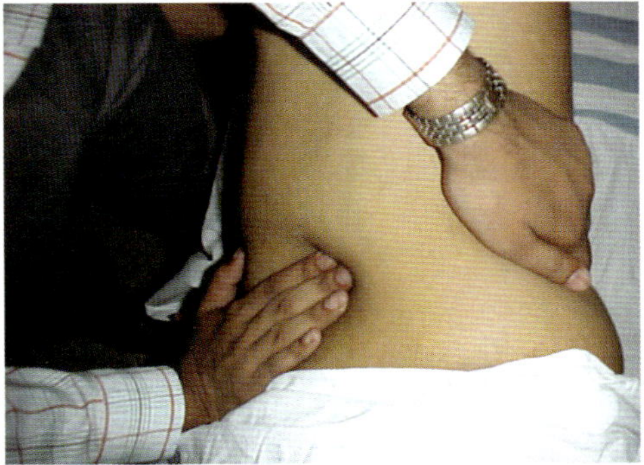

Fig. 4.6: Palpation of just palpable spleen—patient in the right lateral position

- Left hip and knee may be flexed at right angle.
- Tip of the spleen can be palpated with the right hand below the left costal margin.

Hooking method

- Examiner can stand on either side of the patient.
- Place the left hand of the patient under his lower chest.
- Fingers of the examining hand are curled under the left costal margin starting from most lateral aspect.
- Patient is asked to take deep inspiration. Just palpable spleen can be felt with this method.
- Massively enlarged spleen may also be palpated by bimanual method.

Features Favoring Splenic Mass

- Present in the left hypochondrium.
- Enlarges towards the right iliac fossa.
- Notch can be felt.
- Dull to percuss.
- Getting above the mass is not possible.

Features of Splenomegaly

Size: Measure the dimension of splenomegaly from the costal margin along its long axis.

Consistency

- Normally soft
- Acute enlargement of spleen causes soft splenomegaly.
- Chronic enlargement of spleen causes firm splenomegaly.

Edge: Usually regular, occasionally one or two notches may be felt. (Usually over the anteromedial aspect.)

Tenderness

Tender splenomegaly can occur in the following conditions:

- Enteric fever
- Infective endocarditis
- Rupture and infarction of spleen

Massive splenomegaly: Spleen is palpable more than 8 cm below the costal margin.

Bimanual Method of Palpation

- Left hand is placed in the region of loin and the right hand is placed anteriorly in the lumbar region.
- Patient is asked to take deep breaths.
- Two hands are brought together gently.
- Mass will be palpable touching the two hands (e.g. kidney mass, massive splenomegaly).

Different Mechanisms Involved in Splenomegaly

1. Congestive splenomegaly, e.g. CCF, portal hypertension, hepatic outflow obstruction.
2. Reticuloendothelial system hyperplasia, e.g. hemolytic anemias
3. Hyperplasia due to immunological disorders, e.g. collagen vascular disease, infective endocarditis.
4. Infiltrative disorders, e.g. storage disorders, lymphoma.

Ballottement

Keep one hand in the area of loin and place the other hand over the abdominal wall—anteriorly over the mass. Move the mass forwards and backwards between the two hands.

Renal mass is ballottable and bimanually palpable.

Differences between the Splenic Mass and the Renal Mass

Spleen

1. Notch is felt in the lower medial border
2. Direction of enlargement is in the spinoumbilical line
3. Fingers cannot be insinuated between the swelling and the costal margin
4. Not ballottable
5. Mass is dull to percuss

Kidney

- No notch felt
- Direction of enlargement is downwards
- Possible to insinuate the fingers between the swelling and the costal margin
- Ballottable
- Band of resonance will be felt anterior to the mass due to descending colon.

Causes of Splenomegaly

Mild splenomegaly

- Infective endocarditis
- Typhoid fever
- Acute malaria
- Megaloblastic/iron deficiency anemia

Massive splenomegaly

- Chronic malaria
- Chronic myeloid leukemia
- Lymphomas
- Myelofibrosis
- Kala azar

Acute splenomegaly

- Infective endocarditis
- Typhoid fever
- Acute malaria

Chronic splenomegaly

- Portal hypertension
- Chronic malaria
- Chronic myeloid leukemia

Causes of Hepatosplenomegaly

Acute

- Acute viral hepatitis
- Typhoid fever
- Acute malaria

Chronic

- Cirrhosis of liver
- Lymphomas
- Chronic leukemias

Palpation of Kidney (Fig. 4.7)

Occasionally lower pole of the right kidney may be palpable in thin asthenic individuals.

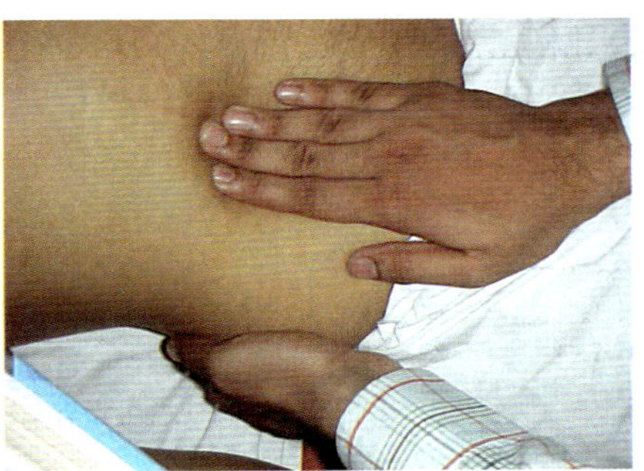

Fig. 4.7: Bimanual palpation of the kidney

- Left kidney is usually not palpable.
- Right kidney is palpated from the right side and left kidney is from the right or left side of the patient.

Kidney mass can be bimanually palpable and ballottable as discussed above.

Unilateral Kidney Enlargement

Causes

- Tumors of the kidney
- Hydronephrosis
- Hypertrophy of one kidney due to atrophy/agenesis of the other kidney.

Bilateral Kidney Enlargement

Causes

- Polycystic kidney—usually bilateral, irregular mass and deeply situated.
- Amyloidosis of the kidney.

Aorta

Aorta is not readily palpable except in thin individuals.

Palpation of Aortic Pulsation

Dip the tips of fingers deeply into the abdomen to the left of umbilicus.

Aortic pulsation is usually felt a little above and to the left side of umbilicus.

Width of aortic pulsation can be made out if the same technique as mentioned above is repeated a few cm to the right of previous site of palpation.

Transmitted pulsation of aorta: There is no separation of 2 fingers which are kept parallel over the area of pulsation.

Expansile pulsation of aorta: There is separation of 2 fingers which are kept parallel over the area of pulsation.

Para-aortic Nodes

- Feel for the aortic pulsation as mentioned above.
- Palpate along the left border of aortic pulsation.
- Nodes are palpable when they are significantly enlarged.
- Para-aortic nodes become palpable when they become significantly enlarged. They are usually found along the left border of aorta in the umbilical region and felt as round firm masses.

Causes of para-aortic lymphadenopathy

- Tuberculosis
- Lymphoma
- Intra-abdominal malignancy
- Germ cell tumors

Urinary Bladder

Normally urinary bladder is not palpable.

Features of urinary bladder enlargements

- History of retention of urine.
- Mass is present in the hypogastrium with regular margin.
- Mass is firm in consistency and usually oval in shape.
- Upper border can be readily made out but lower border cannot be made out.

Differentiate bladder swelling in a female from: Enlarged uterus, ovarian cyst.

Colon

Descending colon may be palpable occasionally in normal persons as a firm tube in the left iliac fossa and also caecum may become palpable occasionally.

Hernial Orifices

Check for inguinal hernia at superficial inguinal ring. It is ideal to ask the patient to stand and look for the cough impulse. Invaginate the finger into the external abdominal ring through the scrotum and ask the patient to cough—early herniation can be made out. Look also for the cough impulse in the epigastrium and umbilical region.

Dipping Method of Palpation

- Dipping method is used for palpation in patients with massive ascites.
- Keep one hand or both the hands (left hand over the right hand) over the area to be palpated.
- Give sudden dipping movements to the fingertips which will displace a quantum of fluid temporarily.
- Displacement of fluid allows the edge of the viscera to come in contact with the fingertips.

PERCUSSION

Percussion is an important aspect of abdominal examination.

Percussion is helpful in detecting following intra-abdominal abnormalities:

1. Ascites
2. Gaseous distension
3. Solid tumor/cyst
4. Enlarged intra-abdominal organs.

Detection of Ascites

a. *Puddle sign:* Detects as little as 120 ml of ascitic fluid within the abdomen.

Key Points

- It is beneficial to carry out light percussion over the abdomen.
- Tympanitic note will be heard while percussing over gas containing viscera.
- Dull note is produced by solid viscera enlargement, fluid collection and solid mass.

Elicitation of puddle sign: Keep the patient in the knee elbow position and maintain it for several minutes.

Percuss around the umbilicus–presence of fluid will result in dull note.

Note: Normally there will be tympanitic note around the umbilicus.

b. Horseshoe-shaped dullness (Fig. 4.8)
  - Helpful in detection of moderate to massive ascites.
  - Fluid usually occupies the area of flanks and hypogastric region.

Method of detection
- Percuss from the umbilical region towards each flank on both sides of the abdomen.
- Percuss also the suprapubic region.
- In the presence of ascites—both flanks and suprapubic areas are dull to percuss due to the collection of fluid.

c. Shifting dullness (Figs 4.9a and b)
  - Shifting dullness indicates presence of free fluid in the abdomen (may detect ascites > 1000 ml).

Method of elicitation
- Ask the patient to lie down flat on his back.
- Examiner percusses from the centre of the abdomen (around the umbilicus) towards one flank till dull note is obtained (normally only lateral abdominal musculature produces dull note).

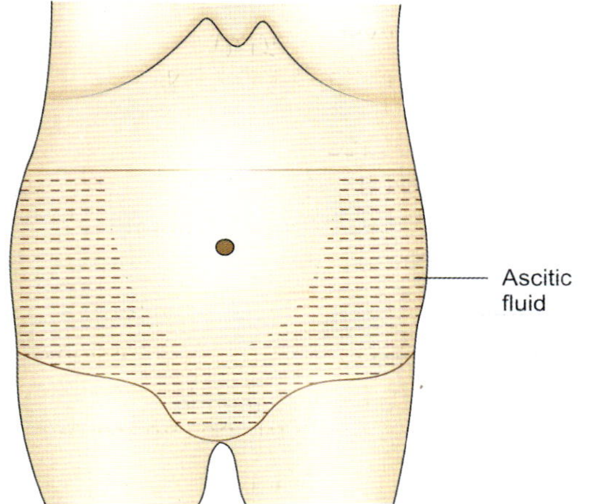

Fig. 4.8: Ascites resulting in horseshoe-shaped dullness

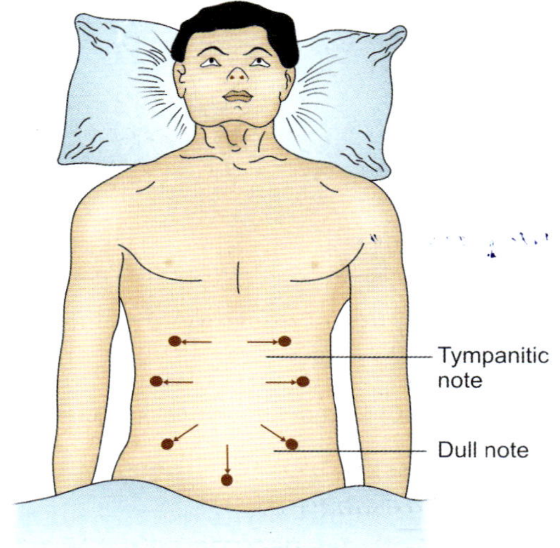

Fig. 4.9a: Demonstration of shifting dullness

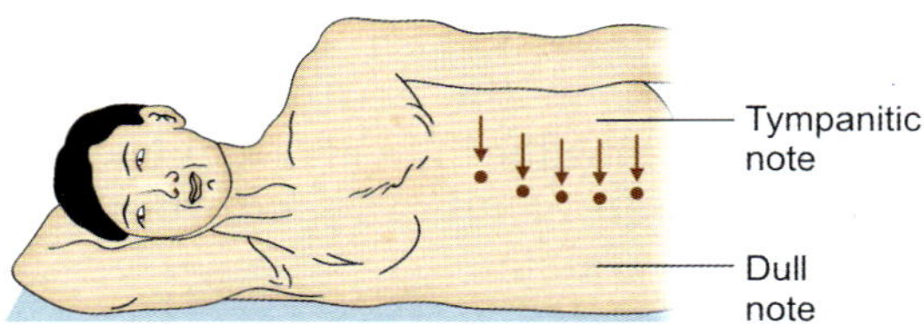

Fig. 4.9b: Shift of dullness to dependant site

- Keep the finger in the area of dull note and turn the patient to the opposite side and wait for few secs.
- Percuss the area of previous dull note and observe for the change of note.
- In the presence of ascites previous area of dull note changes to resonant note due to shift of fluid and floating up of intestinal coils.
- Percuss back towards the midline. Observe for dull note which was previously resonant.

Repeat the above procedure on the other side of the abdomen.

In the following circumstances ascites can be present without shifting dullness:
- Massive ascites
- Adhesions of coils of intestine preventing the fluid to shift.

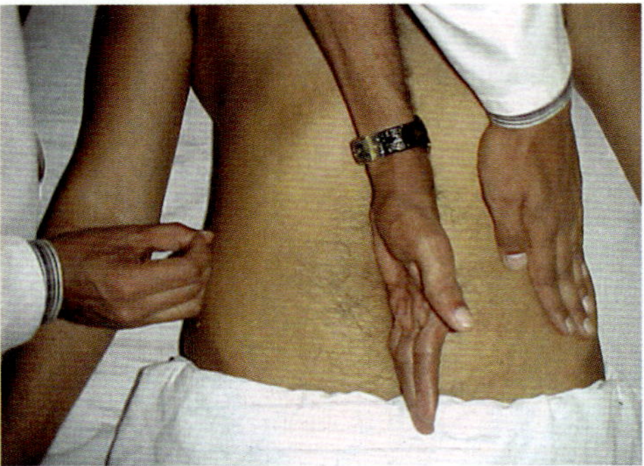

Fig. 4.10: Demonstration of fluid thrill

d. *Fluid thrill:* Fluid thrill usually signifies presence of massive ascites.

Technique of detection (Fig. 4.10)

- Ask the patient to lie flat on his back.
- Ask a bystander to keep the ulnar border of his hand in the centre of patient's abdomen along the linea alba to prevent the transmission of vibrations through the abdominal wall fat.
- Give a tap from one hand to one of the flanks while keeping the flat of the other hand over the opposite flank.
- Appreciate the thrill by the palpating hand when the tap is delivered.

Causes of fluid thrill other than ascites

- Large ovarian cyst
- Large hydronephrosis
- Large hydatid cyst

Percussion of Liver

Upper border

- Start percussing from the right 2nd intercostal space in the midclavicular line till dullness.
- Heavy percussion is beneficial.
- Normally, upper border of liver dullness is at the level of 5th intercostal space.
- Liver dullness will extend down till the lower border.

Lower border: Percuss from the right iliac fossa upwards towards the costal margin till dull note is obtained with light percussion.

Liver span

- Vertical distance measured between upper most and lower most part of liver dullness.
- Normal liver span: Males 10–12 cm, females 8–11 cm.

Causes of decrease of liver dullness

Acute:

- Fulminant hepatic failure (massive liver cell necrosis)
- Air under the diaphragm—perforated hollow viscera in the abdomen.

Chronic:

- Shrunken liver—cirrhosis
- In conditions like emphysema, right pneumothorax, liver dullness may decrease.

Causes of Ascites

Transudate

- Cirrhosis of liver

Differentiating features between ascites and large ovarian cyst

Ascites (Fig. 4.11a)	*Large ovarian cyst* (Fig. 4.11b)
• Umbilicus: Transversely stretched	• Umbilicus: Pushed upwards and may be vertical
• Dullness: Flanks are dull	• Flanks are resonant
• Upper border of dullness will have concavity upwards	• Upper border of dullness will have convexity upwards
• Distance between the umbilicus and anterior superior iliac spine on either side is equal	• Distance between the umbilicus and the anterior superior iliac spine on either side is unequal
	• Maximum girth of the abdomen is below the umbilicus.
	• Getting below the swelling is not possible

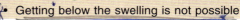

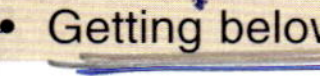

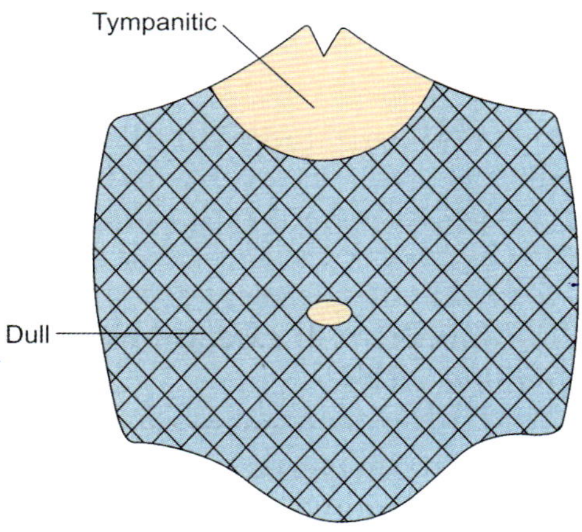

Fig. 4.11a: Massive ascites

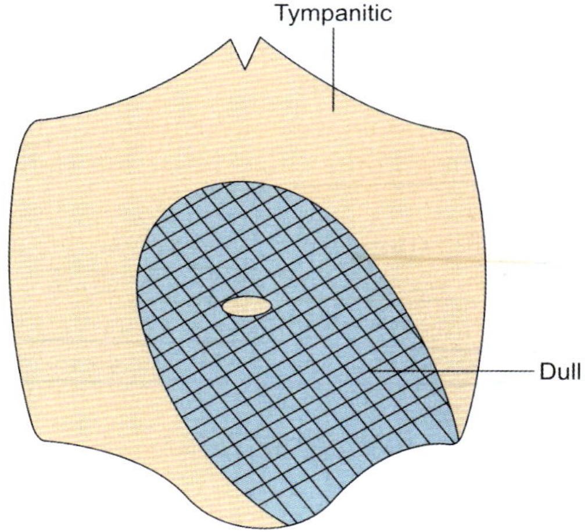

Fig. 4.11b: Large ovarian cyst

- Nephrotic syndrome
- CCF

Exudate

- Pyogenic peritonitis
- TB peritonitis
- Peritoneal malignancy

Points favoring ascites

- Umbilicus is transversely stretched.
- Flanks are dull to percuss.
- Detection of shifting dullness.
- Presence of fluid thrill.

Note: Ultrasound can detect as little as 100 ml of ascitic fluid.

Patients with ascites can have pleural effusion (predominantly right-sided) due to the following mechanisms:

1. *Movements of fluid through the diaphragm:* Through transdiaphragmatic lymphatic channels and Anatomic defects in the diaphragm.
2. Disorders associated with decreased serum albumin and decreased osmotic pressure with fluid leakage.
3. Lymph leakage from thoracic duct channels which are overburdened by ascitic fluid reabsorption.

Splenic Dullness

Significance of splenic dullness:

1. Splenic dullness detection helps in the diagnosis of splenomegaly before becoming palpable.
2. Indicates—the site where the spleen may be palpable.
3. Presence of increase in the area of splenic dullness over the left flank may suggest splenic enlargement in suspected cases of splenomegaly.
4. Detection of traumatic rupture of spleen.
5. Subcapsular hematoma of spleen splenic dullness increases.

Method of detection of splenic dullness

- Keep the patient in the right lateral position.
- Start percussing from the lower part of left lung resonance in the posterior axillary line.
- Percuss towards the left costal margin.
- *Splenomegaly:* Area of dullness of more than 8 cm.

Note: Splenic dullness extends from 10th rib posteriorly from mid-axillary line to the anterior chest.

AUSCULTATION

Normal Bowel Sounds

Auscultate in one area constantly for minimum of one minute (may be at the right of umbilicus).

Peristaltic sounds may appear every 5 secs or every 10 secs in a normal individual.

Minimum of 3–5 minutes of auscultation is required to confirm that peristaltic sounds are absent.

Increased intensity of bowel sounds

Causes

- Massive bleeding into the gastrointestinal tract with rapid intestinal transit of blood.
- Malabsorption syndrome
- Early and acute intestinal obstruction
- Carcinoid syndrome.

Intestinal obstruction: Bowel sounds become greatly exaggerated (Borborygmi) and sounds may have high-pitched twinkling quality.

Absence of peristalsis sounds

- Late stages of intestinal obstruction
- Peritonitis
- Drugs–anticholinergics

Succussion Splash over the Abdomen

- Ask the patient to lie flat on his back.
- Palpate or auscultate for a splashing sound over the epigastrium while the patient is being rocked from side to side.
- Normally, succussion splash may be present up to 2 hours after a main meal.
- Succussion splash heard 4 hours after meal suggests delayed gastric emptying.

Causes of succussion splash over the abdomen, e.g. pyloric obstruction, paralytic ileus, autonomic neuropathy.

Vascular Sounds

Arterial bruits: Sounds produced due to the turbulence of blood flow occurring through narrowed or compressed blood vessel during systole.

Aortic bruit: Auscultated just above and to the left of umbilicus.

Renal bruit

- Can be auscultated on either side of umbilicus.
- May also be over the renal areas posteriorly.

Liver bruit

- Heard in cases of acute alcoholic hepatitis
- Hepatoma
- Hepatic artery aneurysm.

Venous hum over the abdomen: Usually heard in patients with portal hypertension.

Site: Between xiphisternum and umbilicus and increases on inspiration due to the turbulence in the well-developed collateral circulation (like opening of umbilical vein).

Friction Sound (Rubs)

Conditions associated with hepatic rub

- Perihepatitis
- Hepatocellular carcinoma
- After liver biopsy (transiently)

Conditions associated with splenic rub

Splenic infarction

VIRAL HEPATITIS

Clinical Features

- History of fever, body ache and vomiting
- Yellowish discoloration of urine (after about 1 week of development of fever)
- Yellowish discoloration of sclera (jaundice) after about 1 week of development of fever
- Right hypochondrial pain
- Enlarged tender liver

Common virus which cause hepatitis: Hepatotropic viruses—A, B, C , D, and E.

Occasionally viral hepatitis may be due to

- Epstein-Barr virus
- Cytomegalovirus
- Herpes simplex viruses
- Coxsackie B virus infection.

Different Clinical Stages of Acute Viral Hepatitis

- Preicteric/prodromal phase: about 1 week duration
- Icteric stage: 1–2 weeks
- Cholestatic stag: 2–4 weeks (rarely 4–8 weeks)
- Recovery stage

Complications of Viral Hepatitis

Acute

- Fulminant hepatic failure
- Cholestatic hepatitis

Chronic: (Viral hepatitis B, C and D)

- Chronic hepatitis
- Chronic carrier stage
- Cirrhosis of liver
- Hepatocellular carcinoma

Rarer

- Aplastic anemia
- Glomerulo nephritis
- Transverse myelitis
- Polyarteritis nodosa (hepatitis B surface antigen positive in—30% of patients)
- Pancreatitis
- Myocarditis

Cirrhosis of liver: Chronic parenchymal disease of the liver characterized by destruction of architecture of the liver due to necrosis, fibrosis with formation of regenerating nodules.

Complication of cirrhosis

- Portal hypertension resulting in oesophageal varices causing upper gastrointestinal bleed
- Hepatic encephalopathy
- Spontaneous bacterial peritonitis
- Bleeding tendencies
- Systemic infection
- Pulmonary hypertension
- Hepatorenal syndrome

Common cause of chromic hepatitis and cirrhosis

A—Autoimmune disease
B—Hepatitis B/biliary cirrhosis
C—Hepatitis C/cryptogenic
D—Drug induced
E—Ethanol (alcohol)

Diagnosis of Cirrhosis

Symptoms of cirrhosis

- Swelling of feet
- Abdominal distension
- Jaundice

Symptoms of portal hypertension

- Hemetemesis
- Bleeding per rectum

Signs of cirrhosis

- Signs of liver cell failure
- Liver firm may be enlarged and nodular
- Ascites

Signs of portal hypertension

- Dilated tortous veins radiating away from umbilicus
- Splenomegaly

Causes of anemia in a cirrhotic patient

- Hypersplenism
- Massive gastrointestinal bleed
- Malabsorption
- Anemia of chronic disease

Causes of development of fever in a patient of cirrhosis

- Spontaneous bacterial peritonitis
- Systemic infections
- Ongoing hepatitis/hepatocellular necrosis
- Occurrence of hepatocellular carcinoma

Indications of development of hepatocellular carcinoma in a patient of cirrhosis

- Rapid development of massive ascites which becomes hemorrhagic
- Deepening jaundice
- Enlarged liver which is hard in consistency
- Presence of arterial bruit over the liver

Features of hepatic encephalopathy

- Altered sleep rhythm and altered sensorium
- Flapping tremor
- Constructional apraxia

Examination of Inguinal Region and Genitalia

Males: See under urogenital system.
Females: See under urogenital system.

Examination of Anal Canal and Rectum

Prerequisites

- Proper explanation of the procedure to the patient.
- Adequate lighting facilities should be available.

Note: Per rectal examination can cause discomfort to the patient but usually not painful.

Positioning of the patient

- Left lateral
- Buttocks at the edge of the examining couch
- Perineum should be clearly visible (knees are flexed upwards with heels away from the perineum).

Finger used: Index finger of the examining hand (adequately lubricate the gloved fingers).

External Examination of the Anal Canal

Check for the following abnormalities

- Ulcerations, e.g. TB, syphilis, etc.
- Pilonidal sinus—located in the natal cleft (midline posteriorly)
- Hairs may be surrounding the sinus
- Anal fissure—separate the anal ring—look for a tear or a split in the ring
- Anal fistula—depressed area around the anus with surrounding area of granulation tissue
- Warts, e.g. viral (condyloma acuminata)
- Infection—fungal infection, threadworms (may be visible)–causes pruritus
- Pile—thrombosed or may be prolapsed
- Rectal prolapse—may be visible only on straining
- Abscess—perianal abscess, ischiorectal abscess: Tenderness is present between the anus and the ischial tuberosity.

Per Rectal Examination

Indications

General medical indications

- Fever of unknown origin
- Evaluation of bony pain and backache
- Evaluation of blood loss and iron deficiency
- Evaluation of weight loss

Gastrointestinal disorders

- Evaluation of pain abdomen
- Evaluation of altered bowel habit
- All acute abdominal conditions

Urogenital disorders

- Prostatic disorders
- Obstructive uropathy
- Urinary disturbance
- Genital infections

Per rectal examination

- Position of the patient and prerequisites—same as for inspection of anal canal and rectum.
- Introduce the index finger of the examining hand into the anal canal and rectum. Turn the finger all around and palpate all parts of the rectum.

Feel for the following structures while finger is in the anal canal

- Anal sphincter tone and tone of muscles
- Anorectal junction—felt as a thick band of muscle
- Irregularity and ulceration in the anal canal.

Following conditions produce severe pain and tenderness on per rectal examination

- Anal fissure
- Ulcers
- Thrombosed hemorrhoids
- Abscess/fistula

Feel for the following structures while the finger is in the rectum

- Ulcers, growth, narrowing (strictures) and polyps
- Feel the lateral sides of the pelvis and check for the tenderness.

- Lateral wall tenderness may be suggestive of peritonitis.

P/R Examination in a Male

Check for

- Seminal vesicles
- Prostate gland
- Rectovesical pouch

Seminal vesicles

- Lie above the prostate
  - Running upwards from its margins
  - Can be felt only if it is full.
- Thickening of seminal vesicles
  - May be suggestive of tuberculosis.

Prostate

- Felt as firm swelling with smooth and regular surface.
- Malignancy of the prostate is felt as hard and irregular mass.

Prostatic massage: Smears are useful in diagnosis of prostatitis and malignancy of prostate.

Prostatic tenderness: Suggestive of prostatitis

Rectovesical pouch

- Tender swelling lying above the prostate suggests the presence of pelvic abscess.
- Hard nodules in the rectovesical pouch suggest the presence of malignant deposits.

Note: Normally, seminal vesicle and recto-vesical pouch are not palpable.

P/R Examination in a Female

Normal person: Cervix and retroverted uterus can be felt on the anterior wall of the rectum.

Tenderness on the lateral wall may be suggestive of salphingitis.

Abnormalities detectable in the retrouterine pouch (pouch of Douglas)

- Uterine fibroid
- Malignant deposit
- Abscess in the pelvis
- Ovarian cyst

Withdraw the finger after per rectal examination and check the finger for

- Color of stool
- Presence of blood and mucus.

5 Nervous System

CHECKLIST FOR GENERAL PHYSICAL EXAMINATION

- Symptoms and history of present illness
- Symptoms regarding the etiology of neurological deficit
- Past history
- Family history
- Personal history
- Occupational history
- Treatment history
- General physical examination
- Neurocutaneous markers
- Higher mental functions
- Cranial nerves
- Motor system
- Sensory system
- Cerebellum
- Bladder and bowel
- Skull, spine, carotids and gait

History and examination of the nervous system should provide the examiner adequate information so as to arrive at following conclusions:

1. *Clinical diagnosis:* Patient's exact neurological deficit, e.g. hemiplegia.
2. *Anatomical site of lesion:* Exact site of lesion, e.g. internal capsule.
3. *Pathology of the disease:* Pathology responsible for the deficit, e.g. thrombosis.
4. *Aetiology leading on to the neurological deficit:* Cause of the disease, e.g. hypertension.
5. *Functional deficit:* Degree of deficit either temporary, or permanent.

The order of history taking and examination outlined in this chapter may not be followed rigidly.

Scheme of examination may be carried out depending on the clinical circumstances.

History and Approach to a Patient of Neurological Disorder

Scheme of History Taking

Informant: Patient himself or a bystander (in patients with altered mental functions).

History of Present Illness

I. *Symptomatology and History of Present Illness*

a. *Motor disturbances*
   - Weakness or loss of power
   - Stiffness of limbs
   - Wasting or thinning of limbs
   - Involuntary movements
   - Disturbance in walking

b. *Sensory disturbance:* Diminished or altered sensation.

c. *Symptoms of cranial nerve dysfunction.*

d. Symptoms of cerebellar dysfunction.

e. Disturbance of conscious level, altered higher mental functions and speech.

f. Symptoms of bladder and bowel dysfunction.

II. *Symptoms Regarding the Aetiology of Neurological Deficit*

- Headache, vomiting and blurring of vision
- Convulsions
- Fever
- Cardiovascular symptoms

- Respiratory symptoms
- Trauma to the head and spine
- Details of medication taken
- Any vaccination in the recent past
- Other systemic illnesses like diabetes mellitus, hypertension and tuberculosis.

Past History

- Birth history and childhood illness
- Intracranial infection/operations
- TIA/any other neurological disturbance before
- Head or spine injury
- History of convulsions before
- History of diabetes mellitus, hypertension, coronary artery disease and medications.

Family History

Any other members suffering from similar neurological disturbance.

Personal History

- Loss of weight/appetite, bowel or bladder dysfunction.
- Smoking
- Alcoholism
- Diet and nutritional history
- H/o exposure to sexually transmitted diseases.

Occupational History

History of exposure to toxins and chemicals.

Menstrual History and Previous Pregnancies

In a female patient.

Treatment History

Details of treatment taken.

APPROACH TO A PATIENT WITH NERVOUS SYSTEM DYSFUNCTION

Significance of onset, duration and progression of symptoms in a nervous system disease:

Sudden/acute onset of symptoms suggest

- Cerebrovascular disease
- Traumatic disease
- Epileptic disorder

Onset hours to days to weeks

- CNS infections
- Inflammatory disorders
- Demyelination
- Spinal cord compression

Recurrent attacks of neurological disturbance (recovery is complete)

- Epilepsy
- TIAs
- Migraine
- Periodic paralysis
- Myasthenia

Recurrent exacerbations and remissions

- Multiple sclerosis
- Cerebrovascular disease
- Some types of peripheral neuropathy

Subacute or chronic duration of symptoms—progression of symptoms in months

Intracranial space-occupying lesion (ICSOL).

Progression of neurological deficit in years

Degenerative disorder.

Symptom Analysis of Nervous System Disorders

Motor Symptoms

Weakness or loss of power is the most common motor symptom and is analysed as follows:

Part involved (paralysed)

- Paralysis of one limb—monoplegia
- Paralysis of upper and lower limb on one side—hemiplegia
- Paralysis of both lower limbs—paraplegia
- Paralysis of all four limbs—quadriplegia.

Cruciate Hemiplegia

Weakness of one upper limb with opposite lower limb weakness.

Crossed Hemiplegia

Weakness of one half of the body with cranial nerve palsy on the opposite side—crossed hemiplegia.

Cerebral Diplegia

Cerebral diplegia is a form of cerebral palsy affecting the lower limb which causes spasticity of lower limbs.

Note: Partial loss of power is called paresis.

Distribution of Weakness

Distal weakness of upper limb—suggested by difficulty in holding the objects or objects falling off the hand.

Distal weakness of lower limb—suggested by difficulty in gripping the footwear.

Causes of predominant distal weakness

Pyramidal disease and peripheral neuropathy.

Proximal weakness

- *Upper limb*: Suggested by difficulty in lifting the limb above the shoulder/difficulty in combing the hair.
- *Lower limbs*: Suggested by difficulty in getting up from squatting position/difficulty in climbing, going down the staircase.

Causes of predominant proximal weakness

Painless proximal weakness	*Painful proximal weakness*
Myopathies	Osteomalacia
Guillain-Barré syndrome	Polymyositis
Muscular dystrophies	Diabetic amyotrophy

Other symptoms of motor system disease

- Wasting or thinning of limbs—usually signifies lower motor neuron disease or muscle disease.
- Stiffness of limbs—suggests increased tone.
- Involuntary movements like tremors and twitching of muscles (fasciculations).

Patient with spinal cord disease may give history of

- *Sudden involuntary extension of lower limbs—extensor spasm*: Suggests pyramidal tract involvement.
- *Sudden involuntary flexion of lower limbs—flexor spasm*: Suggests pyramidal and extrapyramidal involvement (indicates poor prognosis).

Note: Muscle weakness which is increasing on prolonged use may suggest myasthenia. Some patients may describe slowness of movement rather than weakness suggesting an extrapyramidal disorder.

Apart from muscle weakness disturbance in walking may be due to sensory disturbance, cerebellar ataxia, labyrynthine disease or apraxia of gait.

Sensory symptoms

- Onset
- Duration
- Progression
- Aetiological factors will be same as discussed under motor system.

Different Types of Sensory Disturbances

- Total loss of sensation—anaesthesia.
- Partial loss of sensation—hypoaesthesia.
- Loss of pain sensation—analgesia.
- *Paraesthesia*: Feeling of abnormal sensation (actual stimulus does not exist), e.g.: Feeling of pins and needles and numbness.
- *Dissociated anaesthesia:* Loss of pain and temperature with preservation of touch, e.g. intramedullary lesion of the spinal cord—tumors/syringomyelia.
- *Hyperpathia:* Severely painful or unpleasant sensation to stimulation (associated with increased threshold for stimulation), e.g. thalamic syndrome.
- *Hyperaesthesia:* A general term given to increased sensitivity of the skin to mild stimuli.
- *Hyperalgesia:* Sensitivity to pain is increased (associated with decreased threshold).
- *Allodynia:* Increased reaction to all stimuli. Even a non-painful stimulus such as light touch can produce pain.
- *Glove and stocking type of sensory disturbance*: Sensory disturbance like paraesthesia

involving predominantly extremities like hands and feet, e.g. peripheral neuropathy.

Root pain: Electric shock-like sensation in the distribution of the nerve root that may increase on coughing, sneezing and movement of spine. Indicates nerve root compression, e.g. sciatica.

Patient who has got difficulty in walking or swaying while walking more at night (at dark) or swaying while washing the face suggests the possibility of posterior column disease: loss of proprioceptions "Rombergism".

Tight band like sensation: May be present in patients with posterior column disease.

Lhermitte's symptom: Flexion of neck results in shock like sensation or paraesthesia radiating up to the limbs, e.g.: Cervical spondylosis, multiple sclerosis.

Symptoms of Cranial Nerve Dysfunction

1. *1st (olfactory) nerve:* Disturbance of smell like decrease of smell/loss of smell (anosmia) or altered smell.

Note: Parosmia suggests altered smell.

2. *2nd (optic) nerve:* Patient may complain of decrease acuity of vision, field of vision and disturbed color vision.
3. *3rd (occulmotor) 4th (trochlear) and 6th (abducens) nerve:* These cranial nerve dysfunctions will produce disturbed extra ocular movements. Patient may complain of diplopia and squint.
4. *5th (trigeminal) nerve:* It serves both motor and sensory functions. Motor disturbance will produce difficulty in chewing and mastication. Sensory disturbance will produce loss or decrease sensation over one half of the face (excluding the angle of the jaw).
5. *7th (facial) nerve:* Patient will have following disturbances:
   - Dribbling of saliva from the affected side of the mouth
   - Deviation of angle of the mouth to one side (to the normal side)
   - Collection of food on the affected side of the mouth
   - Inability to close the eye (in patients with LMN facial palsy) slurring of speech, Hyperacusis and taste loss over the anterior 2/3rds of tongue occurs in patients with LMN facial palsy
6. *8th (vestibulocochlear) nerve:* Vestibular dysfunction may produce:
   - Dizziness
   - Vertigo (sensation of rotation)
   - Nausea
   - Vomiting
   - Cochlear dysfunction may produce:
   - Tinnitus, ringing in the ear and decreased hearing or deafness.
7. *Glossopharyngeal (9th) vagus (10th) and cranial (11th) accessory:* Dysfunction may produce:
   - Nasal regurgitation of food
   - Difficulty in swallowing
   - Nasal twang to the speech
8. *Hypoglossal (12th) nerve:* Dysfunction will produce difficulty in movement of the tongue, difficulty in mixing the food in the mouth and slurring of speech.

Symptoms' of Cerebellar Dysfunction

Person will have difficulty in walking or swaying while walking and difficulty in taking food to mouth, difficulty in shaving, writing and incoordination of speech.

Above symptoms are also present in patients with decreased muscle power. So symptoms of cerebellar dysfunction should be assessed proportionate to the grade of muscle power.

Symptoms of Bladder and Bowel Dysfunction

- Affected persons may have incontinence or retention of urine.
- Urgency, frequency and incontinence may be due to bilateral UMN lesions especially involving the spinal cord.
- Retention/dribbling incontinence may be due to cauda equina lesion.

- Compression of spinal cord can result in rapid loss of sphincter control requiring immediate treatment.
- Spinal cord/cauda equina lesion can also cause erectile impotence.

Symptoms of higher mental function dysfunctions like altered conscious level and disturbance of speech (*see* examination of an unconscious patient)

Following details are important in patients with altered conscious level and other altered higher mental functions:

- Onset and evolution of symptoms
- Associated neurological symptoms like headache, convulsions, weakness, vomiting and trauma to the head
- Details of drug ingestion like sedative hypnotics, alcohol and other intoxications

Symptoms suggestive of hepatic, renal, cardiovascular, endocrine and other systemic illness.

Speech Disturbance

Speech disturbance may be due to

- Defective production of speech
- Defective articulation of speech
- Defective voice production

Enquire whether

- Patient has difficulty in understanding or defective word output (central speech defect—aphasia).
- Patient understands the spoken speech with normal word output but has got defective articulation (slurring)—peripheral defect—dysarthria.
- Patient has normal understanding, word output and articulation but defective voice production—dysphonia.

Symptoms Regarding Etiology of Neurological Deficit

Headache and vomiting: **May be indicative of raised intracranial tension.** Headache due to raised intracranial tension:

- Deep-seated bursting type of headache may persist for few minutes to hours.
- Headache will be of longer duration as the disease advances.
- Person may wake up from sleep due to headache.
- Headache may be severe on early morning hours.
- Activity or change of position intensifies the headache.
- Raised intracranial tension is usually associated with projectile vomiting—unexpected forceful vomiting without proceeding nausea. (Projectile)—more in the morning due to high CSF pressure in the morning.
- Neurological headache may also be due to stretch of meninges, vascular structures and diseases of cranial nerves 5, 7 and 10 carrying pain sensation.

Convulsion: Generalised or focal (Jacksonian) seizures are common with cortical lesions, e.g.: Encephalitis, supratentorial mass lesions, cerebrovascular accidents.

Convulsion may also occur due to hepatic, renal, endocrine or metabolic disturbances.

Fever

Fever is usually associated with infective or inflammatory disorders of nervous system like meningoencephalitis.

Febrile systemic illness can secondarily affect the nervous system, e.g. malaria, typhoid, etc.

Symptoms of Cardiovascular Disease

Enquire the symptoms of cardiac disease like chest pain, palpitation and dyspnoea.

Significance of cardiac disease in nervous system disorder

- Mitral valve disease with atrial fibrillation and left atrial myxoma can cause embolic stroke.
- Vegetations of infective endocarditis may result in systemic vascular occlusions including cerebrovascular accident. Infective endocarditis can also cause

mycotic aneurysms of circle of Willis and its consequences.

- Acute myocardial infarction with hypotension can precipitate CVA (cerebrovascular accident).
- Atherosclerosis can involve both coronary and cerebral circulations.

Respiratory Symptoms

Enquire the symptoms of respiratory disease like cough, sputum and haemoptysis.

Respiratory disorders may involve the nervous system in the following ways: Pulmonary tuberculosis may be associated with:

- TB meningitis and endoarteritis causing CVA
- Tuberculoma of brain
- TB spine

Bronchogenic carcinoma may be associated with—secondaries in the nervous system/ paraneoplastic nervous system disease.

Cerebral abscess may be a complication of bronchiectasis.

Respiratory disorders like COPD can result in polycythemia, which is a risk factor for stroke.

Patient with altered sensorium can aspirate and develop aspiration pneumonia.

Trauma to the head and spine

Enquire the history of present and previous trauma to the head, neck and spine.

Acute head and spine injury can cause concussion, contusion of brain and spinalcord compression.

Details of previous medication

Persons taking anti-epileptics and aspirin may be having chronic convulsive disorder or previous thromboembolic stroke respectively. Patients on anticoagulant therapy may bleed into the nervous system. Persons on oral contraceptive pills have got an increased incidence of developing thrombotic CVA.

History of vaccination in the recent past

Significant in patients with demyelinating nervous system disorder. Common with vaccines like nervous tissue anti-rabies vaccine.

Symptoms of Associated Systemic Illness

- *Diabetes mellitus*
  - Risk factor for atherosclerotic CVA
  - Cranial nerve palsy (due to microvascular disease)
  - Autonomic neuropathy
  - Peripheral neuropathy
- *Hypertension causes*
  - Hypertensive encephalopathy
  - Arteriosclerotic CVA
  - Intracerebral and subarachnoid bleed
- *Ischemic heart disease*—suggests the presence of atherosclerotic vascular disease including cerebral vessels.

Past History

Enquire the previous history of:

- Birth trauma, childhood epilepsy/head injury
- Childhood intracranial infections
- Transient ischemic attack
- Neurological illness
- Epilepsy
- Exposure to toxins and chemicals

Birth trauma/injury: can cause neonatal brain damage.

Childhood epilepsy and intracranial infection: An adult epileptic may give childhood history of epilepsy. Previous intracranial infection can give rise to future neurological deficit.

Transient Ischemic Attack

- Sudden onset of ischemic neurological deficit totally recovering within 24 hours (usually lasts 5–20 minutes).
- Suggests transient decrease of cerebral blood flow.
- It is a minor form of stroke and may be a warning symptom for future major CVA.

Deficits are usually confined to a part of the brain perfused by a specific artery.

Different mechanisms of TIAS

- Low flow TIA—tight stenosis or occlusion of an artery with decreased cerebral blood flow.
- Embolic TIA—embolic occlusion of a cerebral vessel.

Source of embolus

- Left heart-mitral stenosis with atrial fibrillation; IHD
- Stenotic or ulcerated atherosclerotic plaque at the origin of the internal carotid artery.

Lacunar TIA: Precede lacunar stroke—may occur several times a day.

TIA can occur in the carotid system or vertebrobasilar system.

TIA of carotid system

Manifests as:

- Transient weakness
- Aphasia
- Transient uniocular blindness (Amaurosis Fugax due to occlusion of ophthalmic artery).

Vertebrobasilar T/A: Manifests as—vertigo, dysarthria, dysphagia, diplopia, etc.

Previous History of Trauma to the Head and Spine

- Details of previous trauma to the head, neck and spine should be enquired.
- Previous trauma may be responsible for variety of neurological dysfunction.
- Examples of previous trauma induced neurological dysfunction:
  - Chronic subdural hematoma
  - Repeated head injury—Parkinsonism
  - Post-traumatic syringomyelia
  - Post-traumatic arachnoiditis
  - Post-traumatic headache and epilepsy.

Exposure to Toxins, Chemicals and Drugs

Exposure to certain toxins and chemicals may be responsible for disturbance in neuronal function.

Examples of drugs, toxins and chemical induced neurological dysfunction:

Acute intoxication

- Ethyl and methyl alcohol
- Organophosphorus compounds

Chronic exposure

- Peripheral neuropathy: Lead, arsenic and thallium, vincristine, phenytoin
- Amiodorone and organophosphates
- Toxic myopathy: Zudovudine, penicillamine, etc.
- Parkinsonism: Exposure to manganese and MPTP (methylphenyl-tetrahydropyridine).

Previous History of Epilepsy

In persons presenting with convulsions enquire the past history of epilepsy. Recurrent attacks of epilepsy may occur either due to improper drug therapy or stoppage of drugs. Anti epileptic drugs like phenytoin can cause peripheral neuropathy and cerebellar dysfunction.

Previous Neurological Illness

Disorders like multiple sclerosis, chronic inflammatory demyelinating neuropathies can have recurrent exacerbations and remissions. Previous history of such episodes should be enquired in suspected patients of demyelinating diseases.

Personal History

Loss of weight and appetite: Significant weight loss and loss of appetite can be associated with disorders like tuberculosis, malignancy or HIV infection with nervous system involvement either primarily or secondarily.

Smoking: Incidence of cerebrovascular disease is increased in persons who are smokers.

Alcoholism: Intake of alcohol can cause following neuromuscular dysfunctions:

Acute effects

- Intoxication
- Hypoglycemia
- Traumatic head injury
- Wernicke's encephalopathy and Korsakoff's psychosis.

Chronic effects
- Chronic subdural hematoma
- Dementia
- Cerebellar dysfunction
- Peripheral neuropathy
- Myopathy

Due to the effect of alcohol on the liver
- Hepatic encephalopathy
- Hepatocerebral degeneration
- Myelopathy

Exposure to syphilis and HIV injection

Sexually transmitted disease like syphilis and HIV infection can involve the nervous system.

Enquire the history of intravenous drug addiction and contact with different sexual partners.

Nervous system manifestations due to syphilis

Meningovascular syphilis
- Syphilitic meningitis
- Endoarteritis and CVA

Parenchymatous syphilis
- Tabes dorsalis
- General paresis of insane
- Syphilitic gumma
- Spinal cord involvement.

Nervous system manifestations due to HIV infection
- Dementia
- Tuberculosis
- Cryptococcal infection
- Toxoplasmosis
- CNS lymphoma

Family History

Certain neurological disorders may be present in more than one family members.

Examples of neurological disorders with familial occurrence
- Migrainous headache
- Stroke
- Familial tremors
- Dementias
- Huntington's chorea
- Hereditary neuropathies
- Epileptic disorders
- Degenerative disorders

It is also important to enquire the consanguinity between parents in suspected cases of familial neurological disorders.

Occupational history: Exposure to toxins and chemicals (*see* above).

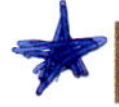

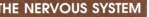

EXAMINATION OF THE NERVOUS SYSTEM

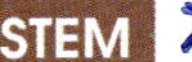

SCHEME OF EXAMINATION

General Physical Examination

- Build—pallor
- Nourishment
  - Icterus
  - Cyanosis
  - Clubbing
  - Lymphadenopathy
  - Edema of feet

Vital signs
- Pulse
- Blood pressure
- Temperature
- Respiratory rate

Presence of Neurocutaneous Markers

Systemic Examination of the Nervous System

a. *Higher mental functions*
   - Consciousness level
   - Orientation to time place and person
   - Intelligence
   - Memory
   - Emotional disturbances
   - Hallucinations and delusions
   - Disturbance of speech
   - Handedness
   - Mini mental scale examination

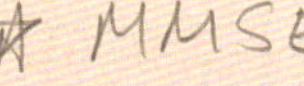

b. *Cranial nerves* 1–12

c. *Motor system*
   - Attitude of limbs
   - Nutrition
   - Tone
   - Power
   - Coordination
   - Involuntary movements

d. *Sensory system*
- Lateral spinothalamic tract: Pain and temperature sensation
- Posterior spinothalamic tract:
  - Touch
  - Vibration
  - Joint sense
  - Pressure sense
- Cortical sensations:
  - Tactile localisation
  - Two point discrimination
  - Stereognosis
  - Graphaesthesia.

e. *Reflexes*
- Superficial reflexes
  - Corneal
  - Conjunctival
  - Abdominal
  - Cremasteric
  - Plantar
- Deep reflexes:
  - Jaw jerk
  - Biceps
  - Triceps
  - Supinator
  - Knee
  - Ankle

- Primitive reflexes
- Visceral reflexes
- Examination of cerebellum
- Signs of meningeal irritation
- Examination of peripheral nerves
- Examination of skull and spine
- Carotid examination
- Examination of gait

Examination of other systems
- Cardiovascular system
- Respiratory system
- Gastrointestinal tract
- Other related systems

EXAMINATION OF THE NERVOUS SYSTEM

Build and nourishment

Should be assessed as in any other systemic examination (*see* general physical examination).

Vital signs

Pulse: Record the rate, rhythm, volume, character and palpability of the vessel wall.

Importance of Peripheral Pulse Examination in Nervous System Disease

Rate: Raised intracranial tension may be associated with bradycardia.

Rhythm: Irregularly irregular pulse may be suggestive of atrial fibrillation with possible emboli, stroke.

Thickening of vessel: Suggests atherosclerosis of blood vessels with cerebrovascular disease

Palpate dorsalispedis, brachial, superficial temporal and carotids for evidence of atherosclerosis.

Blood Pressure

- Hypertension is an important risk factor for atherosclerosis and can cause CVA. Record the blood pressure on the non-paralysed side (to avoid false interpretation of blood pressure due to vasomotor paralysis on the paralysed side).
- Systolic pressure increase and bradycardia occur in patients with increased intracranial tension (Cushing's response) as a result of compression on the medullary centers (distortion of lower brainstem).

Respiration (Table 5.1)

Temperature

Neurological disturbance with fever may be due to infective disorders of the nervous system.

Systemic disease with fever can also cause nervous system dysfunction, e.g. typhoid encephalopathy, cerebral malaria.

Hyperpyrexia may be associated with
- Pontine hemorrhage
- Neuroleptic malignant syndrome
- Cerebral malaria

Pallor

Anemia may be a part of systemic illness which may involve the nervous system.

Vitamin B_{12} deficiency can cause
- Peripheral neuropathy

Table 5.1: Respiration: *See* examination of an unconscious patient

Rate and depth of respiration may vary with different types of neurological lesions as given below:	
Supratentorial lesions Deep seated cerebral lesions Metabolic brain disorders	Waxing and waning of breathing at regular intervals with short periods of apnea
Lower midbrain and upper pontine lesion Lower pontine lesion	Central neurogenic hyperventilation Apneustic breathing—a pause of 2–3 seconds after full inspiration
Dorsomedial medullary lesion	Biot's breathing. Breathing is irregularly interrupted Each breath is varying in rate and breath

Further details on abnormal respiratory rhythms is discussed under the chapter on examination of an unconscious patient.

- Sub acute combined degeneration of spinal cord
- Dementia

Note

- Severe Niacin deficiency can also cause dementia. Pyridoxine, folic acid and thiamine deficiencies can cause peripheral neuropathy.
- Severe anemia may be associated with anemic encephalopathy.
- Occasionally polycythemia may be associated with cerebellar hemangioblastoma and polycythemia may be a risk factor for stroke.

Icterus

Liver disease can cause encephalopathy, myelopathy and neuropsychiatric manifestations. Patients with Wilson's disease can have hepatic and extra-pyramidal dysfunction.

Cyanosis and Clubbing

Indicates cardiovascular and respiratory disorders with secondary involvement of nervous system.

Lymphadenopathy

Disorders associated with generalised lymphadenopathy like lymphoma, leukemia, tuberculosis and HIV infection can involve the nervous system.

Pedal Edema

Patients with paralysis of one side can have edema on that side due to altered vasomotor tone and venous stasis.

Neurocutaneous Markers

Adenoma Sebaceum

Are actually angiofibromas, reddish pink greasy nodules.

Common sites: Cheek and nasolabial folds.

Found in patients with tuberous sclerosis.

Café au lait Spots

Dark brown or light colored patches associated with generalized neurofibromatosis. Presence of either more than 6 spots (5 mm) or a single spot exceeding 1.5 cm in diameter is clinically significant.

Shagreen Patch

Plaque like lesions usually present in the lumbosacral area varying from 1 to 10 cm. Found in patients with tuberous sclerosis.

Neurofibroma

Firm discrete nodules attached to a nerve.

Telengiectasia

Telengiectasiae present in the skin, mucosa, gastrointestinal tract, spinal cord and brain can be associated with familial telengiectasia (Osler-Weber-Rendu disease).

Telengiectasia in the bulbar conjunctiva is associated with cerebellar degeneration (ataxia telengiectasia).

Vascular Nevus

Nevus covers the large part of face and cranium associated with angiomas of brain (Sturge-Weber syndrome).

Low Hairline

Posterior hairline is below the C_4 vertebra, associated with craniovertebral anomalies.

Short Neck

Ratio of the length of the body to the length of the neck is more than 13:1.

Short neck is associated with cranio-vertebral anomalies.

Pes Cavus and Kyphoscoliosis

Associated with hereditary neurological disorders (e.g. Freidrich's ataxia) and also intraspinal disorders like syringomyelia.

Presence of Hairs, Lipoma or Dimple in the Skin over the Spine

Associated with spina bifida occulta.

SYSTEMIC EXAMINATION OF THE NERVOUS SYSTEM

Higher Mental Functions

1. *Conscious level:* Conscious level is graded as follows:
   a. Fully conscious
   b. Drowsy: Easily arousable by touch or noise—alertness will persist for a short period.
   c. Stupor: Arousable only by vigorous stimulation.
   d. Coma: Not arousable by any form of stimulus.
2. *Orientation to time place and person*
   - *Orientation to time*: Enquire the exact time during the period of examination.
   - *Place*: Enquire where the patient is present at the time of examination.
   - *Person*: Identification of the relative or a bystander at the time of examination.
3. *Intelligence:* Ask the patient to do simple mathematical calculations.
4. *Memory:* Test the memory for:
   a. *Immediate memory*
      - Memory of events occurred within 30 seconds.

        Ask the patient to recall memory of digits forward and backward (digit span).

        Center for immediate memory: Frontal lobe, perisylvian cortex
   b. *Recent memory*: Memory of events occurred within minutes, weeks and months. Patient is asked to recall and repeat 3 words after 3–5 minutes of telling.

      Center: Mamillothalamic tract, hippocampus. Causes of recent memory loss, e.g. Korsakoff's psychosis.
   c. *Remote memory:* Memory of events occurred years back–like memory of school days in adult patients.

      Center: Possibly in the association cortex, limbic system.

      Causes of memory loss: Alzheimer's disease, multi infarct state, alcoholism, Wernicke's encephalopathy.
5. *Emotional labilities*
   - Episodes of spontaneous weeping or laughing (without provocation)
   - Occurs in conditions like pseudobulbar palsy and frontal lobe disorders.
6. *Hallucinations and delusions*
   - Hallucination: Patient will have false feelings without any appropriate stimulus/cause.
   - Delusion: Person will have false beliefs, which are held despite against to the prevailing circumstances.
   - Hallucination and delusions are commonly associated with temporal and occipital lobe lesions.

Speech Disturbances: Examination of Speech and Language

Test the following aspects

- Comprehension
- Spontaneous speech
- Naming
- Repetition
- Reading
- Writing

- *Comprehension*: Ability to understand the conversation and questioning
- *Spontaneous speech*: Observe for word output, melody and length of speech
- *Naming*: Asking to name the objects
- *Repetition*: Ask the patient to repeat short sentences or single words
- *Reading*: Assessing for defect in reading
- *Writing*: Assess grammar, word order and spelling.

Approach to a patient of speech defect

While assessing comprehension, commands which involve axial movements like showing the tongue, closing or opening of eyes should not be used as such commands can be performed by the person even with significant defect with comprehension (sensory aphasia).

Central Speech Defects (Aphasia/Dysphasias)

a. Broca's (motor) aphasia:
- Word output is decreased
- Speech is non-fluent and usually dysarthric
- Comprehension is intact
- Site of lesion: Broca's area: Posterior part of inferior frontal gyrus with surrounding cortex.
- Vascular territory involved: Occlusion of superior division of left middle cerebral artery.
- *Causes*: Head injuries, CVA, intracranial space-occupying lesion (ICSOL).

b. Wernicke's (sensory) aphasia
- Understanding for spoken and written language is impaired.
- Word output is normal but with large number of inappropriate words (paraphasias).
- Site of lesion: Wernicke's area—posterior third of superior temporal gyrus and surrounding cortex.
- Vascular territory involved: Occlusion of inferior division of left middle cerebral artery.
- Causes: Head injuries, CVA, ICSOL

c. Global aphasia
- Word output and understanding of spoken and written speech is grossly decreased.
- Site of lesion: combined involvement of Broca's and Wernicke's areas.
- Vascular territory involved: stem occlusion of left middle cerebral artery.
- Causes: Head injury, CVA , ICSOL

d. Conduction aphasia
- Understanding is intact. Word output is intact but with wrong words, repetition and memory are impaired.
- *Site of lesion:* Around auditory cortex and arcuate fasciculus
- Connection between the Wernicke's and Broca's areas are impaired.

e. Anomic aphasia: Naming and word findings become impaired.
- *Site of lesion:* Language areas in the left hemisphere including middle and inferior temporal gyrus.
- *Causes:* Alzheimer's disease, head injury, metabolic encephalopathies.

Aprosodia

Impairment of melody and stress of speech, e.g. it is raining and it is raining?

Note the difference between the messages conveyed between the above two sentences.

Site of lesion: Perisylvian area in the right hemisphere.

Aphemia

Features: Fluency of speech is severely impaired with normal comprehension, reading and writing.

Lesion: Partial involvement of motor speech area (Broca's area)

Transcortical sensory aphasia

Features: Behaves like Wernicke's aphasia with intact repetition.

Site of lesion: There is defective connection between speech areas and temporal cortex.

Vascular territory involved: Posterior watershed zone infarct.

Transcortical motor aphasia

Features: Behaves like motor aphasia with intact repetition.

Site of lesion: Defective connection between speech areas and prefrontal areas.

Vascular territory involved: Watershed zone between anterior cerebral and middle cerebral circulation.

Isolation aphasia

Features: Severely impaired comprehension with parrot-like repetition of heard conversation (echolalia).

Site involved: Pathologically language area is isolated from other parts of brain.

Causes

- Infarction of watershed zones
- Carbon monoxide poisoning
- Anoxic encephalopathy

Subcortical aphasias

- May have combination of different types of speech defects–due to defective:
  - Subcortical language network.
  - Subcortical aphasia occurs in lesions of thalamus and head of caudate nucleus of left side.

Additional speech disturbances

Alexia: Difficulty in reading and understanding simple words and sentences.

Agraphia: Spelling and grammar are impaired in the written form of language.

Echolalia: Spoken speech is repeated without meaning.

Palilalia : Repeated repetition of same words, phrases and syllables.

Echolalia and palilalia are manifestations of Alzheimer's disease.

Additional Signs of Cortical Dysfunction

Hemineglect and Anosognosia

- Occurs in patients with damage to the non-dominant hemisphere (usually right)
- Person has disability in the form of denial of existence of one side of the body or denial of disability.

Constructional Apraxia

Occurs due to lesion in the right hemisphere. Person will have difficulty in constructing elements in the correct fashion to form meaningful structures.

Dysarthrias

Disordered articulation of speech. *Due to:*

a. Defect in the vagal, hypoglossal, facial nerves and their connections and muscles supplied by them.

b. Disorders of cerebellum.

Normal articulation of speech is due to contraction of pharynx, palate, tongue and lip muscles.

Production of labials (m, b, p)—by the lip muscles—supplied by facial nerve.

Production of linguals (i and t): By tongue movement—supplied by hypoglossal nerve

Production of guttarals (k and g): By palate movement—supplied by 9th and 10th cranial nerves.

Different Types of Dysarthrias

Lesions of lower motor neurons

- 7th nerve palsy—labial dysarthria
- 12th nerve palsy—lingual dysarthria
- 9th and 10th nerve palsy—nasal twang to speech

Cortical dysarthria: This is a form of Broca's aphasia with lesions involving the Broca's area. Person may have other language disorders.

Extrapyramidal disorders

- Slurred rapid speech
- Low pitched monotonous speech, e.g. Parkinsonism.

Cerebellar disease: Scanning speech with separation of syllables.

Bilateral pyramidal disease: Spastic thick speech.

Disorders like myasthenia gravis and dystonias can also have dysarthria.

Dysphonia

Phonation or voice production is the function of vocal cords.

Disturbed voice production or dysphonia may be due to the following causes

- Vocal cord paralysis—due to recurrent laryngeal nerve palsy
- Respiratory muscle paralysis
- Spasm of the glottis—tetanus and tetany
- Local causes in the larynx—acute or chronic laryngitis
- Laryngeal polyp and growth
- Occasionally hoarseness of voice may be due to cigarette smoking and steroid inhalation.

Importance of Handedness

Handedness is decided by the hand/foot which is preferentially used for skilled movements, e.g. eye which is preferentially used to see through a hole.

- Foot which is preferentially used to kick a football.
- Majority of persons are right-handed.

In right-handed individuals, language function is in the left hemisphere. Majority (70%) of left-handed individuals also have language representation in the left hemisphere.

Other left-handed individuals may have diffuse language function.

Note: In patients with altered conscious level testing of orientation, memory, intelligence, etc. may not be relevant.

Mini Mental Scale Examination (Table 5.2)

EXAMINATION OF CRANIAL NERVES

1. Olfactory Nerve

- Conveys sensation of smell.
- Cortical center of smell: Amygdaloid body, hippocampus and pyriform cortex.

Tests for smell sensation

- Rule out the local nasal pathology like rhinitis, which may interfere with smell sensation.
- Patient is asked to close the eyes.
- Close the nostril, which is not being tested.
- Use familiar objects of smell (e.g. coffee powder, oil of peppermint).
- Avoid irritant smells like liquor ammonia—irritants may stimulate the trigeminal nerve endings in the nasal mucosa, which may interfere with interpretation of smell.

Causes of Ist nerve paralysis

Intra cranial tumors compressing the olfactory tract. Chronic meningeal inflammation.

2. Optic Nerve

- Subserves the function of vision
- Cortical center of vision: Visual cortex (occipital lobe).

Area Nos—17, 18 and 19.

a. Acquity of Vision

Distant vision: Tested by finger counting at 6 meters distance or using Snellen's chart (*see* chapter on disorders of eye).

Near vision: Jaeger type card with different sizes are used.

Average near vision acquity lies between Jaeger 1 to 4.

Causes of diminished visual acquity

- All refractory errors
- Cataracts

Table 5.2: Mini mental scale examination

Patient's name	*Name of the examiner*
	Date:
Orientation	Score
What is the date, day, month, year, season	5 (1 for each correct answer)
What is the name of this ward, floor, hospital district, state	5 (1 for each correct answer)
Registration	
Ask the patient to name 3 objects and ask him to repeat.	3 (1 for each object)
Attention and calculation	
Ask the patient to subtract 7 from 100 serially 5 times	5 (1 for each correct answer)
Recall	
Ask the patient to repeat 3 objects mentioned above	3 (1 for each under registration correct answer)
Language and copying	
Ask the patient to name a pencil and watch	2 (1 for each)
Repeat the following: No ifs, ands or buts following a 3 stage command	1
Picking up a paper with the right hand, fold it in half and place it on the floor	3 (1 for each command)
Read and obey the following	
Close your eyes	1
Asking the patient to write a sentence	1
Asking the patient to copy a design (like two intersecting pentagons)	1
	Total score = 30
Less than 23 score suggests an organic brain disorder	

- Corneal and vitreal opacities
- Retinal and optic nerve disease.

b. Field of Vision

Average field of vision (in around figures)

- Lateral field 100°
- Upwards—60°
- Medial field—60°
- Lower—75°
- Binocular field of vision 200° laterally
- 140° vertically

Visual field testing

Confrontation method

- Test each eye separately.
- Examiner sits opposite to the patient at a distance of about 1 meter.
- For testing the patient's right eye, ask the patient to cover his left eye with left hand and to look at the examiners left eye.
- Examiner covers his right eye with the right hand and looks at the patient's right eye.
- Examiner holds his left index finger to the side in between himself and the patient.
- Examiner brings the index finger into the field of vision from laterally and the patient is asked to respond as soon as he sees the moving finger.
- Movements should be tested in all directions upwards, downwards, to the right and to the left. Patient's field of vision is compared with the examiners own field of vision (assumed it to be normal).

Different Types of Field Defects

Hemianopia: Loss of vision in one half of the visual field.

Homonymous hemianopia: Loss of vision of the identical half on both sides of field of vision.

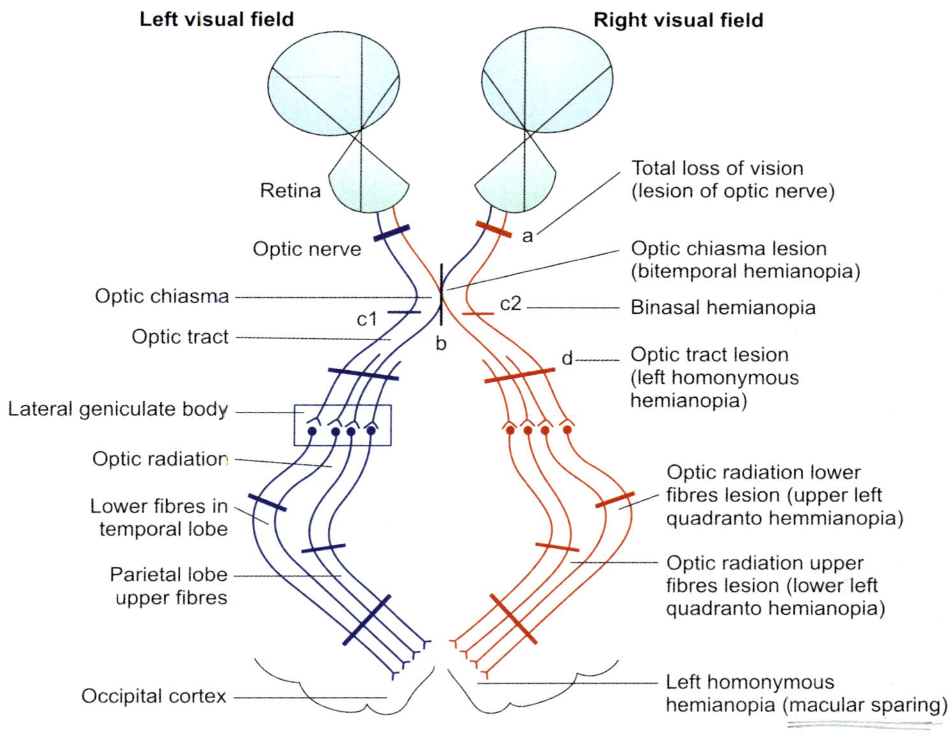

Optic pathway and lesions

On the side of lesion, there will be:

- Nasal hemifield defect
- Contralateral eye: Temporal hemifield defect

Lesion: Optic tract—complete (no macular sparing)

Lesion of occipital cortex/occipital radiation—macular sparing present with homonymous hemianopia.

Heteronymous hemianopia: Loss of vision of the non-identical half of the both sides of field of vision.

Quadrantanopia

- Loss of vision limited to one quadrant of a field.
- Upper quadrantanopia: Found in patients with temporal lobe lesion.
- Lower quadrantanopia: Lesion in the parietal lobe.
- *Bitemporal hemianopia*
  - Loss of vision in the temporal halves of both fields of vision
  - Lesion: Central optic chiasma, e.g. pituitary tumor.

Binasal hemianopia

- Loss of vision in the nasal (inner) half of both sides of vision.
- Lesion: Bilateral lesion involving each side of optic chiasma.

c. Colour Vision

See Chapter 10 on disorders of eye.

3. 3rd, 4th and 6th Cranial Nerves

Oculomotor (3rd) nerve

Extraocular muscles supplied by the 3rd nerve:

- Levator palpabrae superioris
- Superior rectus
- Inferior rectus
- Medial rectus
- Inferior oblique

Nucleus of the 3rd nerve: Situated in the mid-brain

Parasympathetic components of the 3rd nerve (Edinger-Westphal nucleus):

- Situated in the mid brain
- Supplies parasympathetic fibers to pupil. Parasympathetic stimulation produces pupillary constriction.

Trochlear nerve (4th): Muscles supplied—superior oblique, supplied by the nucleus of the opposite side.

Nucleus—situated in the midbrain.

Abducens nerve (6th): Muscles supplied—lateral rectus. Nucleus situated in the pons.

Action of extraocular muscles

- *Super rectus:* Upward movement of eye when it is outward turned
- *Inferior rectus:* Downward movement of eye when it is turned outwards
- *Lateral rectus:* Outward horizontal movement
- *Medial rectus:* Inward horizontal movement
- *Superior oblique:* Downward movement when the eye is turned inwards
- *Inferior oblique:* Upward movement when the eye is turned inwards.

Sympathetic supply to the pupil

Descending sympathetic pathway in the brainstem

↓

Superior cervical ganglion

↓

Long ciliary nerves

↓

Dilator pupillae

Sympathetic stimulation produces pupillary dilatation.

Movements of Eyes

Conjugate Movements

Symmetrical movements of the two eyes in the same direction and visual axis meet at the point at which eyes are directed. Conjugate movements of eyes require integrated action of 3rd, 4th and 6th nerve nuclei and their cortical connections.

Cortical center for conjugate eye movements—frontal eye fields (area No. 8).

Saccadic movements: Eye movements are conjugate and rapid.

Pursuit movement: Slow and smooth movement of eyes following a target.

Cortical center: Parieto-occipital cortex.

Supranuclear Paralysis of Eyeball Movement

Paralysis of lateral conjugate gaze : Lower brainstem lesion.

Brainstem center for horizontal gaze: Parapontine reticular formation.

Internuclear Ophthalmoplegia

Median longitudinal fasciculus (MLF) connects abducens nucleus on one side to the oculomotor nucleus on the opposite side. Lesion of MLF results in internuclear ophthalmoplegia.

Characteristics

- On attempted lateral gaze: Adducting eye fails to adduct and abducting eye shows nystagmus (ataxic nystagmus).
- Left lnternuclear ophthalmoplegia: Left eye fails to adduct.
- Conditions associated with internuclear ophthalmoplegia: Multiple sclerosis.

One and half syndrome

- Due to the lesion involving both MLF and Abducens nucleus on the same side.
- Only possible movement: Abduction of eye on the other side.

Nuclear Paralysis of 3rd, 4th and 6th Cranial Nerves

In nuclear paralysis individual eyeball movements are paralysed due to paralysis of individual extra ocular muscles.

Examination of 3rd, 4th and 6th Cranial Nerves

- Ask the patient to look at a clear point—point of a pen or pencil.

- Examiner moves the point in all 4 directions in the midline, i.e. right, left upwards and downwards.
- Patient should follow the point with his eyes.
- Patient should hold the deviation for 5 seconds in each position (deviation of more than 10 seconds may normally elicit nystagmus).
- Check for defective movement of one or other eye and nystagmus.

Characteristic Features of 3rd Nerve Palsy

- Lateral or divergent squint (due to unopposed action of lateral rectus)
- Ptosis
- Dilatation of pupil
- Eye is down and out

Causes of Isolated 3rd Nerve Paralysis

In the midbrain: Stroke, demyelination

Compression of the nerve along its course:

- Posterior communicating artery aneurysm
- Tumors of the base of the skull
- *Other conditions:* Diabetes mellitus, vasculitic conditions.

> *Note:* Diabetes Mellitus causing microangiopathy involves the central part of the third nerve.

As a result pupil is usually spared (pupillodilator fibers are superficially placed in the nerve) and patient presents with external ophthalmoplegia.

Trochlear (4th) Nerve Paralysis

Affected person will have defective downward movement of the involved eye.

Examination: Person is asked to look downwards in the mid position of gaze.

Characteristics of 4th Nerve Palsy

- Outward rotation of eyeball by the unopposed action of inferior rectus (on attempted downward gaze).
- Vertical diplopia—diplopia when the eyes are turned medially
- Visible squint is rare.

Head Tilt Produced by the 4th Nerve Palsy

Persons with lesion of trochlear nerve will have diplopia when he tilts the head towards the side of paralysed muscle. In order to avoid diplopia—person tilts the head away from the side of paralysed muscle.

Examples of isolated 4th nerve palsy—head injury.

> *Note:* Nuclear lesion of the 4th nerve—opposite superior oblique is paralysed. Lesion along the course of the nerve: Ipsilateral superior oblique is paralysed.

Paralysis of 6th Nerve

Characteristics

- Inability to move the eye laterally with diplopia on lateral gaze
- Person will have medial squint
- Isolated 6th nerve paralysis occurs with pontine lesions.

False localising signs of 6th nerve

- This type of 6th nerve palsy occurs in patients with raised intracranial tension.
- Paralysis of 6th nerve may be due to the downward displacement of the brainstem.
- 6th nerve paralysis recovers on treating the raised intracranial tension.

Causes of combined 3rd and 4th and 6th nerve palsies

- Cavernous sinus thrombosis
- Superior orbital fissure syndrome
- Diabetes mellitus

Ptosis

Ptosis is defined as drooping of upper eyelid. It may be unilateral or bilateral.

Causes of ptosis

- *Neurogenic:* 3rd nerve paralysis (pupil is dilated)

  Horner's syndrome (pupil is constricted)
- *Myogenic:* Myasthenia gravis, ocular myopathy
- *Mechanical:* Trauma, inflammation and tumors of the upper eyelid.

Complete Ptosis

Complete ptosis occurs in patients with oculomotor paralysis.

Due to the paralysis of levator palpabrae superioris, person is not able to look upwards even with effort.

While attempting to look upwards, frontal belly of occipitofrontalis stands prominent producing wrinkling of forehead as a compensatory mechanism.

Partial Ptosis

- Partial ptosis occurs in patients with Horner's syndrome.
- Person can voluntarily look upwards with effort.

Squint and Diplopia

Squint (Strabismus)

Squint occurs as a result of paralysis of one of the extraocular muscles, with deviation of eye to the opposite side (due to the action of normal extraocular muscle).

Types: Acquired (paralytic) squint:

Characteristics

- May be of sudden onset with a known cause
- Causes diplopia but blindness is absent
- Visual axes and images are separated
- Individual eyeball movement is abnormal
- Diplopia is greatest in the direction of action of paretic muscle
- Vertigo may be an associated feature
- Tilting of head involuntarily to the side of action of paralysed muscle can occur to avoid diplopia.

Concomitant Squint

Characteristics

- Occurs due to defective binocular vision
- Manifests in childhood
- Individual eyeball movement is normal
- Diplopia is not present
- Vertigo is absent

Diplopia (Double vision)

Patients with paralytic strabismus complain of double vision (diplopia). Images of two eyes do not fall on the identical portion of the retina due to defective movement of one eye and cortex interprets as two images.

Image which is formed on the macula of normal eye will be distinct (true image).

- Image which is formed outside the macula of the affected eye will be indistinct and blurred (false image).
- Diplopia will be maximum in the direction of action of weak muscle.
- False image is always present in that part of the visual field into which the paralysed eye should normally move the eye.

Pupil

Inequality in the Size of the Pupil

Causes

- Physiological anisocoria
- Pathological—oculomotor paralysis
- Horner's syndrome

Irregular pupil: Occurs due to synechiae as a result of iritis.

Hippus: Alternate contraction and dilatation of pupil, which occurs independent of exposure to light.

Depends on rhythmic activity of neuronal centers.

Conditions associated with hippus multiple sclerosis.

Pupillary Reflexes

Light reflex

Light is thrown on the cornea from the lateral aspect.

Observe for the constriction of the pupil on the same side (direct) and also on the other side (consensual).

Pathway of light reflex

- *Afferent*: Via the optic nerve up to the pretectal area in the midbrain.
- *Efferent:* From the Edinger-Westphal nucleus supplying the constrictor pupillae via the ciliary ganglion (3rd nerve).

Accommodation reflex

Ask the patient to look at an object which is brought suddenly in front of the nose from a distance.

Observe for convergence of two eyes and pupillary constriction.

Suggested pathway for convergence and accommodation

- Afferent fibres from medial rectus → via 3rd nerve → mesencephalic nucleus of 5th nerve → pretectal area (convergence center) → Edinger-Westphal nucleus → 3rd nerve → sphincter pupillae–pupillary constriction.
- Visual fibres → occipital cortex → occipito mesencephalic tract → pontine centre for convergence → Edinger-Westphal nucleus → 3rd nerve.

Different Types of Pupillary Abnormalities

Pinpoint pupil

Size of the pupil will be less than 1 mm.

Causes

- Organophosphorus poisoning
- Pontine hemorrhage
- Opium poisoning

Argyl Robertson pupil

Characteristics: Accommodation reflex is present with absence of pupillary reflex

Site of lesion: Pretectal area

Causes: CNS syphilis, diabetes mellitus

Myotonic pupil of Adie

Characteristics

- Slow and delayed reactions of the pupil to light
- Absent deep tendon reflexes in the lower extremities
- More common in females.

Note: In persons with myotonic pupil dysautonomia is supposed to be responsible for the pupillary abnormalities and defect may be in the ciliary ganglion.

Other causes: Amyloidosis, diabetes mellitus

Marcus Gun Pupil

Technique of elicitation: Shine the light into the normal eye and quickly change it to the abnormal eye (swinging flash light test).

Observation: Pupillary dilatation instead of constriction in the impaired eye due to insufficient afferent stimulus to constrict the pupil.

Deflect: Partial injury to the retina or optic nerve on the affected side (afferent pupillary defect).

Causes: Retrobulbar neuritis and other optic nerve diseases.

Horner's Syndrome

Defect: Lesion of the descending sympathetic chain (at pons, medulla or cervical sympathetic chain).

Causes

- Trauma to the neck
- Carotid occlusion
- Brainstem lesion
- Pancoast's tumor

Components

- Ptosis
- Anhydrosis
- Miosis
- Enophthalmos
- Loss of ciliospinal reflex
- Red eye
- *Ptosis:* Occurs due to the paralysis of tarsal (Müller's) muscles supplied by sympathetics.
- *Enophthalmos:* Inward movement of eyeball—apparent retraction of the eyeball probably due to narrowing of palpebral fissure and ptosis.
- *Miosis:* Occurs due to loss of sympathetic supply to dilator pupillae with overaction of constrictor pupillae supplied by parasympathetics.
- *Anhydrosis:* Loss of sweating on one side of face.
- *Loss of sweating of whole of one side of face:* Lesion at common carotid.

- Loss of sweating only on side of the nose and medial aspect of forehead.
- Lesion distal to carotid bifurcation.
- Loss of ciliospinal reflex: Absence of pupillary dilatation on stimulation of the neck.

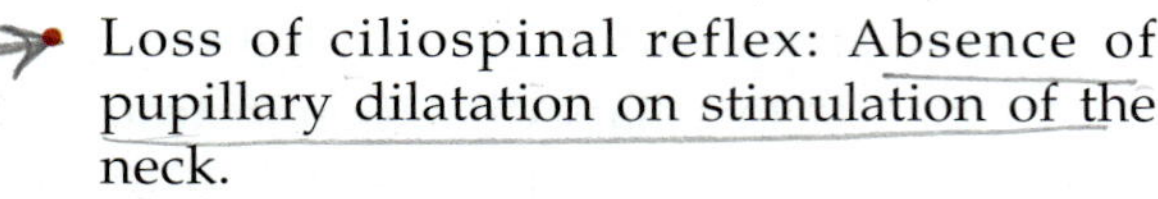

4. Trigeminal Nerve (5th)

Motor nucleus: Situated in the pons. Components of 5th cranial nerve:

- Ophthalmic—purely sensory
- Maxillary—purely sensory
- Mandibular—motor and sensory

Sensory supply

Supplies full one half of the face except near the angle of the mandible (supplied by C_2 dermatome).

Sensory supply takes origin from neurons in the trigeminal ganglion (Gasserian ganglion) and fibers concerned with light touch enter the pontine nucleus.

Fibers concerned with pain and temperature descend up to C_2 segment (descending tract) and fibers join medial lemniscus and ascend. Lower part of the descending tract contains fibers representing the upper part of the face.

Motor supply: Supplies muscles of mastication like

- Temporalis
- Tensor tympani
- Masseter
- Tensor veli palatini
- Lateral and medial pterygoids

Examination of Trigeminal Nerve

Sensory Part

1. Testing the sensation of one half of the face for touch, pain and temperature.
2. Corneal and conjunctival reflex.

Corneal Reflex

Touch the cornea with wisp of cotton from the lateral aspect and observe for the closure of the eye on the same side and also the opposite side.

Pathway of corneal reflex

- *Affarent:* Via the ophthalmic division of the trigeminal nerve
- *Efferent:* Via the facial nerve supplying the orbicularis oculi
- *Center*: Pons

Absence of corneal reflex suggests: Lesions of 5th or 7th cranial nerve and loss of connection between the 5th and 7th cranial nerves.

Vth Nerve Lesion

Unilateral loss of corneal sensation.

No response on corneal stimulation (afferent defect).

But on stimulation of opposite cornea there will be closure of both eyes.

Note: Lesion in the cervical cord can cause loss of sensation of upper part of face–due to the involvement of descending tract of 5th nerve. Long-term trigeminal nerve paralysis can produce ulceration of the cornea and dryness of mouth.

Motor Component of Trigeminal Nerve

Testing the Muscles of Mastication

Temporalis and masseter: Palpate the muscles above and below the zygomatic arch, when the patient is clenching the teeth and compare the differences between the strength of the muscles on two sides.

Lateral pterygoids: Check the lateral movement of jaw against resistance. Jaw can be moved towards the affected side and cannot be deviated towards the normal side.

Key Points

- In unilateral lesion of the Vth cranial nerve, jaw will be deviated to the side of lesion.
- In persons with lower motor neuron type of Vth nerve palsy, there will be atrophy of the Temporalis and Masseter muscles leading onto hollowing of the temple and face.
- Bilateral weakness of muscles of mastication will produce the jaw to open and hang loosely.

Jaw Jerk (see deep reflexes)

Causes of trigeminal nerve paralysis

- Cerebellopontine angle tumor
- Infarction or demyelination of pons
- Meningioma of sensory ganglion.

Facial (7th) Nerve

Supplies muscles of facial expression.

Carries taste fibers from anterior 2/3rds of tongue (via chorda tympani nerve).

Nucleus of the facial nerve is situated in the pons.

Examination of the Facial Nerve

Testing the Muscles of Facial Expression and Features of Facial Palsy

1. *Frontal belly of occipitofrontalis*
   - Ask the patient to look upwards
   - Observe for the wrinkling of forehead
   - Wrinkling will be absent in patients with LMN facial palsy.
2. *Orbicularis oculi*
   - Examiner tries to open the eye which has been tightly closed by the patient.
   - In patients with LMN facial palsy, the patient cannot close the eye or examiner can easily open the eye.
3. *Buccinator:* Ask the patient to blow the cheek against resistance (not possible if the buccinator is paralysed).

Note: Paralysed cheek balloons more than normal if the cheeks are puffed out.

4. *Platysma:* Ask the patient to show the teeth with open mouth against resistance. Observe for the fold of platysma which stands prominent.
5. Nasolabial fold will be obliterated on the affected side of facial palsy.
6. Angle of the mouth will be deviated to the normal side, while the patient is asked to show the teeth.
7. Patient will have labial dysarthria (slurring of speech).

Types of Facial Palsy

1. Upper motor neuron facial palsy:
   - Volitional type
   - Mimitic type
2. Lower motor neuron facial palsy

Upper Motor Neuron Facial Palsy Volitional Type

Characteristics

- Facial palsy will be on the opposite side of the lesion.
- Only lower part of the opposite side face is involved. So patient will have intact wrinkling of forehead and eye closure.
- Usually associated with ipsilateral hemiplegia.

Causes

- Cerebrovascular accident including the cortex, corona radiata and internal capsule
- Encephalitis
- Cerebral tumors (supratentorial)
- Head injury
- Upper part of the face receives bilateral representation in the cortex making it less vulnerable to be involvement in unilateral UMN lesions.

Note: Occasionally, in acute severe UMN facial palsy, transiently upper part of the face may be involved.

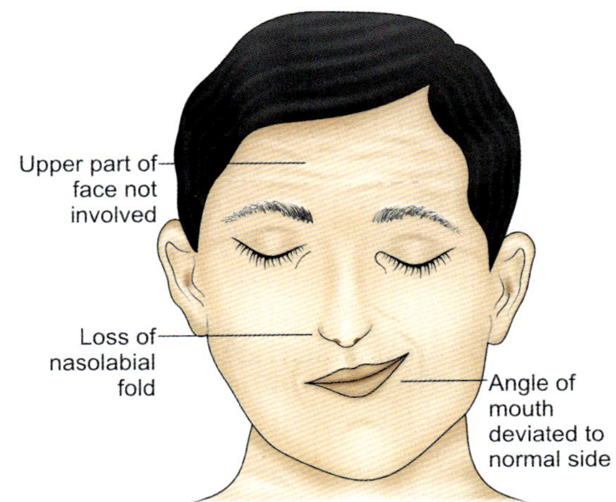

Upper motor neruron lesion of facial nerve on right side

LMN course of the facial nerve and manifestations of different levels of lesion

Site of lesion	*Characteristics*
• At pons	– LMN 7th nerve palsy Long tract signs (opposite side)
• Internal auditory meatus	– LMN 7th nerve palsy, Taste loss, anterior 2/3rds tongue Decrease of salivation and lacrimation. 8th nerve involvement
• Between internal auditory meatus and geniculate ganglion (facial canal)	– LMN 7th palsy, taste loss anterior 2/3rds of tongue loss of tears, hyperacusis
• At geniculate ganglion	– LMN 7th palsy, taste loss, hyperacusis, decrease lacrimation and salivation.
• Between geniculate ganglion and nerve to stepidius	LMN 7th palsy, hyperacusis, decrease salivation and taste (no decrease of lacrimation)
• After nerve to stepidius and before nerve to chorda tympani	LMN 7th palsy, taste loss, decrease salivation
• After chorda tympani	– LMN 7th palsy
• In the parotid gland	– Only branch of 7th nerve can be involved.

Bilateral UMN Facial Palsy

Features

- Occurs in patients with pseudo bulbar palsy
- Emotional incontinence
- Brisk jaw jerk and bilateral UMN signs

Mimitic Type of UMN Facial Palsy

In this type of facial palsy voluntary movements are normal.

Facial palsy is visible only on emotional movement (like smiling or weeping).

There will be mask like face with lack of expression.

Significance of mimitic facial palsy: Suggests defect is in the central pathway controlling the emotional movements like frontal lobe anterior to pre central gyrus and extra-pyramidal, thalamic and hypothalamic connections.

Lower Motor Neuron Type of Facial Palsy

Site of lesion: Anywhere from the nucleus of the nerve in the pons up to its lower motor neuron course.

Characteristics

- Whole of the face on the side of the lesion will be paralysed.
- Due to the involvement of the upper part of the face, wrinkling of the forehead is lost and eye closure will not be possible.

Note: Involvement of lacrimation is due to the involvement of greater superficial petrosal nerve.

Hyperacusis (painful hearing or unpleasant quality to louder intensity sounds) is clue to the involvement of nerve to stapedius.

Decrease taste and salivation are due to the involvement of nervus intermedius (travelling via chorda tympani).

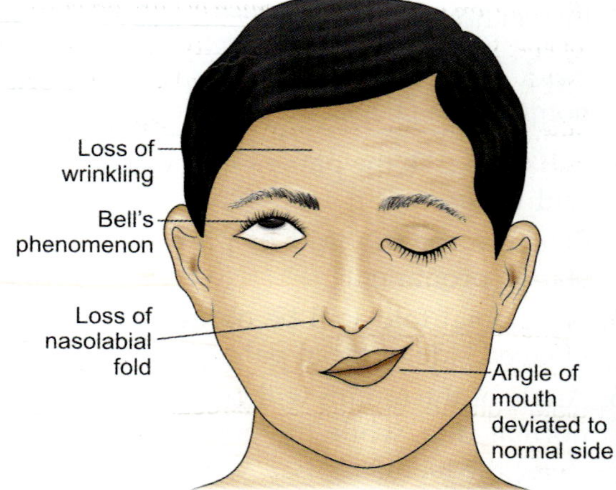

Lower motor neruron lesion of facial nerve on right side

Bell's Phenomenon

This is the visible upward movement of the eyeball, which occurs in patients with LMN facial palsy, when the patient is asked to close the eye.

Causes of LMN facial palsy

- Pontine lesions
- Cerebellopontine angle lesion
- Bell's palsy
- Ramsay hunt syndrome
- Diabetes mellitus
- Parotid tumor and parotid surgery, etc.

Causes of bilateral LMN facial palsy

- Guillain-Barré syndrome
- Diabetes mellitus
- Sarcoidosis

Face in bilateral LMN facial palsy: No voluntary movement of face. Sclera will be visible on attempted eye closure.

Consequences of Long-standing Facial Palsy

- *Hemi facial spasm:* Occurs with every facial movement and persists indefinitely.
- *Crocodile tears:* Tearing which occurs while eating, due to the fibres, which are originally connected with muscles of face later, innervate lacrimal gland.
- *Retraction of the mouth which occurs on closure of eye:* Fibres, which originally connected to orbicularis oculi, innervate orbicularis oris.
- *Jaw-winking:* Involuntary closure of eye on lateral movement of jaw.

Examination of Taste Sensation

Different taste sensations to be tested

Taste sensation	*Substance used*
Sweet	Sugar
Salt	Common salt
Sour	Vinegar
Bitter	Quinine

Method of Testing

- Patient is asked to keep the tongue protruded to one side throughout the test (closing the eyes).
- Hold the tip of the tongue with a gauze piece and moisten the tongue with the taste substance solutions (tip of the tongue—for sweet and salt, sides of the tongue for sour and posterior aspect of the tongue for bitter taste).
- Patient should indicate the taste by pointing to the card, in which different tastes are written.
- Patient should rinse the mouth in between each test.

Note: Tip of the tongue can sense all forms of taste sensations.

Detection of early facial palsy

- Examiner tries to open the closed eyelids of the patient against resistance.
- Normal contraction of orbicularis oculi can be felt as vibrations.
- Early facial palsy, there will be absence of vibrations of orbicularis oculi contraction.

Pathway of taste

Anterior 2/3rds of tongue → chorda tympani → Posterior 1/3rd of tongue → glossopharyngeal → Palate—greater superficial petrosal Larynx, epiglottis and oesophagus → vagus →	PONS Nucleus of tractus solitarius	PONS Parabrachial nucleus	→ Dorsal nucleus of thalamus → INSULA → Directly to cortex Amygdala → Hypothalamus Ventral forebrain

Vestibulocochlear nerve

- Nucleus situated at pontomedullary junction.
- Cochlear part of the nucleus situated in the pons.
- Vestibular part of the nucleus situated in the medulla.

Vestibular connections

Vestibular apparatus → semicircular canals → vestibular nerve → nucleus in the medulla → connected with midbrain, cerebellum, spinal cord and temporal lobe.

Examination of vestibular component: Look for positional nystagmus, Doll's eye movement (*see* chapter 11 on unconscious patient).

Elicitation of positional nystagmus

- Patient is sitting on the bed and his head is turned to one side by about 30°.
- Patient is suddenly made to lie on his back with the head projected beyond the bed and head is brought below the horizontal plane by about 30°.
- Observe for nystagmus and enquire the patient for vertigo.
- If no response occurs head can be turned to the opposite side.

In benign positional vertigo

- Nystagmus occurs after a latency of 5–10 secs.
- Fast phase of the nystagmus is towards the lower ear.
- Rapid adaptation with failure of response to immediate stimulation.

Central vertigo: Nystagmus occurs immediately and without adaptation.

Nystagmus

Definition: Conjugate usually rhythmic involuntary movement of eyeballs.

Checking for nystagmus

- Ask the patient to follow the finger or an object starting from midline.
- Move the finger in all four directions.
- Maintain deviation of eyes for 5 secs in each direction of gaze.
- Look for the direction of nystagmus while holding the eyes open.

Causes and characteristics of different types of nystagmus

Cause	Characteristics
• Congenital and if visual defect in early age	Pendular (equal rate and amplitude of nystagmus)
• Brainstem dysfunction, e.g. alchohol, phenytoin therapy	Vertical up and down nystagmus other signs of brainstem dysfunctions
• Cervicomedullary lesion	Down beating vertical nystagmus
• Vestibular lesion	Horizontal nystagmus and rarely rotary type. Fast component away from the side of lesion, may have a torsional component Nystagmus decreases by gaze fixing or lying quiet in neutral position
• Peripheral vestibular lesion	Associated with vertigo nausea, vomiting, deafness and tinnitus Quick adaptation of nystagmus
• Central vestibular lesion	Persistent nystagmus (vertical, rotary/multidirectional No effect of visual fixation
• Cerebellar lesion	Horizontal nystagmus with its fast—component occurs in the direction towards the side of lesion (gaze evoked nystagmus). Other signs of cerebellar dysfunction will be associated
• Lesion of cerebellar vermis	Vertical nystagmus with upbeat component
• Ataxic nystagmus (*see* MLF lesion)	

Direction of nystagmus: Direction of nystagmus is described by the faster component of the nystagmus.

Grades of nystagmus

- Grade I: Nystagmus only when eye is deviated to one side (faster component is towards the side of gaze)
- Grade II: Nystagmus while looking straight.
- Grade III: Nystagmus with its faster component opposite to the direction of gaze.

Nystagmoid jerk: On extreme lateral deviation of eyes 2 to 3 jerky movements occur (no clinical significance).

Optokinetic Nystagmus

- Physiological phenomenon.
- Present whenever the person follows a rapidly moving scene (railway carriage nystagmus).
- Eye will be following a moving object and when they cannot follow it any longer, eyes move back to fix on a new object. Regular repetition of this process will produce nystagmus.

Significance: Loss of optokinetic nystagmus to one side indicates opposite parietal lobe pathology.

Cochlear component of 8th nerve: Cochlea is responsible for hearing.

Acoustic pathway

Organ of Corti (end organ of hearing) → Fibres originate and form cochlear nerve → reach pontine nucleus → lateral leminiscus → medial geniculate body → auditory radiation → superior temporal gyrus of opposite hemisphere.

Air conduction: Sound traverses the outer and middle ear to reach cochlea and stimulate organ of Corti.

Bone conduction: Sound traverses skull bones to reach organ of Corti.

Normally, air conduction is better than bone conduction.

Tests of Hearing

Rinne's Test

Strike the tuning fork of 512 frequency and keep it near the external auditory meatus of the patient.

When the patient is still hearing the tuning fork sound, change the position of the fork and keep it on the mastoid process till he stops hearing. Keep back the tuning fork again near the patient's external auditory meatus (normal person still hears the sound).

Interpretation: Normally air conduction is better than bone conduction. This is called **Rinne positive** (can also occur in sensory neural deafness). In middle ear disease bone conduction is better than air conduction. This is called **Rinne negative**.

Weber's Test

Vibrating tuning fork is placed over the center of the forehead.

Patient is asked to tell whether he can hear the sound on both ears equally or in one ear better than the other.

Normal: sound is heard equal on both sides/midline.

Nerve deafness: Sound is better heard in the normal ear.

Middle ear disease: Sound is better heard in the affected ear.

Causes of 8th nerve disease

Cochlear division

- Pontine lesion
- Aminoglycoside toxicity
- Cerebellopontine angle tumor
- Temporal lobe disease

Vestibular division

- Minier's disease
- Aminoglycosides
- Brainstem disease
- CP angle tumor
- Temporal lobe disease

Glossopharyngeal (9th), vagus (10th) and accessory (11th) cranial nerves.

Nucleus and supply of 9th and 10th and 11 cranial nerves.

Glossopharyngeal

Sensory supply: Posterior 1/3rd of tongue taste sensation and pharyngeal mucosa.

Afferent from baro-and chemoreceptors and parotid secretions.

Sensory fibers terminate in tractus solitarius

Motor supply: From nucleus ambiguous in the medulla, supplies stylopharyngeus.

Vagus

Sensory supply: From pharynx, larynx, trachea, oesophagus, thorax and abdominal viscera.

Sensory fibers terminate in the nucleus of tractus solitarius.

Motor supply: Nucleus ambiguous supplies voluntary muscles of palate, larynx and pharynx.

Dorsal motor nucleus: Parasympathetic supply to thoracic and abdominal viscera.

Accessory

Cranial part: From lower part of nucleus Ambiguous supplies through vagus (intrinsic muscles of larynx and pharynx).

Spinal part: From C_1 to C_5 cervical segments supplying trapezius and sternomastoid.

Examination of 9th, 10th and 11th cranial nerves.

Glossopharyngeal (9th) Nerve: Supplies

Taste sensation of posterior 1/3rd of tongue:

Tested by applying a weak electric current to the back of the tongue. This will produce an acid taste if sensation is intact.

Motor part: Clinical motor abnormality of 9th nerve may not manifest and cannot be satisfactorily tested.

Causes of 9th nerve palsy: Usually 9th nerve will be involved along with cranial nerves 10th and 11th, e.g. fracture base of skull, invasive tumors of base of skull.

Vagus (10th) and Accessory (11th) Nerves

Tests for 10th and 11th cranial nerves:

Position of uvula: Normally, uvula is at the center. In unilateral 10th and 11th nerve paralysis uvula will be shifted to the opposite side.

Palate movement: Ask the patient to say "Ah" and look for the palate movement. Normally both sides move equally.

Unilateral paralysis: Affected side palate does not move. Affected side palate may be pulled to the normal side.

Gag Reflex

Touch the posterior pharyngeal wall separately on either side with a swab stick and cotton.

Normal: Immediate gagging on touching the posterior pharyngeal wall.

Unilateral gag absent: Suggests unilateral sensory/motor/both abnormality of 9th and 10th nerve.

If only sensory defection one side: Opposite side stimulation produces normal response.

If motor defect on one side: Absent palate movement on saying "Ah".

Combined lesion on one side: Uvula to opposite side, palate drawn to opposite side, no response on touching the pharynx.

Note: In cases of recurrent laryngeal nerve lesion (branch of vagus)—person will have hoarseness of voice.

In cases of bilateral vocal cord paralysis person will have stridor and bovine cough.

Causes of 10th nerve paralysis

- Unilateral—as mentioned under IX nerve
- Bilateral—bulbar palsy

Note: Occasionally, gag reflex may be absent bilaterally, but palate movement on both sides are normal on telling "Ah".

Causes of 9th, 10th and 11th Cranial Nerve Palsies

Unilateral (LMN)

- Jugular foramen syndrome
- Lateral medullary syndrome

Bilateral (UMN)

- Motor neuron disease
- Pseudobulbar palsy

Bilateral (LMN)

- Progressive bulbar palsy
- Poliomyelitis

Testing the Spinal Part of Accessory Nerve

Trapezius: Paralysis of trapezius will produce flattening of muscle with drooping of arm.

Ask the patient to raise his shoulder towards his ear again resistance. Not possible if the trapezius is paralysed.

Sternomastoid: Turn the patient's neck to one side against resistance.

Observe for the contraction of sternomastoid of the opposite side.

Hypoglossal (12th) Nerve

Nucleus: Medial medulla

Supplies intrinsic muscles of tongue.

Examination of 12th nerve

- Ask the patient to move the tongue side-to-side slowly and then rapidly.
- Ask the patient to protrude the tongue. Test the movement of the tongue on either side against resistance (movement of tongue towards the cheek while giving resistance from outside).

Interpretation

- In unilateral paralysis of the 12th nerve tongue will be deviated to the affected side due to the action of opposite genioglossus.
- Palpate the tongue with a gauze piece.
- In upper motor neuron paralysis of 12th nerve (usually bilateral) tongue will be small and stiff.
- In lower motor neuron paralysis of the 12th nerve affected part of the tongue will be flabby with fasciculations. (Keep the tongue inside the mouth while looking for fasciculations.)

Causes of 12th Nerve Paralysis

Bilateral UMN lesion

- Motor neuron disease
- Bilateral internal capsular lesion

Bilateral LMN lesion

- Bulbar palsy
- Vascular lesion of medulla

Unilateral LMN

- Medial medullary lesion and
- *Other causes:* As mentioned for 10th nerve.

Note: In acute hemiplegia of internal capsular lesion 12th nerve can be transiently involved.

Motor System

Upper Motor Neuron (UMN)

- Upper motor neuron constitute the following structures:
- Pyramidal tract—corticospinal tract:
  - Consists of fibers which start from the cells in motor cortex (precentral gyrus-area No. 4) connecting with the motor neurons in the spinal cord and brainstem cranial nerve nuclei.

Lower Motor Neuron (LMN)

Lower motor neuron constitute the following structures:

1. Cranial nerve nuclei in the brainstem and their corresponding cranial nerves.
2. Anterior horn cells and their efferent nerve fibers passing via the peripheral spinal nerves.

Features of UMN lesion

- Groups of muscles are involved
- Hypertonia
- Superficial reflexes are absent
- Deep reflexes are exaggerated
- Plantar reflex: On the affected side becomes extensor

Paraplegia in extension: Limbs are held in extension, suggests corticospinal lesion.

Paraplegia in flexion: Limbs are held in flexion—due to flexor hypertonia, suggests progressive lesion of the spinal cord involving bilateral pyramidal and reticulospinal tract.

Note: Smaller and precise movements are usually more and early involved than the gross movements in UMN lesions.

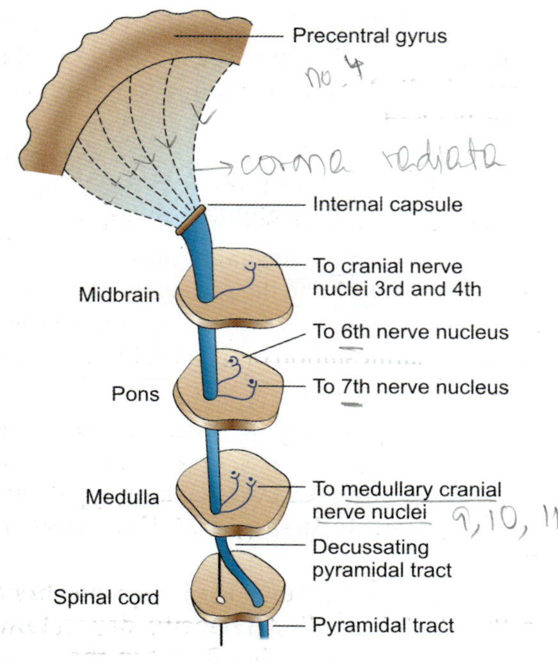

Motor pathway

Features of LMN Lesion

- Affects individual muscle
- Hypotonia
- Wasting of the muscles involved
- Both superficial and deep reflexes become absent depending on the motor root or nerve involved.
- Fasciculations may be present.

Examination of the Motor System

Components of the motor system examination

- Attitude of limbs
- Nutrition
- Tone
- Power
- Coordination
- Involuntary movements.

Attitude of limbs: This is the position of the limbs, which it adopts when the patient is in the resting position.

Attitude of limbs of a hemiplegic: Upper limb will be adducted, flexed and semipronated, and lower limbs will be extended, externally rotated and foot inverted and plantar flexed.

Nutrition: Nutrition is assessed by comparing the muscle bulk on either side of body.

Tests for nutrition

Measure the girth of upper limb: Right and left forearm 10 cm—above and below the olecranon respectively.

Lower limb

- Right and left thigh: 18 cm above the patella
- Right and left calf: 10 cm below the tibial tuberosity.
- In a right-handed individual, right upper limb may be more than the left upper limb by an inch but lower limb girth will be equal.

Wasting and Hypertrophy of Muscles

Causes of muscle wasting

- Lower motor neuron disease
- Muscular dystrophy
- Long-standing UMN disease with disuse atrophy of muscle.

Hypertrophy of muscles: True hypertrophy may be due to excessive continued workload of muscles, e.g. athletic training, myotonic disorder.

Pseudohypertrophy

- Muscle bulk is increased in patients with pseudohypertrophy, but muscles are weaker indicating it is not a true hypertrophy.
- Increase in the bulk of muscles is due to deposition of fat and fibrous tissue.
- Muscles of calves, buttocks and infraspinatus are particularly affected.

Note: Enlargement of calf muscles in patients of Duchenne and Becker types of muscular dystrophies may be due to initial true hypertrophy (hypertrophied muscle fibers) and then replaced by fat and connective tissue with loss of muscle fibers (pseudo-hypertrophy).

Causes of muscle enlargement
- Duchenne and Becker types of muscular dystrophies
- Limb girdle type of muscular dystrophy
- Hypothyroidism
- Polymyositis

Causes of localised muscle swelling
- Cysticercosis
- Muscle infarction/hematoma
- Tropical pyomyositis

Causes of wasting of small muscles of hand
- Motor neuron disease
- Carpal tunnel syndrome
- Syringomyelia
- Pancoast's tumor
- Thoracic outlet syndrome
- Leprosy
- Lead poisoning

Tone

Definition: A state of tension present in the muscle at rest.

Assessed by resistance offered by the muscles for passive movement.

Normal tone: Normally, tone is inhibited by corticospinal, and vestibulo- and reticulo-spinal tract. Tone abnormality occurs in all conditions affecting these tracts.

Tests for Demonstration of Tone

a. Feel of muscles:
   - Hypertonic muscles may be firm to feel and not easily displacable.
   - Hypotonic muscles may be soft to touch and easily displacable.

b. Ask the patient to keep the upper limbs outstretched infront of him.
   - Give a tap to the outstretched limb on each side.
   - Observe for—movement of limbs.
   - Hypotonic limb—undergoes wider range of displacement.

Testing the tone of upper limb: Passively flex/extend the wrist, elbow and note the resistance offered.

Testing the tone of lower limb: Hold the lower limb between the two hands and quickly rotate the limbs. Suddenly lift the knee away from the bed.

Normal person: There will be bending of knee with the heel still touching the bed.

Hypertonia: Whole leg will be lifted as one.

Types of Tone Alteration

Hypertonia (increase of tone): Hypertonia is a classical manifestation of pyramidal and extra-pyramidal disorder.

Spasticity: Spasticity is a manifestation of pyramidal tract disease. Hypertonia is present in only one group of muscles and hypertonia is not present throughout the range of movement.

Degree of tone developed is proportional to the stretch applied (velocity dependant), e.g. flexor hypertonia is present in the upper limb and extensor hypertonia is present in the lower limb.

Clasp Knife Spasticity

Clasp knife spasticity is a classical manifestation of pyramidal tract disease. There is increase in resistance for the initial movement and the resistance decreases if the movement is continued.

Physiological basis of clasp knife spasticity
- Clasp knife spasticity is physiologically due to lengthening reaction.
- When the muscle is subjected to stronger stretch, there will be stimulation of inverse stretch with reflex inhibition of motor neuron.

Distribution of hypertonia in corticospinal lesion

Upper limb
- Shoulder adduction
- Elbow flexion
- Flexors of wrist and fingers

} Flexed and adducted upper limb

Lower limb
- Hip extensors
- Knee extensors
- Plantar flexors of foot

} Extended lower limb planter flexion of foot

Rigidity

Rigidity is a manifestation of extrapyramidal disorder.

Hypertonia is present throughout the range of movement in patients with rigidity.

Types of Rigidity

Cog wheel rigidity: Rigidity is interrupted by jerky feeling. There will be alternate regular and rapid contraction of agonists and antagonists, e.g. Parkinson's disease.

> *Note:* Cog wheeling may occur without tremor (tremor may contribute and exacerbate the cog wheeling).

Phenomenon of gegenhalten

- Gegenhalten is a manifestation of frontal lobe disease.
- Flexors and extensors are equally affected. Tone varies irregularly.
- Patient appears to be voluntarily resisting the movement or appears to aid the movement.

Hysterical tone alteration: Tone appears to increase as more effort is applied by the examiner to passively move the limb.

Paraplegia in extension: Limbs are held in extension—bilateral pyramidal disease.

Paraplegia in flexion: Limbs are held in flexion (flexor hypertonia—due to progressive lesion of the spinal cord bilateral pyramidal and reticulospinal tract involvement) indicates poor prognosis.

Myotonia

Suggests prolonged muscle contraction and relaxation of muscles (more marked on cold temperature).

Demonstration of myotonia

1. Tap the thenar eminence—look for adduction of thumb and appearance of dimpling which will disappear slowly (myotonia can be demonstrated on taping any muscle).
2. Slow relaxation of hand muscles after a strong grip.

Conditions associated with myotonia

- Myotonia congenita
- Occasionally hypothyroidism

Hypotonia

Hypotonia suggests decreased resistance offered for passive movement.

Causes

- Lower motor neuron disease
- Cerebellar disease
- Muscular disease
- UMN disease, in the stage of neuronal shock
- Rheumatic chorea

Power

Power is estimated by testing the strength of muscles.

Grades of muscle power

Grade 0—no movement
Grade I—flicker of contraction
Grade II—movement with gravity eliminated
Grade III—movement against gravity
Grade IV—movement against minimal resistance
Grade V—movement against full resistance–normal power.

> *Note:* In pyramidal disease movements which are acquired later in the process of evolution are first to be lost, e.g. precision grip (opposition of thumb and finger) is more impaired than the power grip.

Distribution of pyramidal weakness:

- *Upper limb*: Weakness of shoulder extension, abduction and dorsi flexors of wrist.
- *Lower limb*: Weakness of hip flexors and dorsi flexion of foot.

Examination of Muscle Power

Neck extension

- Patient lies prone.
- Patient is asked to raise his shoulder away from the bed which is resisted by placing the one hand over the occiput. Contracting

muscles can be seen and felt (stabilise the chest by placing the other hand over the chest).

Neck flexion

- Patient lies supine.
- Place one hand over the upper chest for stabilisation.
- Patient is asked to flex the neck which is resisted by placing the other hand over the forehead.
- Contractions of sternomastoid, platysma and other flexors of neck can be seen and felt.

Rotation and lateral movements can be examined with modification of flexion and extension movements.

Nerve supply of neck muscles: C_1 to C_8 segments.

Trunk and abdominal muscles: Trunk and abdominal muscles are spared in classical

Main movements taking place at each joint and principal muscles involved are given below

Shoulder	
Flexion (forward elevation)	Anterior fibres of deltoid, pectoris major, subscapularis
Extension (backward elevation)	Posterior fibres of deltoid, L. dorsi, teres major
Adduction	Pectoralis major, latissimus dorsi
Abduction	Deltoid and supraspinatus
External rotation	Infraspinatus and teres minor
Internal rotation	Subscapularis and teres major
Elbow	
Flexion	Biceps brachii
Extension	Triceps
Pronation	Pronator teres and quadratus
Supination	Biceps, brachioradialis and supinator
Wrist	
Palmar flexion	Flexor carpii radialis and ulnaris
Dorsiflexion	Extensor carpi radialis and ulnaris and other muscles
Adduction and ulnar deviation	Flexor and extensor carpi ulnaris
Abduction and radial deviation	Flexor and extensor carpi radialis
Hand grip	
Strength of the grip	Patient is asked to squeeze the index and middle fingers of the examiner. Assess the strength of the grip
Hip	
• Flexion	Ileopsoas
• Extension	main muscle involved gluteus maximus
• Abduction	Gluteus medius and minimus
• Adduction	3 Adductors (adductor magnus, medius and minimus)

Note: Gluteus maximus helps in raising from sitting position, straitening from bent to erect position, climbing and also in running.

Knee

- Flexion—hamstrings (biceps femoris, semimembranosus and semitendinosus)
- Extension—quadriceps femoris (3 vasti and rectus femoris)

Ankle

- Plantar flexion—gastrocnemius and soleus
- Dorsiflexion—tibialis anterior
- Eversion—peroneii muscles
- Inversion—tibialis posterior

internal capsular hemiplegia due to their bilateral representation in the cortex.

Examination of Trunk and Abdominal Muscles

Extensors of spine: Segmental supply: All segments of spinal nerves.

Patient lies on his face and then attempts to raise his shoulder off the bed. Muscles of the back can be seen to contract.

Intercostals: Segmental supply: $T_1 - T_{12}$

Observe the movements of intercostal muscles and movements of ribs on inspiration and expiration.

Abdominal muscles: Segmental supply $T_5–L_1$

Patient lies on his back and is asked to raise the head against resistance. Watch for the movements of umbilicus and also palpate the abdominal muscles during contraction.

Beevor's Sign

- Beevor's sign helps in the detection of weakness of abdominal muscles.
- Patient is asked to raise the head against resistance while lying down supine. Observe for the position of umbilicus.
- Umbilicus will be pulled upwards, if the lower abdominal muscles are paralysed.
- Umbilicus will be pulled downwards, if the upper abdominal muscles are paralysed.

Gower's Sign

Person uses the arms to climb up the legs while getting up from sitting or lying down position (due to proximal muscle weakness), e.g. Duchenne muscular dystrophy.

Small Muscles of Hand

Lumbricals

Action: Cause flexion at the metacarpophalangeal joint and extension at the interphalangeal joint.

Testing: Ask the patient to actively extend the inter phalangeal joint with the metacarpophalangeal joint held in flexion.

Interossei

Action: Palmar interossei—adduct the fingers

Dorsal interossei—abduct the fingers.

Testing adduction of the fingers: Ask the patient to hold the card between the extended fingers.

Testing abduction of the fingers: Ask the patient to spread the extended fingers against resistance.

1st dorsal interossei: Patient is asked to abduct the index finger against resistance.

Examination of Individual Muscles

Infraspinatus: CS, C_6—suprascapular nerve

Test: Keep the patient's elbow at 90° and to the side of the body. Offer resistance when the patient tries to carry the flexed forearm backwards and palpate the muscle (Fig. 5.1).

Deltoid: CS, C_6—circumflex nerve (Fig. 5.2).

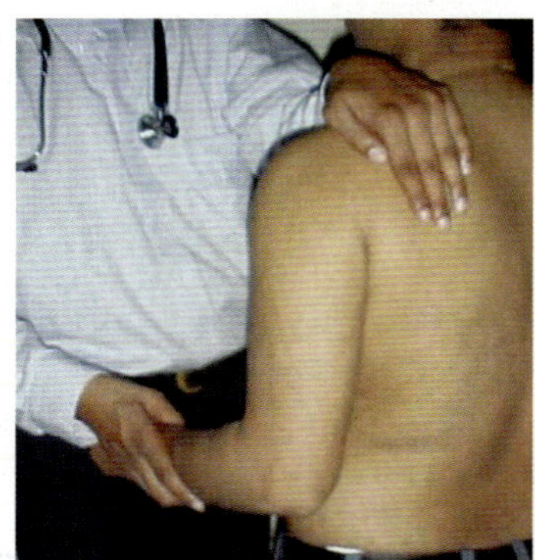

Fig. 5.1: Testing Infraspinatus

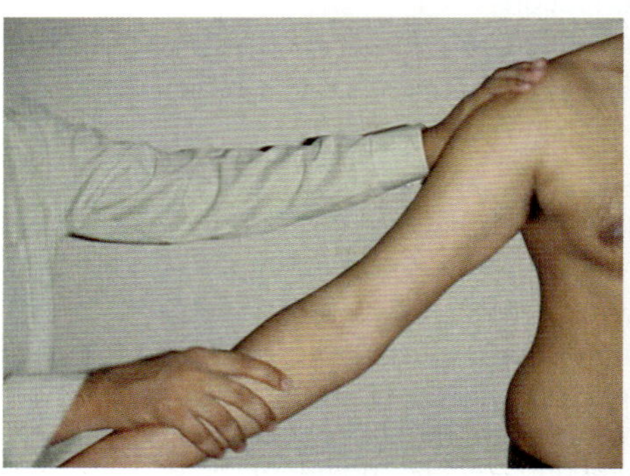

Fig. 5.2: Testing deltoid

Test: Ask the patient to hold the arm horizontally in abduction. Examiner tries to depress the elbow while the patient tries to resist it.

Pectoralis Major

Clavicular part: CS, C_6—lateral pectoral nerve (Fig. 5.3)

Test: Patient is asked to raise the arms above horizontal and is asked to adduct against resistance. Observe and feel for the clavicular part of the muscle contraction.

Sternal part: $C_{6,7,8}$ and T_1—medial pectoral nerve (Fig. 5.4)

Test: Ask the patient to raise the arm to a level below horizontal and is asked to adduct against resistance (Fig. 5.4).

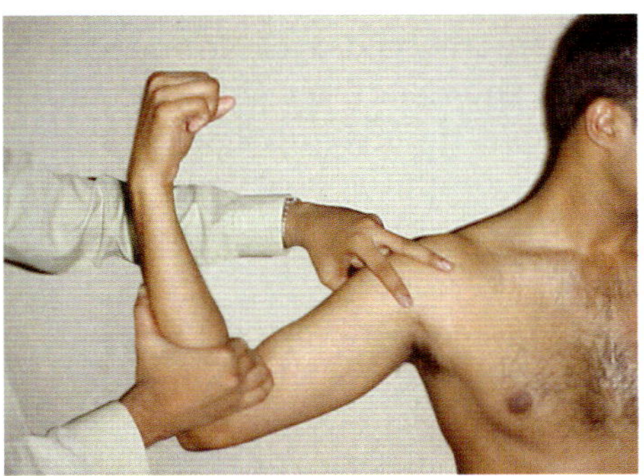

Fig. 5.3: Testing pectoralis major—clavicular part

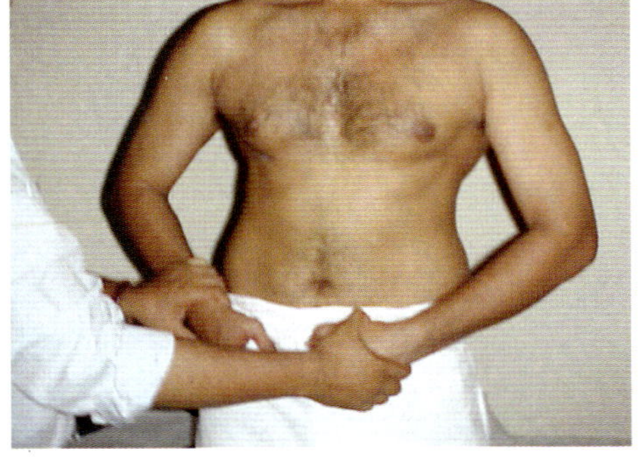

Fig. 5.4: Testing pectoralis major—sternal part

Serratus anterior: CS, 6,7—nerve to serratus anterior (Fig. 5.5)

Test: Ask the patient to push forwards against a wall or against resistance applied by the examiner.

Winging of scapula occurs when the muscle is paralysed. Patient is not able to elevate the arm above right angle.

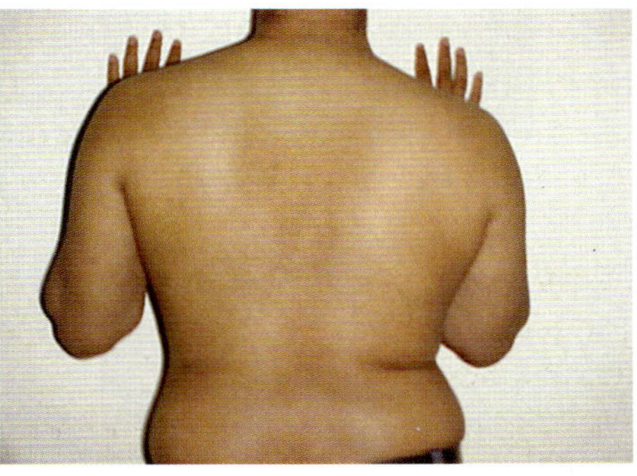

Fig. 5.5: Testing serratus anterior

Supraspinatus: C_5, C_6—suprascapular nerve (Fig. 5.6)

Test: Patient is asked to raise the upper limb straight at right angles from the side of the body against resistance. Supraspinatus carries out initial 30° of this movement (deltoid helps to carry out further 60" of this movement).

Rhomboids: C_5—nerve to rhomboids (Fig. 5.7)

Test: Ask the patient to keep the hands on his hip and ask him to carry his elbow forcefully backwards against resistance. Palpate the muscle belly medial to the scapula.

Elbow flexion: Biceps: $C_{5,6}$—musculocutaneous nerve (Fig. 5.8)

Test: Ask the patient to pull the forearm against resistance. Feel for the biceps contraction.

Latissimus dorsi: $C_{6,7,8}$—nerve to L. dorsi

Test: Ask the patient to cough and palpate the posterior axillary folds while coughing. OR Patient is asked to carry his hands behind his back while the examiner applies resistance to the backward and downward movement (Fig. 5.9).

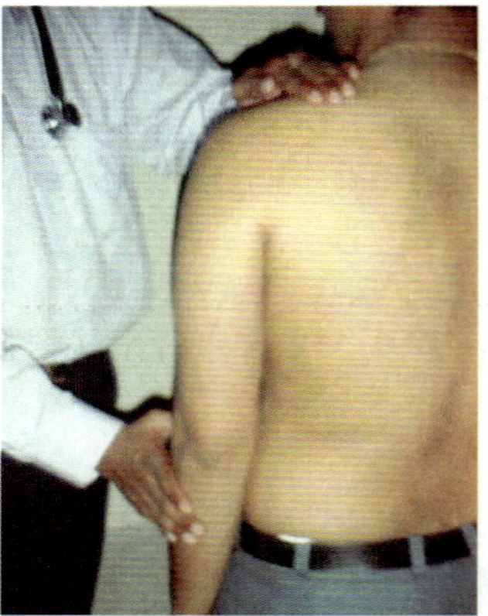

Fig. 5.6: Testing supraspinatus

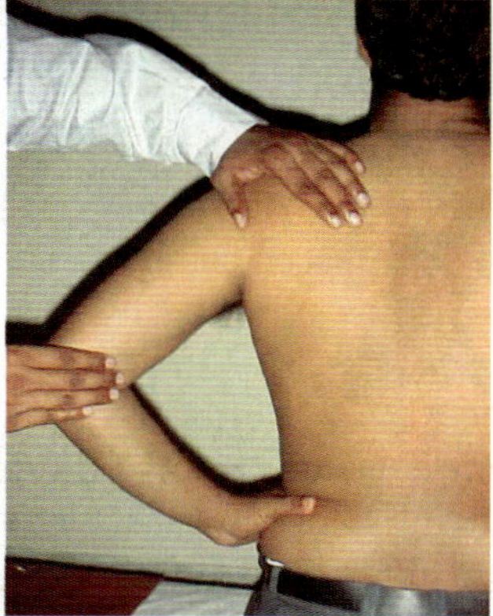

Fig. 5.7: Testing rhomboids

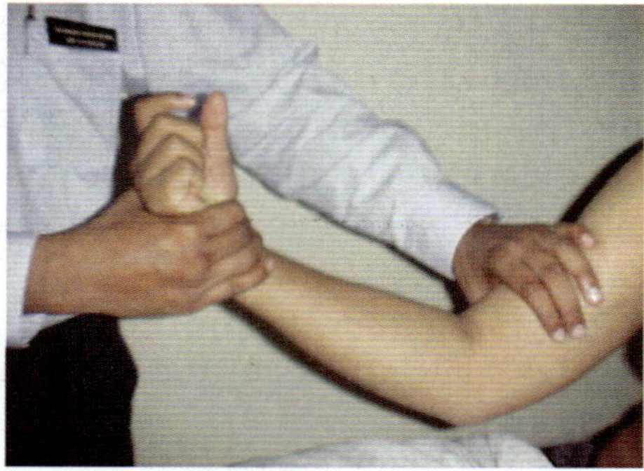

Fig. 5.8: Testing elbow flexion

Elbow extension: Triceps: $C_{6,7,8}$—radial nerve (Fig. 5.10)

Test: Ask the patient to push the forearm against resistance. Feel for the triceps contraction.

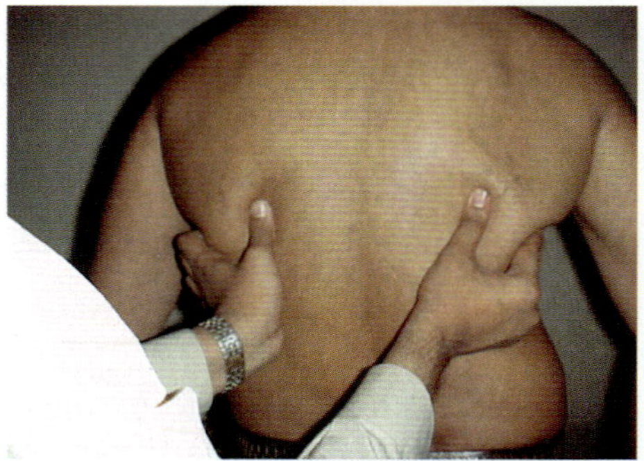

Fig. 5.9: Testing latissimus dorsi

Wrist flexion: $C_{6,7,8}$—median and ulnar nerves

Test: Patient is asked to flex the closed fist. Examiner tries to resist the flexion.

Wrist: Extension: $C_{6,7,8}$—radial nerve

Test: Ask the patient to make a fist and ask him to resist while the examiner is trying to pull his fist downwards.

Hand grip: $C_{7,8}$, T_1.

Test: Patient is asked to squeeze the two fingers of the examiner (middle and index finger) while the examiner is trying to pull them out. Comparison of the grips on both sides can be done by testing them simultaneously.

First dorsal interossei: Ulnar nerve—C_8, T_1

Test: Patient is asked to adduct the index finger against examiner's resistance.

Flexion of hip: Iliopsoas—$L_{1,2,3}$ (Fig. 5.11)

Test: Ask the patient to raise the leg while the examiner is applying resistance by placing hand on the patient's thigh.

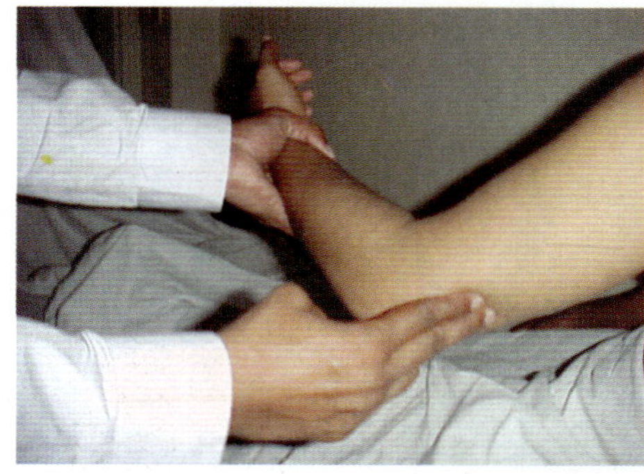

Fig. 5.10: Testing elbow extension

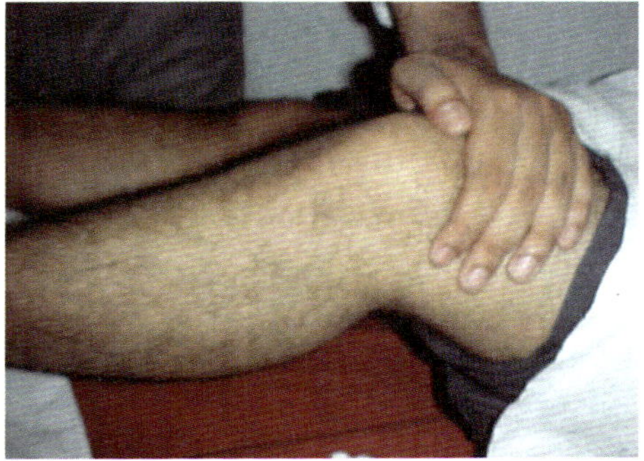

Fig. 5.11: Testing flexion of hip

Hip extension: L_5, S_1

Test: Keep the patient's knee in the extended position and examiner lifts the lower limb away from the bed. Patient is asked to push his lower limb downwards while the examiner tries to resist it.

Adductors of hip: $L_{2,3}$—adductor magnus, brevis and adductor longus

Test: Patient is asked to bring both the knees together while the examiner is applying resistance by placing his hands between patient's knees.

Abductors of hip: Gluteus medius and minimus—$L_{4,5}$, S_1

Test: Patient is asked to spread both legs while the examiner is applying resistance by keeping his hands on the bed firmly outside the knees of the patient.

Knee extension: Quadriceps: $L_{2,3,4}$

Test: Patient's knee is kept in flexion and is asked to straighten it against the resistance offered by the examiner's hand (Fig. 5.12).

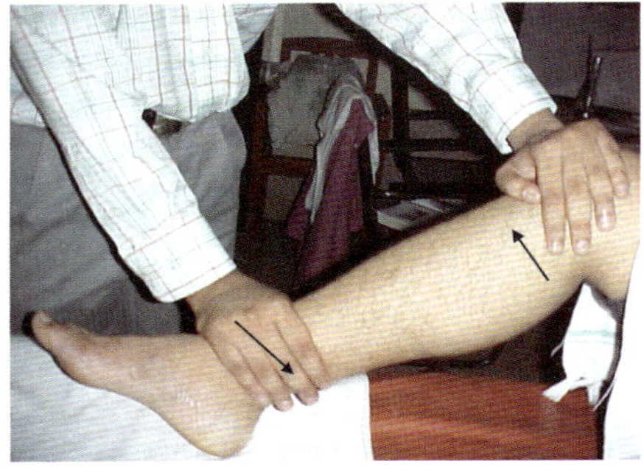

Fig. 5.12: Testing knee extension

Knee flexion: Hamstrings: $L_{4,5}$, S_1

Test: Keep the patient's knee flexed with the foot on the bed. Patient is asked to keep the foot further down while the examiner tries to straighten the ankle (Fig. 5.13).

Ankle: Dorsiflexion: Tibialis anterior—L_4, L_5

Test: Ask the patient to pull up the foot against resistance (Fig. 5.14).

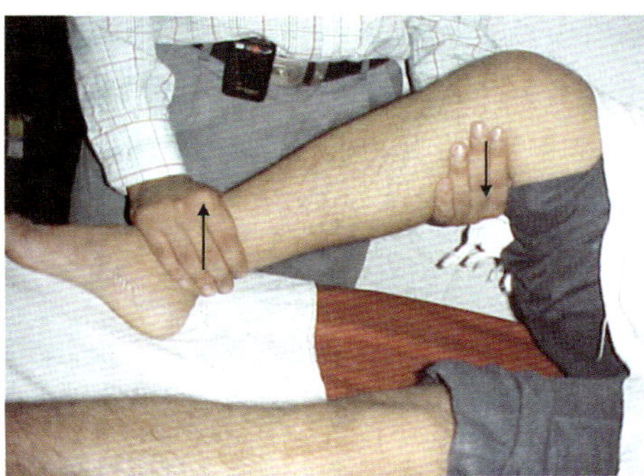

Fig. 5.13: Testing knee flexion

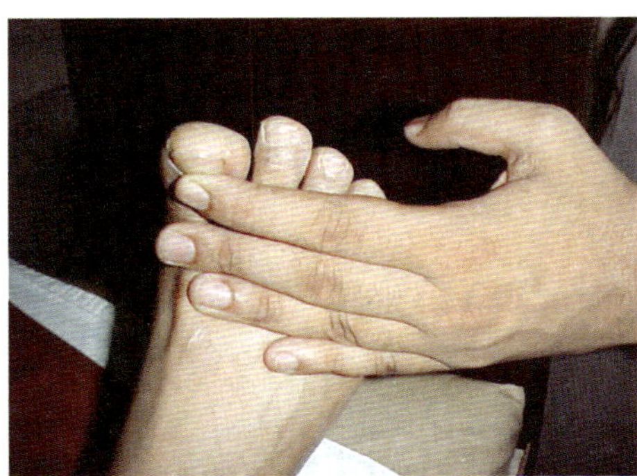

Fig. 5.14: Testing dorsiflexion of ankle

Plantar flexion: Gastrocnemius: S_1, S_2

Test: Ask the patient to push down the foot against resistance (Fig. 5.15).

Eversion foot: Peroneous longus and brevis: L_5, S_1

Test: Ask the patient to evert the foot against resistance.

Inversion of foot: Tibialis posterior: L_4, L_5

Test: Ask the patient to invert the foot against resistance.

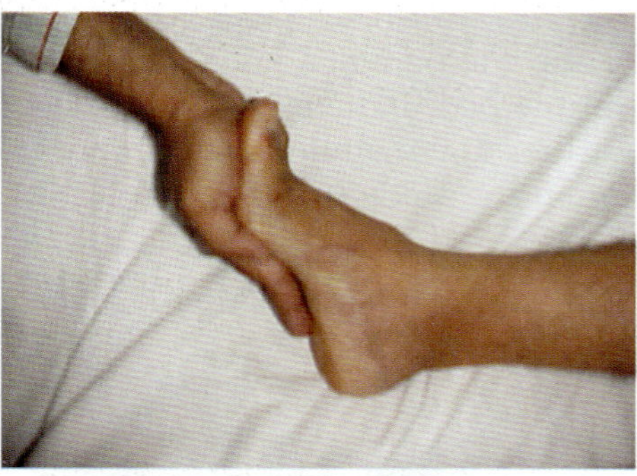

Fig. 5.15: Testing plantar flexion of ankle

Coordination

Details on coordination will be discussed under the chapter on cerebellum.

Note: Coordination should always be assessed proportionate to the muscle power. Patients with less than grade three power may have incoordination due to loss of power itself.

Myasthenia

Myasthenia literally means muscle weakness. Usually the term is used for weakness of muscles in patients with myasthenia gravis.

Characteristics of muscle weakness due to myasthenia gravis

- Weakness varies from time to time.
- Weakness increases with repeated using of muscles.
- Weakness leads to total muscle paralysis.
- Weakness recovers quickly after a very short period of rest.

Bedside tests for myasthenia

1. Maintain upward deviation of eyes (observe for drooping of upper eyelid).
2. Tight eye closure becomes weaker after repetition.
3. Ask the patient to count successively up to 100. Person develops muscle fatigue after counting for few numbers.
4. Out stretch the upper limb horizontally with the palm upwards and maintain the position for around 3 minutes—observe for shaking of limbs and drooping of fingers.
5. Back muscles: Sitting up and lying down repeatedly–observe for the muscle fatigue.

Involuntary Movements

Different types of involuntary movements

- Tremors
- Chorea
- Athetosis
- Ballism
- Myoclonus
- Dystonias
- Fasciculations

Tremors

Definition: Rhythmic movements of a part of a body around a fixed point.

Different types of tremors

Physiological—frequency 8–13 Hz (fine tremors).

Action tremor

- Exaggerated physiological tremor.
- Tremor occurs in certain position of limbs and trunk and during active movements, e.g.
  - Anxiety neurosis
  - Alcohol withdrawal tremor
  - Thyrotoxicosis
  - β_2 agonist therapy
  - Some type of familial or essential tremors.
- *Flapping tremors (asterixis):* Flapping tremor is characterised by lapse in the posture of outstretched hand and arm, e.g. metabolic encephalopathy.
- *Parkinsonian tremor*
  - Coarse and resting tremor (3–5 Hz).
  - Emotional stress increases the amplitude of tremor.
  - Associated with flexion and extension of fingers with adduction and abduction of the thumb—"pill rolling".
- *Intention tremor (ataxic)*
  - Tremor is not present at rest.
  - Present when fine adjustment of the movements are required.

– There will be interruption of forward movement with side wise movement of parts of the body, e.g. cerebellar dysfunction.

Other Involuntary Movements

Chorea (Dance)

Chorea is characterised by non-repetitive, purposeless and jerky movements.

Emotional and voluntary effort may increase it.

Person manipulates them to make them less noticeable.

Disappears during sleep, e.g. Syndenhams chorea (rheumatic), Huntington's chorea.

Site of lesion: Cortex and extrapyramidal system.

Athetosis

Athetosis is characterised by slow writhing purposeless movement. Commonly occurs in digits, hand and tongue, etc.

Site of lesion: Contralateral striatum, e.g. hemiplegia of long duration–infantile hemiplegia.

Hemiballism

Hemiballism is characterised by wide swinging movements predominantly involving the proximal limb muscles.

Site of lesion: Contralateral sub-thalamic nucleus of Luys.

Myoclonus

Myoclonus is characterised by sudden shock like movement producing recurring muscle jerks.

Generalised or may involve only one part of the body.

Site of lesion: Diffuse neuronal degeneration involving cerebrum, cerebellum.

Minipolymyoclonus

Small jerky movements of distal muscles may result in individual movements of fingers.

This term was originally described in patients with motor neuron disease. Minipolymyoclonus can also have central origin.

Dystonia

Dystonia is characterised by abnormal persistent posture or attitude in one or other part of the body, e.g. overextension or overflexion of the hand, inversion of foot and torsion of spine, etc.

Site of lesion: Contralateral striatum.

Tics

Repetitive brief contractions of a muscle or groups of muscles in the same region.

Patient is able to mimic tics and can suppress it with intense concentration, e.g. sniffing, lip movement, etc.

Fasciculation

- Fasciculation is characterised by irregular twitching or contraction of muscle fibers supplied by a single motor neuron either visible or palpable.
- Suggests degeneration of lower motor neuron (spinal motor neurons and cranial motor neurons).
- Fasciculation initially occurs in shoulder girdle, upper arms and chest muscles and disappears with extensive atrophy.
- Normally, few fasciculations can be present especially after fatigue.
- Persistent fasciculations associated with atrophy and muscle weakness is significant
- Fasciculations are better elicitable by minimal mechanical stimulation of the muscle and cold exposure.

Conditions associated with fasciculations:

- Motor neuron disease
- Thyrotoxic myopathy
- Syringomyelia and bulbia
- Syphilitic amyotrophy
- Organophosphorus poisoning

Fibrillation

Fibrillations cannot be made out through intact skin and made out only on EMG recording.

Fibrillation represents an isolated activity of denervated individual muscle fiber due to defective stabilisation of its membrane potential. Fibrillations occur in conditions associated with lower motor neuron degeneration.

Effects of long-standing muscle paralysis

Contracture: Contracture occurs due to progressive fibrotic changes in the paralysed muscle and tendons.

Considerable force may be required to overcome the contracture.

Sensory System

Receptors and fibers of different modes of sensation

- *Touch*
  - Receptors—naked nerve endings, mechanoreceptors in the skin
  - Nerve fibers—large and small nerve fibers
- *Pain*
  - Receptors—nociceptors
  - Nerve fibers—small fibers
- *Temperature*
  - Receptors—thermoreceptors for heat
  - Nerve fibers—small fibers
- *Vibration*
  - Receptors—pacinian corpuscles
  - Nerve fibers—large fibers
- *Joint sense*
  - Receptors—muscle spindles and tendon endings
  - Nerve fibers—large fibers

Sensory Pathways

Posterior spinothalamic tract carries following sensations:

Posterior spinothalamic tract carries following sensations:

- Well localised touch
- Vibration
- Joint position

Lateral spinothalamic tract: Lateral spinothalamic tract carries the following sensations: Pain and temperature.

Examination of Sensory System

Lateral spinothalamic tract

1. Test the pain sensation by pinprick.
2. Temperature

Temperature sensation is tested by using two test tubes of different temperatures.

Cold sensation: Test tube containing water around 5°C to 10°C.

Hot sensation: Test tube containing water around 37°C to 47°C.

Extremes of hold and cold temperatures should be avoided as they evoke pain response.

Temperature sensation may be lost early in leprosy.

Pain and temperature sensations are selectively lost in the intrinsic spinal cord lesions.

Posterior Column Sensations (Proprioception)

Touch

Touch the different dermatomes with a wisp of cotton or a blunt object.

Vibration

- Tested with a tuning fork of frequency of 128 Hz.

Key Points for sensory examination

- Patient should be fully conscious and cooperative.
- Patient should clearly understand the test procedure and closes the eyes throughout the examination.
- Preferable to test the sensation in dermatomal pattern.
- Start testing an area of sensory loss as noted by the history.

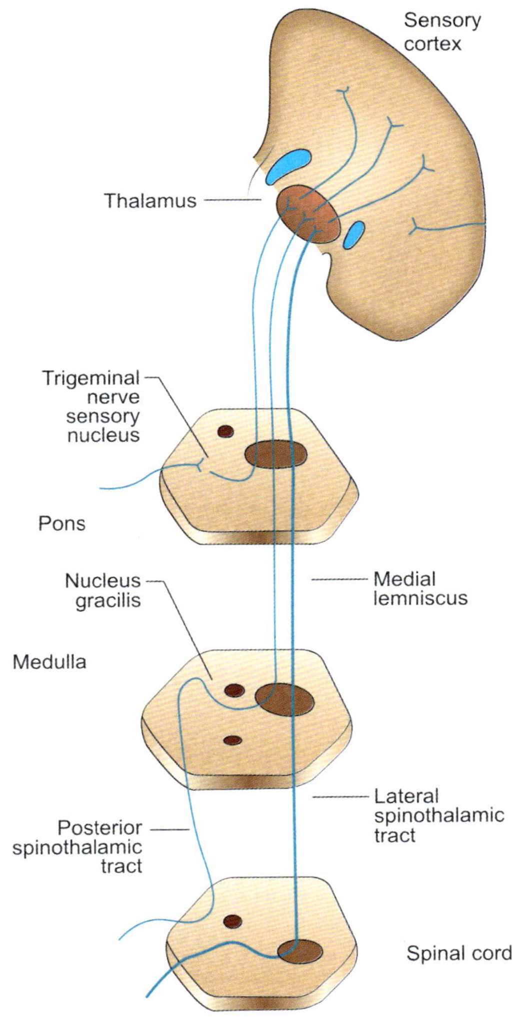

Sensory pathway

- Tuning fork of 128 Hz gives slow quantitative stimulation because of the slow decaying of vibrations.
- Strike the tuning fork of 128 Hz with a knee hammer and keep it on the patient's forehead.
- Patient should be able to appreciate the vibration and not the touch of the fork. Keep the vibrating tuning fork, starting from the distal most bony prominence and proceed proximally (including the spinous processes).
- Enquire the patient about the feeling of sensation of vibration.
- Early vibration sense loss: Elderly and diabetes mellitus.

Joint Sense (Fig. 5.16)

Test the distal most joint—for the upper limb-distal interphalangeal joint of the finger. For the lower limb-distal interphalangeal joint of toes.

Clearly explain the procedure to the patient with the eyes open.

*Hold the joint to be tested on its lateral aspect (patient is closing his eyes).

Neighboring toes or fingers should not be touched.

Hold and stabilise the proximal phalanx with the other hand.

Move the joint up and down repeatedly and ask the patient about the position of the joint.

If there is impairment in the sensation of the distal joint proceed to the more proximal joint.

If the patient fails to recognise the joint position consistently, it is an indication of posterior column disease.

Note: *Note:* Direction of movement can be sensed by the patient if the joint is held from its dorsal and ventral aspect instead of on its lateral aspect.

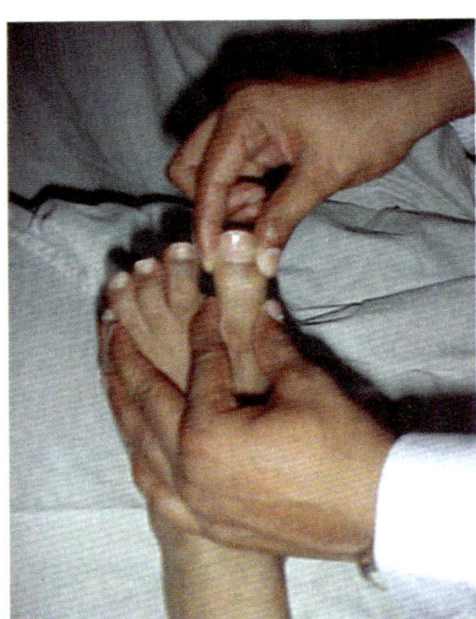

Fig. 5.16: Testing joint sense

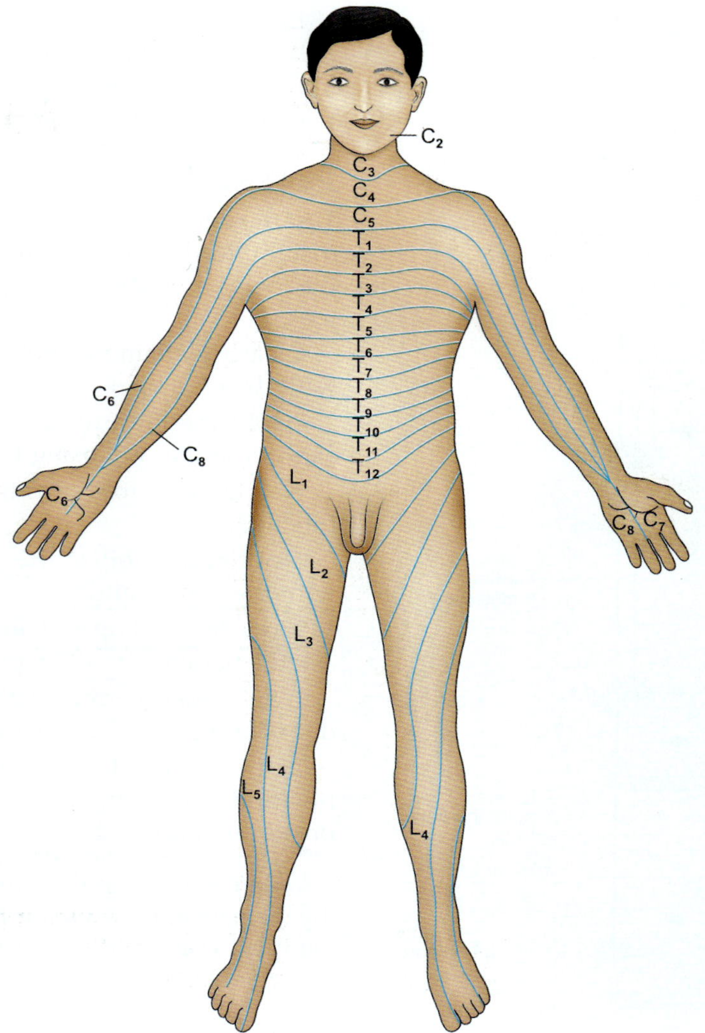

Anterior view
Distinct dermatomes of the body representing innervation by different spinal nerves
C_1—no cutaneous distribution

Normal joint movement appreciation

- Upper limb—fingers: 2–3 mm.
- Lower limb—toes: 3–5 mm.

Position Sense

Ask the patient to close his eyes.

Keep the limb in one particular position and ask the patient to keep his opposite limb in the same position as the other limb. Patients with abnormal position sense on one side will not be able to keep the opposite limb in the same position as the limb on the diseased side.

Romberg's Sign

This is a sign of posterior column dysfunction. Patient is asked to stand upright with the feet together when the eyes are closed. Patient with sensory loss (posterior column disease)

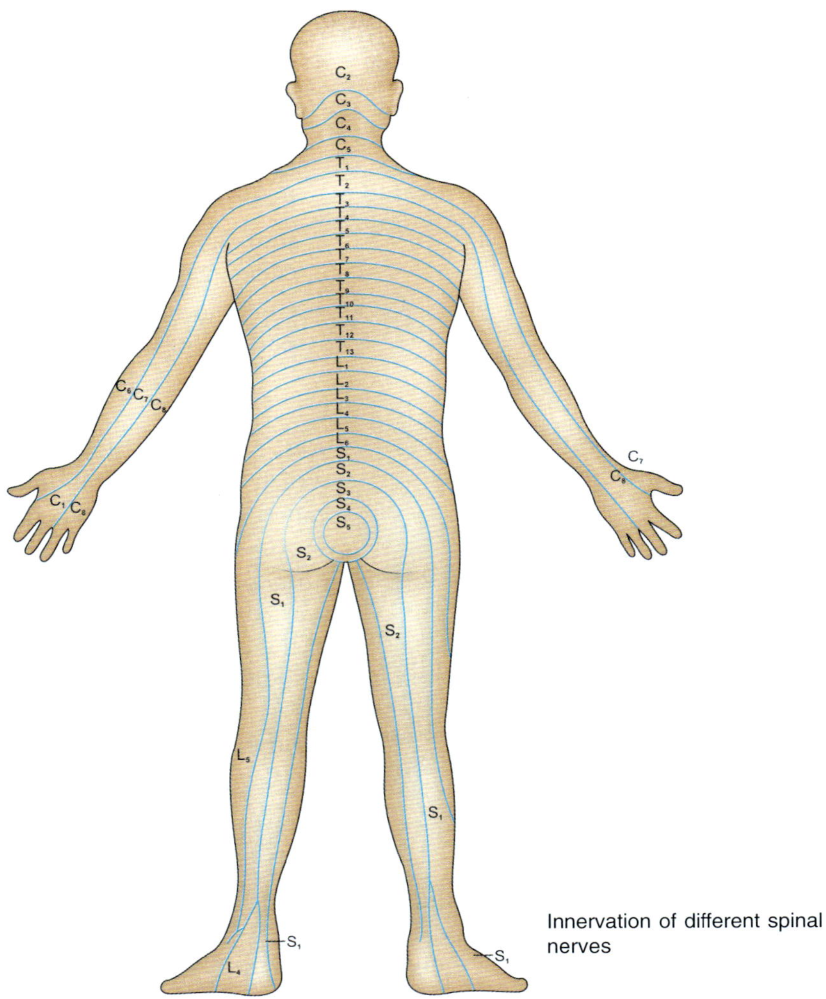

Innervation of different spinal nerves

Posterior view

will sway markedly. (Minimal swaying may be normal.)

Pseudoathetosis

A sign of posterior column dysfunction.

Slow writhing movements of fingers occur with closure of eyes when upper limb is held extended. Movements are absent when the person is watching the movements.

Pressure Pain

Elicited by squeezing the muscle (biceps, triceps) or tendons (Tendo Achilles). Pressure pain is lost in tabes dorsalis.

Causes of posterior column disease

- Tabes dorsalis
- Spinal cord compression
- Vitamin B_{12} deficiency causing subacute combined degeneration of spinal cord.

Saddle Anaesthesia

Saddle anaesthesia occurs in cauda equina or conus medullaris lesion.

Sensation over the lower sacral segments are impaired.

All forms of sensations are impaired, lower limb reflexes and bladder control are usually lost in patients with saddle anaesthesia.

Sacral Sparing

Sensation is preserved in the distribution of sacral dermatomes.

Occurs due to intramedullary lesion in the upper thoracic or cervical cord.

There will be sparing of laterally located fibers in the spinothalamic tract carrying sensation from the sacral segments.

CORTICAL SENSATION

Examination of Cortical Sensations

Tactile Localisation

Touch the point on the skin and patient is asked to localise it with closure of eyes.

Two Point Discrimination

Touch two separate points on a part of the body simultaneously, first wide apart and then as close distance as possible (while closing the patient's eyes). Note the ability of the patient to distinguish two separate points.

Normal person can distinguish two points separately as close a distance of around 2 mm over the fingertips.

Sensory Inattention

This is a test for parietal lobe dysfunction.

Person should identify his right and left hand normally while testing for sensory inattention.

Examination: Touch two identical parts on each side of the patient's body simultaneously, while patient is closing his eyes.

Patients with sensory inattention will identify only on normal side (routine testing of sensation is normal).

Significance: Patients with sensory inattention on one side will have opposite parietal lobe pathology.

Key Points

- Cortical sensation testing is to know the function of parietal lobe.
- Primary modalities of sensation should be intact before testing cortical sensation.

Stereognosis

- Ability to recognise the dimension of an object is called stereognosis.
- Patient should be able to recognise the familiar objects given to him by the feel of its size and shape while closing his eyes.
- Inability to recognise the dimension is called **astereognosis**.
- Cortical sensations will be impaired in parietal lobe dysfunction.

Graphesthesia

Ability to recognise the numbers of letters which are drawn on any part of the body is called **graphesthesia**.

Ask the patient to close the eyes. Write a number or a letter of sufficient size on different parts of the body and compare it on two sides of the body. Normal person should be able to recognise the number written.

Examination of Reflexes

Superficial Reflexes

- Superficial reflexes are polysynaptic reflexes.
- They require intact cortical center for their reflex action.
- In upper motor neuron lesion they are lost.

Superficial reflexes are

- Corneal reflex
- Conjunctival reflex
- Abdominal reflex
- Cremasteric reflex
- Plantar reflex
- Corneal and conjuctival reflex (*see* trigeminal nerve).

Abdominal Reflex (Fig. 5.17)

Lightly stimulate the part of the abdomen from outside inwards in different parts of the abdomen preferably on expiration as shown in Fig. 5.17 and look for muscle contraction.

Segmental innervation $T_7 - T_{12}$

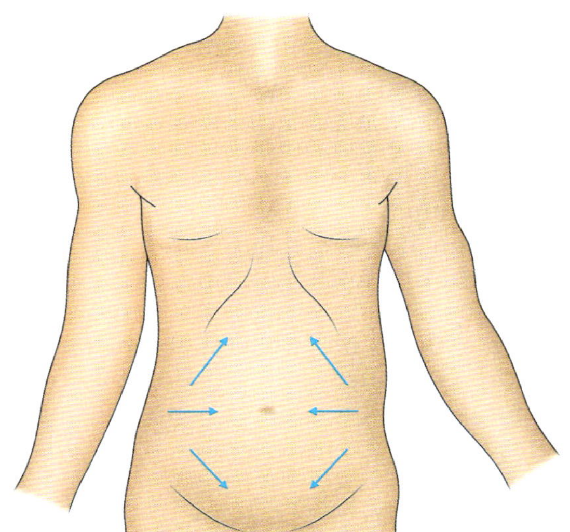

Fig. 5.17: Elicitation of abdominal reflexes

Abdominal reflexes may not be elicitable in elderly, obese and after repeated pregnancies.

Abnormalities

- Loss of abdominal reflexes.
- UMN lesion on that side.
- LMN lesion—loss of reflex in the corresponding dermatome.
- Abdominal reflexes are lost early in patients with multiple sclerosis.
- Abdominal reflexes are preserved till late in patient with motor neuron disease.

Cremasteric Reflex

- Segmental supply L_1, L_2
- Stimulate inner and upper part of thigh.
- Observe for the pulling up of scrotum and testis on the side of the stimulus (due to contraction of the cremasteric muscle).
- Loss of cremasteric reflex—UMN lesion on that side—L_1, L_2 lesion.
- Cremasteric reflex may not be elicitable in elderly persons.

Plantar Reflex

Segmental supply S_1.

Method of Elicitation

Classical method (Fig. 5.18)

Strike the outer aspect of the sole of the foot with a non-painful object and move towards the ball of small toes. Observe for the movement of the foot, toes and lower limb.

Note: Medial aspect of the sole should not be used for elicitation as it may elicit grasp reflex.

Normal response: Plantar flexion of the foot and toes.

Abnormal response

- Most important component:
  - Dorsiflexion of great toe
- Associated components:
  - Fanning of other toes.
  - Flexion of knee
  - Contraction of tensor fascia lata
  - Dorsiflexion of ankle

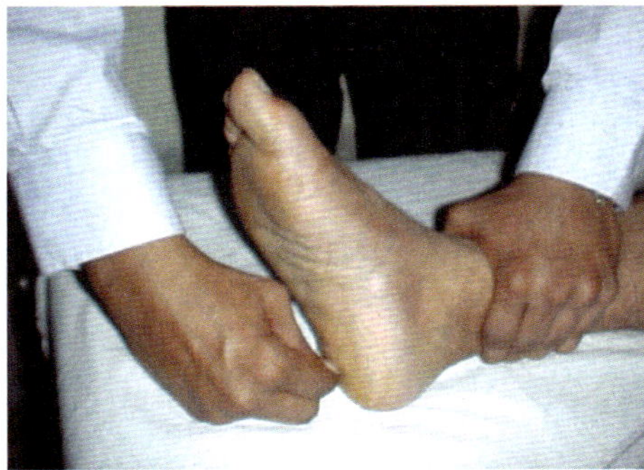

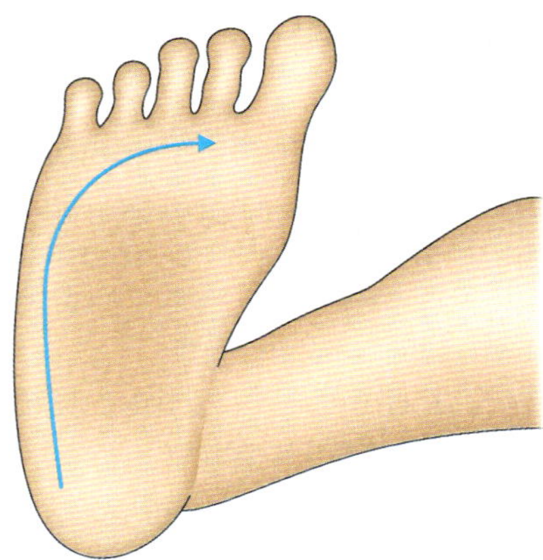

Fig. 5.18: Elicitation of plantar reflex

Key Points

- Move the great toe and observe for any evidence of osteoarthritis of great toe (hallux rigidus) before eliciting plantar reflex. Stabilise the lower limb by holding it above the ankle to prevent withdrawal response while eliciting plantar response.

Abnormal plantar response is called Extensor plantar or Babinski sign present or positive.

Extensor plantar response is the most important sign of UMN disease.

Plantar reflex may be absent or not elicitable under following circumstances

- Cold feet
- Relevant muscle paralysis
- Anesthesia of skin of feet
- Fixation of great toe

Causes of extensor plantar response apart from UMN disease

a. Infants below the age of one year
b. Comatose patients
c. After an epileptic fit
d. Deep sleep

Note: If there is no movement of great toe observe for contraction of Hamstrings and Tensor fascia lata.

Occasionally, turning the patient's head to the opposite side may reinforce the plantar reflex.

Different Methods of Eliciting Plantar Reflex

Oppenheim's method: Apply pressure with the finger and thumb from above downwards on either side of the anterior surface of the tibia and look for plantar response.

Gordon reflex: Firmly squeeze the calf muscles and look for the plantar reflex.

Chaddock reflex: Strike the outer aspect of the foot below the lateral malleolus and observe for the response.

Deep Reflexes

- Deep reflexes are monosynaptic reflexes.
- Deep reflexes are under the inhibitory control of the pyramidal tract (UMN).
- In lesion of pyramidal tract, inhibitory control is lost and deep reflexes become exaggerated.
- Occasionally, deep reflexes are hyperactive in patients with anxious person and Tetanus.
- Deep reflexes may remain absent for few hours/days after acute stroke or spinal cord injury—called a state of neuronal/spinal shock.

a. *Jaw Jerk* (*Fig. 5.19*)

- Center: Pons
- Pathway: Sensory and motor components of trigeminal nerve.
- Ask the patient to open the mouth slightly and keep the finger below the lower lip.
- Tap the knee hammer on the finger in a downward direction and observe for the movement of jaw.
- Jaw jerk may not be elicitable in normal persons.
- Brisk jaw jerk: Indicates bilateral UMN lesion above the pons, e.g.: pseudobulbar palsy.

b. *Biceps Jerk* (*Fig. 5.20*)

- Segmental supply C_5, C_6
- Position of the elbow: At right angle with forearm semipronated.

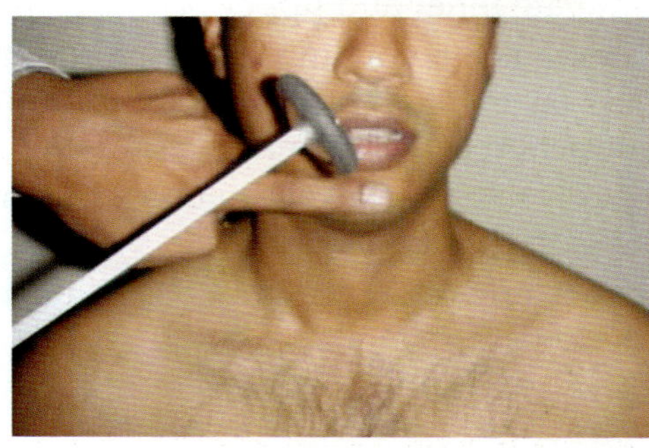

Fig. 5.19: Jaw jerk

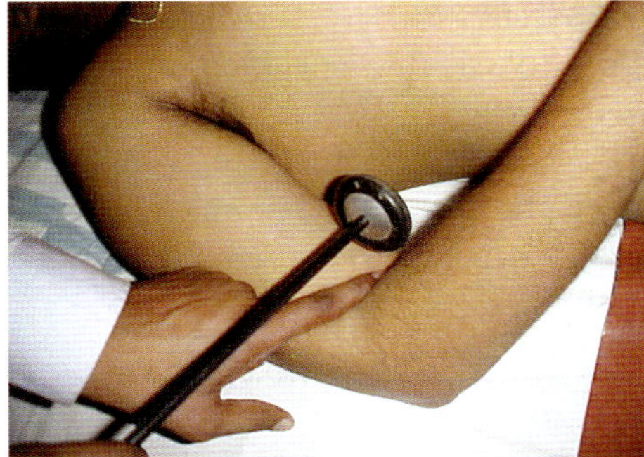

Fig. 5.20: Biceps jerk

- Examiner taps his own finger which is kept on the patient's biceps tendon and observe for the contraction of biceps with flexion of elbow.

c. *Triceps (Fig. 5.21)*

- Segmental supply C_6, C_7
- Position of the elbow: Keep the forearm of the patient on his own trunk loosely and tap the triceps tendon (about 5 cm above the elbow).
- Observe for the contraction of triceps with extension of elbow.

d. *Pectoral Jerk*

- Segmental supply (C_5 through T_1, segment).
- Examiner strikes his finger, which is kept on the anterior axillary margin (lateral border of pectoralis major).
- Observe for adduction of arm due to contraction of pectoralis major (C_5–T_1).

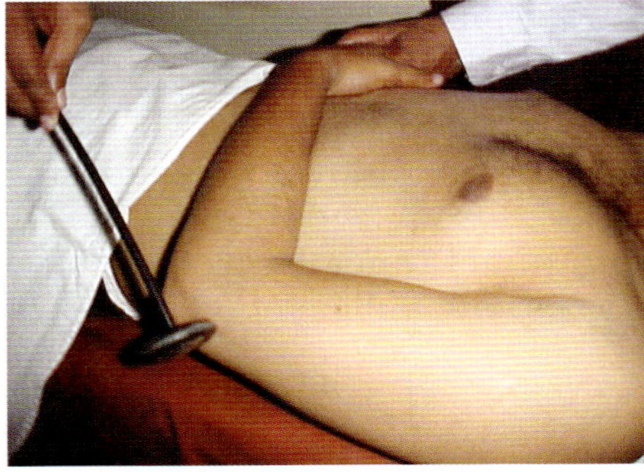

Fig. 5.21: Triceps jerk

e. *Supinatory (Brachioradialis) reflex (Fig. 5.22)*

- Segmental supply: C_5, C_1
- Tap the lower end of radius 5 cm above the wrist or tap the styloid process of radius.
- Observe for supination of forearm, flexion of elbow and minimal flexion of fingers.

f. *Inverted Supinator Jerk*

- On eliciting the supinator jerk—there will be only flexion of fingers without flexion of elbow and supination of forearm.
- Inverted supinator jerk suggests lesion at C_5 and hyperreflexia below C_5 level.

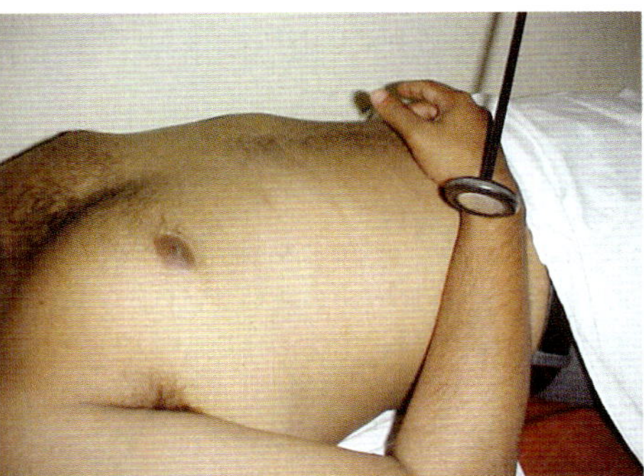

Fig. 5.22: Supinator jerk

g. *Knee Jerk (Fig. 5.23)*

- Segmental supply: L_2, L_3
- Patient is lying on his back. Place the left hand under the knee (to be tested) or under both the knees.

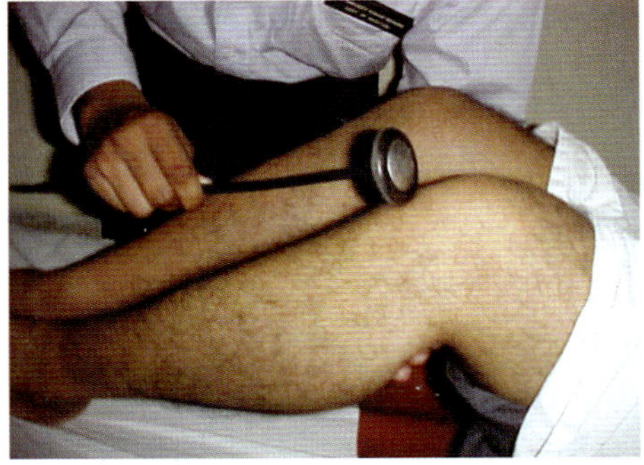

Fig. 5.23: Knee jerk

- Tap the tendon of quadriceps (4 heads: Vastus medialis, lateralis, intermedius and rectus femoris) with the knee slightly flexed.
- Observe for the extension of knee.

h. *Ankle jerk* (*Fig. 5.24*)
- Segmental supply S_1, S_2
- Percuss the Tendo Achilles with foot dorsiflexed and knee minimally flexed.
- Observe for plantar flexion of foot and contraction of calf muscles.

Alternative method for eliciting ankle jerk
- Patient is standing with his back facing the examiner. Keep the flexed leg of the desired side on a chair with the foot projecting over the edge of the chair.
- Strike the Tendo Achilles from above and observe for contraction.

i. *Hung up Reflex*
- Elicit the ankle jerk—there will be normal response with delayed return to resting position (delayed relaxation)–found in patients with hypothyroidism due to slow relaxation of muscle fibers (a form of pseudo myotonia).
- Normal half relaxation time: Mean value 320 to 340 millisecs.
- Slow relaxation of muscle fibers occurs due to slow reaccumulation of calcium ions with disengagement of actin and myosin components.

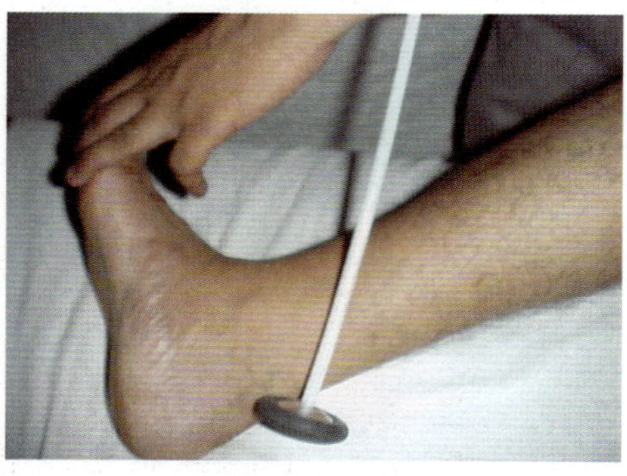

Fig. 5.24: Ankle jerk

Grading Reflexes
- Grade '0'—reflex absent (even with reinforcement)
- 1 (+)—elicitable only on reinforcement (sluggish or like normal ankle jerk)
- 2 (++)—brisk or like normal knee jerk
- 3 (+++)—exaggerated
- 4 (++++)—presence of clonus

Reinforcement of deep reflexes

If the deep reflexes are not elicitable, it can be made elicitable with reinforcement.

Method of reinforcement

For upper limb reflexes: Ask the patient to clench the teeth, while simultaneously eliciting the deep reflex.

For lower limb reflexes: Jendrassik's maneuver.

Ask the patient to interlock the flexed fingers of his hands and pull one against the other while simultaneously eliciting the deep reflex.

Mechanism of reinforcement

At the level of muscle spindles: Increased sensitivity of muscle spindles.

At the level of spinal cord: Excitability of anterior horn cells is increased.

Clonus

Definition: Series of involuntary contraction of muscles in response to sudden rapid and constant stretch. Clonus signifies hyperreflexia and hypertonia associated with increased gamma efferent activity.

Patellar Clonus (*Fig. 5.25*)

Patient lies supine with the knee extended and supported by the bed.

Push the patella briskly downwards towards the foot.

Observation: Repeated contractions of quadriceps with pulling of patella upwards.

Ankle Clonus (*Fig. 5.26*)

Support the slightly bent knee with one hand above the knee. Hold the forefoot and

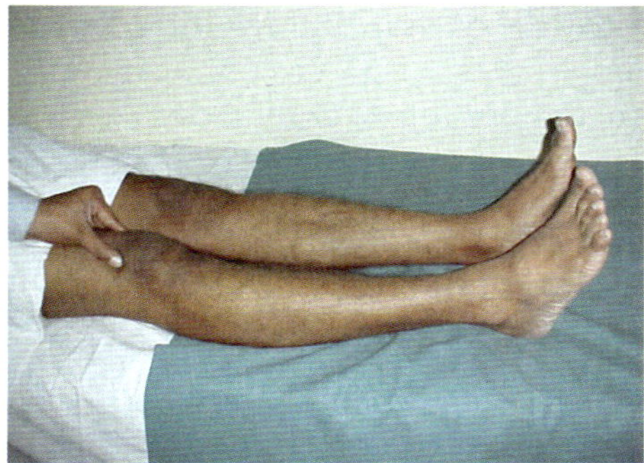

Fig. 5.25: Patellar clonus

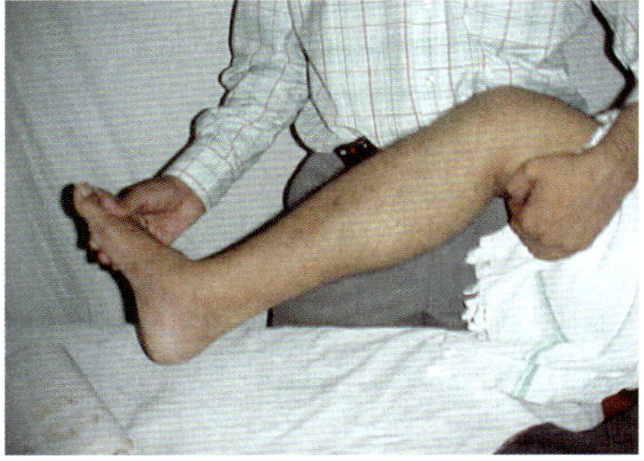

Fig. 5.26: Ankle clonus

suddenly dorsiflex the ankle while maintaining the stretch for sometime.

Observation: Repeated contractions of ankle.

Primitive Reflexes

- Primitive reflexes are not elicitable in healthy adults.
- May be present in infancy.
- Elicitable in persons with cerebral dysfunction.

Glabellar Tap Reflex (Myerson's sign)

- Tap the glabella repeatedly.
- Normal person blinks for 2–3 times and then stops blinking.
- Abnormal, persistence of blinking till the stimulus persists.
- Conditions associated—extrapyramidal disease—Parkinson's disease.

Snout Reflex

Give a minimal tap to the upper or lower lip. Observe for puckering and protrusion of lips. Significance: Associated with corticospinal disease.

Suckling Reflex

Common in infant disappears after infancy.

Touch the comer of the mouth and observe for sucking movements of lips, tongue and jaw.

Significance: Associated with diffuse cerebral disease.

Palmomental Reflex

Stimulate (scratching across) the thenar aspect of the palm.

Observe for the contraction of the ipsilateral mentalis and dimpling of the chin.

Significance: Positive palmomental reflex (especially unilateral) suggests corticospinal or diffuse cerebral disease.

Grasping Response

Patient tries to grasp the object or the examiners hand, when an object is introduced between patient's thumb and forefinger.

Significance: Positive grasp reflex suggests contralateral frontal lobe disease.

Avoiding Response

Stimulate the ulnar aspect of the patient's hand. Patient's hand tries to move away from the stimulus.

Significance: Positive avoiding response suggests contralateral parietal lobe disease.

Miscellaneous Signs of Pyramidal Tract Disease

Hoffman's Sign

Distal phalanx of the middle finger is flexed and then suddenly released.

Significance: In pyramidal tract disease—tips of the other fingers flex with adduction of thumb. If the sign is present unilaterally it is more significant.

Watenberg's Sign

Examiner interlocks the flexed fingers of the patient with his own fingers of one hand and tries to flex further/pull apart.

Normal response: Thumb remains abducted and extended.

Cortical spinal lesion: Thumb flexes and adducts.

Physiological basis for Hoffman's and Watenberg's sign: Thumb abduction is a later acquirement in the process of evolution which will be lost in pyramidal tract disease.

Finger Flexion Reflex

Keep the patient's arm with the palm upwards.

Examiner taps his fingers with the knee hammer which are kept over the fingers/palm of the patient.

Significance: Hyperreflexia is associated with increased flexion of fingers.

Miscellaneous Reflexes

Anal reflex

Stimulate the perianal skin gently and observe for the contraction of external anal sphincter.

Segmental supply: S_2 to S_5.

Bulbocavernous Reflex

Segmental supply: S_3 and S_4 nerves

Pinch the dorsum of glans penis.

Observation: Place the finger on the perineum behind the scrotum and palpate for the bulbocavernous contraction.

Mass Reflex

Mass reflex is observed in patients with severe spinal cord lesion.

Method of elicitation: Stimulate (pinprick or stimulating the sole of foot) any portion below the level of lesion especially in the midline.

Response

- Flexion of lower limbs.
- Extensor plantar
- Sweating of skin below the level of the lesion
- Evacuation of bowel/bladder.

Anatomy, Nerve Supply of the Urinary Bladder and Different Types of Neurogenic Bladder Dysfunction

Cortical center: Paracentral lobule—pathways descend into the spinal cord.

Brainstem center

- Tegmentum of midbrain (facilitatory)
- Tegmentum of pons (inhibitory).

Spinal cord

- *Parasympathetic supply:* S_2, S_3 and S_4 segments
- *Stimulation produces:* Contraction of detrusor and relaxation of internal sphincter.

Sympathetic supply: Upper lumbar spinal cord via the inferior hypogastric plexus (T_{10}–T_{12} segments).

Stimulation produces: Relaxation of detrusor and contraction of internal sphincter.

(Somatic) supply: S_2, S_3 and S_4 segments—to the external sphincter via the pudendal nerve.

Different Types of Neurogenic Bladder

Cortical Bladder

Due to involvement of frontal lobe and its descending pathways.

Characteristics: Patient will have loss of awareness of bladder fullness.

Person can have incontinence and loss of social control of micturition.

Spinal Cord Damage above the Lumbo-sacral Segments (Automatic bladder)

Characteristics

- Hypertonic or spastic bladder.
- Bladder will have small capacity.
- Person will have frequency, urgency and urge incontinence.

Disorders of Cauda Equina, Conus Medullaris, Sacral, Pelvic and Pudendal Nerves (Autonomous bladder)

Characteristics

- Flaccid or atonic bladder.

- Distension of bladder occurs with overflow incontinence.
- Loss of sensation over S_2 to S_4 segments.

Sensory Bladder

Due to loss of bladder sensation.

There will be large volume of urine in the bladder with large residual urine.

Note: In acute severe spinal cord lesion initially there will be acute retention of urine with later development of reflex voiding of urine.

Bowel

Constipation or bowel incontinence may accompany the corresponding disorder of micturition in neurological disturbances.

CEREBELLUM AND CEREBELLAR DYSFUNCTION

Anatomy and Connections of Cerebellum

Functions of Cerebellum

- Control of regulation of muscle tone.
- Control of gait and posture and balance.
- Coordination of voluntary movements especially like skilled movements.

Anatomy

Flocculonodular lobe (archicerebellum): Concerned with the equilibrium with the body.

Anterior vermis and paravermian cortex (anterior lobe–paleocerebellum): Concerned with determination of posture and muscle tone.

Posterior lobe (middle portion): Vermis and cerebellar hemisphere–neocerebellum.

Concerned with coordination of skilled movements.

Connections of Cerebellum

Inferior cerebellar peduncle (restiform body): Connects cerebellum to medulla oblongata.

Affarents to Cerebellum

- Spinocerebellar, olivocerebellar and vestibulocerebellar
- Reticulocerebellar fibres

Efferent from Cerebellum

To vestibular nuclei, reticular formation and olivary nuclei.

Middle Cerebellar Peduncle (Brachium pontis)

Connects cerebellum to pons.

Only afferent fibres: To cerebellum from pontocerebellar tract.

Part of frontopontocerebellar tract from opposite cerebellar cortex.

No efferent fibres

Superior cerebellar peduncle (Brachium conjunctivum): Connects cerebellum to midbrain.

Afferent fibres to cerebellum: Tectocerebellar tract.

Efferent fibres from cerebellum: Dentato rubrothalamic and dentato thalamocortical tract (to opposite red nucleus and thalamus) from one side dentate nucleus to opposite olivary nucleus.

Manifestations of abnormalities of different parts of cerebellar dysfunction

a. Nystagmus and abnormalities of ocular movement
   - *Site of lesion:* Flocculonodular lobe
b. Abnormality of gait and truncal ataxia
   - *Site of lesion*—of the vermis
c. Incordination of limbs
   - *Site of lesion:* Cerebellar hemisphere.

Note:
- Fibers from cerebellum also reach the opposite cerebral cortex via the thalamus.
- Fibers from opposite cerebral cortex also reach cerebellum.
- Cerebellum has no direct connections with the lower motor neurons.
- Cerebellum also receives inputs from reticular formation of the brainstem.

Clinical Signs of Cerebellar Dysfunction

Extensive lesions of one cerebellar hemisphere produces: Hypotonia, ataxia and postural abnormalities on the same side of the lesion.

Lesion of the vermis: Produces disorders of equilibrium, gait and truncal ataxia.

Important Clinical Signs of Cerebellar Dysfunction

Dysmetria

Occurs due to defective adjustment of force and amplitude of movements.

There will be overshooting when the object is reached, e.g. past pointing

Dyssynergia

Occurs due to breaking up of movements into their components whenever movements involving multiple joints are attempted. Movements become jerky.

Titubation

Oscillation of head in the anteroposterior direction with frequency of 3–4 per second.

Titubation occurs in patients with midline cerebellar lesions, e.g. multiple sclerosis.

Nystagmus

See also under nystagmus.

Occurs due to defective postural fixation of conjugate gaze. There will be increase in the amplitude of the nystagmus with decrease in the rate when the eyes are turned towards the lesion. Other ocular signs in cerebellar dysfunction: Ocular flutter and Opsoclonus

Speech

Scanning type: Speech is scanned so that words are broken up into syllables. Each syllabus may be expressed with varying force after an involuntary interruption. Speech becomes slurred and explosive (staccato).

> *Note:* Speech disturbance in patients with cerebellar dysfunction may be due to dyssynergy and incoordination of muscles of articulation and phonation. There will be poor control of volume of the sound.

Key Points

- Abnormal physical signs of cerebellar dysfunction are more common with acute lesions. Compensatory mechanisms decrease the severity of abnormal physical signs in chronic cerebellar lesions.
- Physical signs of cerebellar dysfunction occur due to defective coordination of voluntary movements, defective regulation of muscle tone and balance.

Hypotonia

- Hypotonia is more apparent with acute cerebellar lesions.
- In severe cerebellar lesions body can tilt to the side of lesion.
- There will be decrease of cerebellar facilitation of motor cortex due to defective tonic output from cerebellar nuclei.
- Hypotonia is predominantly due to decrease of alpha and gamma motor neuron activity.
- There is decrease in the fusimotor activity with defective function of muscle spindles.
- Hypotonia may be responsible for ataxia and intention tremor.

Rebound Phenomenon

Patient's forearm is flexed against resistance and suddenly released. Patient may strike his face with the forearm. (Examiner keeps his hand near the patient's face—to protect it.)

Normally, triceps contracts and arrests overflexion of the forearm which becomes defective in cerebellar lesions (impaired check reflex).

Dysdiadochokinesis

This is due to irregular force and speed of movement with defective voluntary movement and incoordination of muscles.

Rapid alternating movements are not possible to perform.

Patient is asked to rapidly pronate and supinate the out stretched hands alternatively (becomes irregular in patients with cerebellar disease).

Manifestations of Improper Coordination (Ataxia)

Persons with cerebellar dysfunction will have abnormality in the rate, range and force of movements.

Finger Nose Test

Patient is asked to touch the tip of his nose with the tip of his index finger of each out stretched hand in turn. Observe the movement pattern and intention tremor.

Cerebellar dysfunction: As the patient approaches the nose there will be side to side oscillation and over shooting of fingers.

Knee Heel in Coordination

Patient is asked to touch each of his knee with the opposite heel and then run it down the shin repeatedly.

Observation

- Patients with incoordination will have jerky movements and over shooting of the limb while approaching the target.
- Finger nose and knee heel in coordination may be due to hypotonia, defective postural fixation of joints and defective checking of velocity and force of movement. Each movement will be fragmented into constituent parts.

Pendular Knee Jerk

Elicit the knee jerk while the leg is hanging freely.

In patients with cerebellar dysfunction there will be swinging movement of foot and leg, to and fro several times (more than 3 times) before coming to rest. Pendular knee jerk is a manifestation of hypotonia and lack of restrictive effect of the muscles on each other (quadriceps and hamstrings).

Other tests for incoordination: Draw a small circle and ask the patient to put numerous dots inside the circle.

Cerebellar lesion: Dots will be outside the circle and more to the side of the lesion.

Tandem Walking

Tandem walking is the test for the vermis of the cerebellum.

Patient is asked to walk heel to toe in a straight line. Patients with cerebellar dysfunction will have gross swaying.

This is a manifestation of defective maintenance of balance and posture.

Cerebellar gait (*see* under gait).

Causes of Cerebellar Dysfunction

Unilateral

- Cerebellopontine angle tumor
- Lateral medullary syndrome
- Cerebellar abscess
- Cerebellar infarct

Bilateral

Different types of cerebellar degenerations.

Examination of the Autonomic Nervous System

Bedside tests

1. *Skin:* Person will have impaired sweating. Complete sympathetic lesion will have absence of sweating.
2. *Pupillary abnormalities*
   - Pupil may become immobile to light and accommodation.
   - Evidence of Horner's syndrome may be present.
3. *Pulse rate and heart rate*
   - Autonomic neuropathy causes abolition of sinus arrhythmia.
   - Heart rate on standing.
   - Change of position from lying down to standing position normally produces increase of heart rate and then relative bradycardia.
   - In parasympathetic lesions above response is decreased or lost.
4. *Blood pressure response*
   - Postural hypotension: Check the supine blood pressure after about 15 minutes of resting.

- Measure the standing blood pressure after 3 minutes.
- Normal response: Decrease of about 10 mm of systolic blood pressure.
- Autonomic dysfunction: Decrease of 20–30 mm of Hg of systolic BP after 3 mins and diastolic BP drop of more than 10 to 15 mm of Hg.

5. *Hand grip test*
   - Patient lies supine and grips the sphygmomanometer cuff as hard as possible for about 5 minutes and record the blood pressure.
   - Normal response: Increase of BP by 10 to 15 mm of Hg.
   - Autonomic dysfunction: Diastolic BP increases by less than 10 mm of Hg.
6. *Skin tests*
   - Skin temperature: Record the skin temperature by the thermometer.
   - Autonomic paralysis: Vasodilatation will cause increase of skin temperature.
7. *Cold pressor test*
   - Immerse the hand in ice water for 60 seconds.
   - Normal response: Systolic BP increases by around 10–20 mm of Hg.
   - Diastolic BP increases by around 10–15 mm of Hg.
   - Autonomic dysfunction: Less increase of blood pressure.
8. *Valsalva test:* Patient is asked to exhale into a mouth piece connected to a manometer maintaining a pressure of 40 mm of Hg for 15 seconds. Simultaneous ECG records the heart rate.

Interpretation

- 1st phase: Expiration against closed glottis–BP decreases and heart rate increases.
- Valsalva release (opened glottis): Heart rate decreases and BP over shoots the resting value parasympathetic dysfunction: Above responses to valsalva are impaired.

Peripheral Nerve Examination

Palpation of Peripheral Nerves

Posterior Auricular nerve: Turn the neck to one side and feel the nerve posterior to Sterno-mastoid and also as it crosses anteriorly across the neck.

Ulnar nerve: Feel immediately above the olecranon groove.

Lateral popliteal nerve: Feel as it passes around the neck of the fibula.

Signs of Meningeal Irritation

Neck Stiffness

Examiner keeps his hand under the patient's occipital region. Examiner raises the head of the patient with the forward movement until the chin touches the chest.

Patients with meningitis will complain of neck pain and is not able to flex his neck.

Kernig's Sign

Keep the patient supine. Flex the hip fully and try to extend the knee. Patient is not able to extend the knee, because of spasm and pain.

Brudzinski's Sign

Neck sign: Flex the neck of the patient–there will be automatic flexion of both the lower limbs.

Key Points

- Palpate the peripheral nerve trunk in its entire course.
- Fusiform swelling of the nerve may be present in patients with leprous neuritis.
- Beeding of the nerve trunk occurs in patient with amyloid neuropathy.
- Thickening of all peripheral nerve can occur in patient with hereditary neuropathies, e.g.: Déjérine-Sottas disease.
- Neurofibromas are benign neoplasms arising from the neurilemmal sheath of peripheral nerve.
- Longer nerves in their distal parts are more affected. May be due to the decreased energy. failure of protein transport to distal parts of the nerve and more of myelin degeneration.

Leg sign: Flex the patient's hip on one side. There will be flexion of opposite limb at hip and knee.

Note: Above signs of meningeal irritation are due to stretching of the irritated meninges and nerve roots causing muscle spasm.

Examination of Skull and Spine

Palpate the skull and spine for local destructive lesions due to trauma/tumors.

Percussion tenderness over the spine may be due to destructive lesions or occasionally spinal epidural abscess.

Auscultation of the Neck and Over the Skull

Presence of a bruit in the supraclavicular fossa may be due to subclavian or vertebral artery stenosis.

Significance of bruit over the skull: suggests AV fistulas, aneurysms or angiomas.

In patients with significant one sided carotid occlusion, bruit may be heard over the opposite eye due to collateral circulation.

Examination of Carotids

Feel for the common carotid pulsations on either side (it is preferable to feel internal carotid pulsations but always not practicable).

Atheroma at carotid bifurcation results in feeble pulsation on that side.

Presence of a bruit over the carotid may be suggestive of narrowing at its bifurcation.

Gait

Examine the type of gait and its abnormalities in patients with ability to walk.

Different Types of Gait Abnormalities

- *Circumduction gait (hemiplegic gait):* Person walks with upper limb adducted, flexed and lower limb extended with abduction and circumduction of lower limb while walking.
- *Cerebellar gait*
  - Wide based gait with patient swaying from side to side.
  - Patients with unilateral cerebellar lesions will sway to the affected side.
  - Patients with lesion of the vermis will have truncal ataxia.
- *High stepping gait:* Patient takes the foot high up in order to clear the ground and is then brought down, e.g. patients with foot drop.
- *Stamping gait:* Patient raises the leg high up and brings down the heel first with a slapping sound on the ground, e.g. posterior column disease.
- *Wadding gait*
  - Body sways from side to side (like of a duck) and feet are kept wide apart. There will be backward movement of shoulders with forward movement of the abdomen, e.g. proximal muscle weakness.
  - Waddling is due to defective stabilisation of hip by gluteal muscles (gluteus medius).
- *Parkinsonian gait:* Short, rapid and shuffling steps. Patient is stooped forwards without swinging of arms, e.g.: Parkinson's disease.
- *Apraxic gait:* Sequence and composition of movement is lost. Short shuffling of steps may be present, e.g., bilateral frontal lobe disease.
- *Spastic paraplegia:* Lower limbs are stiff and knees may cross over each other "scissoring" of gait.

Examination of Other Systems

Examination of CVS, RS, GIT and other related systems should be examined for evidence of abnormalities.

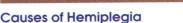

COMMON CLINICAL TOPICS IN NEUROLOGY

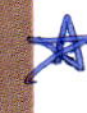

Causes of Hemiplegia

- *Sudden onset*
  - Cerebrovascular accident
  - Encephalitis
  - Head injury

- *Slow onset*
  - Cerebral tumor
  - Cerebral abscess
  - Chronic subdural hematoma

Cause of Upper Limb Weakness (Brachial monoplegia)

- Faciobrachial monoplegia (CVA)
- Encephalitis
- Space occupying lesion involving the cerebral cortex
- Brachial plexus lesion

Causes of Lower Limb Weakness (Crural monoplegia)

- Lesions of cauda equina
- Compression of sciatica nerve
- Cortical lesion–occlusion of paracentral artery.

Causes of Nervous System Disorders with Predominant onset in the Upper Limb

- Syringomyelia
- Motor neurone disease
- Cervical cord compression

Causes of Nervous System Disorders with Predominant onset in the Lower Limb

- Peripheral neuropathy
- Guillain-Barré syndrome
- Thoracolumbar spinal cord disease

Causes of Paraplegia

Spastic paraplegia (UMN lesion)

- Transverse myelitis
- Spinal cord compression
- Anterior spinal artery occlusion
- Subacute combined degeneration
- Syringomyelia
- MND
- Multiple sclerosis

Flaccid paraplegia (LMN lesion)

- Anterior poliomyelitis
- Guillain-Barré syndrome
- Muscular dystrophies

Localising the Level of Lesion in a Nervous System Disorder

Cortical Lesion

- Usually causes monoparesis
- May be flaccid
- Cortical sensory loss
- Aphasia occurs with left cortical involvement
- Convulsions may occur

Internal Capsular Lesion

- Commonest site of cerebrovascular disease.
- Marked spasticity is present.
- Convulsions and unconsciousness are not present
- UMN facial palsy associated with ipsilateral hemiplegia
- Hemianopia and hemianaesthesia may be associated.

Brainstem Lesion

In brainstem lesions, cranial nerve palsy occurs on the side of the lesion with hemiplegia on the opposite side. This is called crossed hemiplegia. Cranial nerve palsy is of LMN type, e.g.

- Midbrain lesion—3rd nerve palsy with crossed hemiplegia.
- Pons—6th or 7th nerve palsy with crossed hemiplegia.
- Medulla—9th, 10th, 11th and 12th cranial nerve palsy with opposite sensory or motor loss.
- Lateral medullary lesion (Wallen Berg syndrome)—9th, 10th and 11th cranial nerve palsy with ipsilateral facial sensory loss with contralateral limb anesthesia.
- Medial medullary lesion—LMN 12th nerve palsy on one side with contralateral hemiplegia.

Spinal Cord Lesion

- Cranial nerves are not involved except at high cervical cord lesion.
- LMN signs at the level of lesion.
- UMN signs are present below the level of lesion.

- Bladder involvement is usually present.
- Definite level of sensory loss.

(dermatomal)

Important Causes of Paraplegia without Urinary Bladder Involvement

- Guillain-Barré syndrome
- Myopathies
- Motor neuron disease

Paraplegia in Extension

- Due to involvement of pyramidal tract
- Associated with extensor spasms (sudden involuntary extension of lower limbs)
- Carries better prognosis

Paraplegia in Flexion

- Indicates progressive lesion of spinal cord
- Due to involvement of extra pyramidal structure like reticulospinal and rubrospinal tract
- Associated with bad prognosis and flexor spasms (sudden involuntary flexion of lower limbs).

Features of Different Types of Spinal Cord Lesions

Extradural extramedullary compression

Causes

- Secondary metastases
- TB spine (Pott's disease)
- Interverterbral disc prolapse
- Disorders of vertebra
- Trauma to the spine
- Chordomas, sarcomas

Features

- Pain in the back with root pain.
- Bilaterally symmetrical involvement.
- Bilateral weakness, sensory complaints and autonomic dysfunction.
- Percussion tenderness over the spine may be present.

Extramedullary Intradural Compression

Causes

- Secondary metastases
- Adhesive arachnoiditis
- Meningiomas, neurofibromas

Features

- Many features are similar to extradural compression.
- May have asymmetrical involvement and symptoms may persist unilaterally for a long time.

Intramedullary Lesions

Causes

Syringomyelia, gliomas, ependymomas.

Features

- Root pain not common.
- Late pyramidal signs
- LMN signs prominent (segmental amyotrophy may be present).
- Associated with dissociated anaesthesia.
- Early sphincter involvement.

Causes of Spinal Cord Compressions at Multiple Levels

- Multiple intervertebral disc prolapses
- Multiple neurofibromatosis
- Adhesive arachnoiditis
- Multiple secondaries in the vertebra
- Arteriovenous malformations
- Multiple vertebral fractures

Causes of Cervical Cord Lesions (Causes quadriplegia)

Compressive

- Craniovertebral anomalies
- Cervical spondylosis
- Trauma to the cervical cord

Non-compressive lesions causing quadriplegia

- Motor neuron disease
- Peripheral neuropathy
- Myasthenia/muscular disease
- Multiple sclerosis

Ellseberg's Phenomenon

This phenomenon is a manifestation of extradural compression of the cervical spinal cord.

In Ellseberg's phenomenon distribution of symptoms start in a U shaped pattern.

Symptoms start as weakness of ipsilateral upper limb, then ipsilateral lower limb and spreads to opposite side lower limb and then involves the opposite side upper limb in a U shaped manner. This occurs because of lamination of fibers in the spinal cord.

Whole of cauda equina lesion

- Severe pain in the back with root pain
- Lower limb muscle weakness
- Sensory loss involving the saddle area
- Absent deep reflexes in the lower limb and absence of plantar reflex
- Loss of sphincter control

> *Note:* Muscle involvement sensory loss and reflex loss may be variable in patients with partial cauda equina lesions.

Conus Medullaris Lesions

Features

- Usually pain in the low back.
- Early and prominent sphincter (urinary and faecal) disturbance.

Due to involvement of the lowermost part of the spinal cord: Pyramidal signs in the lower limb—brisk reflexes and extensor plantar.

Due of involvement of the lumbosacral roots

- Symmetrical saddle anesthesia.
- Loss of ankle jerk.
- Loss of bulbocavernous and anal reflexes.

Different Terminologies used while Describing Stroke Syndromes

Blood supply of internal capsule:

Anterior limb of internal capsule

- Superior-half is supplied by lenticulostriate branches of middle cerebral artery.
- Inferior-half is supplied by recurrent artery of Heubnere's (branches of anterior cerebral artery)
- Genu of internal capsule is supplied by lenticulostriate branches of middle cerebral artery.

Posterior limb of internal capsule is supplied by

- Superior half is supplied by—lenticulostriate branches of middle cerebral artery.
- Inferior half is supplied by—anterior choroidal artery branch of internal carotid artery.

TIA (transient ischemic attack)

Ischaemic neurological deficit lasting less than 24 hours (usually 5–20 minutes).

RIND (reversible ischemic neurological deficit)

Ischemic event which resolves over 24–72 hours or may last for a week.

Stroke in Evolution

Ischemic neurological deficit with stepwise increase in deficit over a period of hours to days.

Completed Stroke

Cerebro vascular accident which results in maximum neurological deficit occurring over few hours.

Ischemic Penumbra

A zone of hypoperfusion with viable cells remaining for few hours surrounding an area of severe ischemia.

Lacunar Infarct

Small infarcts in the cerebral white matter/ brain stem occurring as a result of pathological changes in the small penetrating arteries either due to arteriosclerosis or lipohyalinosis caused by hypertension.

FEATURES OF CEREBRAL EMBOLISM, THROMBOSIS AND HEMORRHAGE

Features of Cerebral Embolism

- Sudden onset of neurological deficit.
- Neurological deficit is maximum at the onset.
- Symptoms like headache, vomiting and altered consciousness are less common compared to cerebral hemorrhage.

- May be associated with features related to the source of embolism, e.g. mitral valve disease with atrial fibrillation.
- Carotid atheroma.

Features of Cerebral Thrombosis

- Gradually progressive neurological deficit.
- May occur when the patient is at rest (sleep).
- History of TIA preceding thrombosis is common.
- Headache, vomiting and altered consciousness are less compared to cerebral hemorrhage.
- Usually associated with history of hypertension and features suggestive of atherosclerosis.

Features of Cerebral Hemorrhage

- Sudden onset of neurological deficit.
- May occur when the person is physically active/having emotional stress.
- Usually associated with severe headache, vomiting altered consciousness and convulsions.
- Hypertension is the most important risk factor.
- Carries bad prognosis.

DIFFERENT TYPES OF CEREBROVASCULAR ACCIDENTS WITH EXAMPLES

Example 1: Cerebral Embolism

30-year-old female presented with history of sudden onset of weakness of right half of the body with deviation of angle of the mouth to the opposite side.

There was history of minimal headache without vomiting or convulsions. There was history of slurring of speech. Patient is a known case of rheumatic heart disease on penicillin prophylaxis.

On examination

Patient had UMN facial palsy on the right side with decrease power on the right half of the body patient had irregularly irregular pulse with mid diastolic murmur at the mitral area.

Possible Neurological Diagnosis 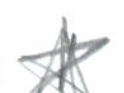

Cerebro vascular accident, right-sided hemiplegia, right UMN facial palsy due to embolic occlusion of the left middle cerebral artery (at the level of internal capsule) with rheumatic heart disease—mitral stenosis with atrial fibrillation.

Cerebrovascular accident is evidenced by

- Sudden onset of neurological deficit pertaining to a vascular territory.
- Possible mitral stenosis with atrial fibrillation may be the cause of embolism.

UMN facial palsy on the right side is evidenced by—deviation of angle of the mouth to left side.

Other features of UMN facial palsy on the right side

- Person is able to close the eye on the right side.
- Preservation of wrinkling of forehead on looking upwards on the right side.
- Nasolabial fold obliteration on the right side.
- Buccinator and platysma weakness on the right side.

Slurrring of speech in this patient is due to Labial dysarthria occurring as a result of facial palsy.

Right sided hemiplegia is evidenced by Decreased power on the right upper limb and lower limb

Other features

- Increased tone on the right side causing spasticity flexor hypertonia in the upper limb and extensor hypertonia in the lower limb. 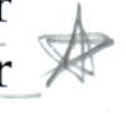
- Loss of superficial reflexes with plantar extensor on the right side.
- Deep reflexes are exaggerated on the right side.

Evidence for embolic nature of CVA in this patient

- Sudden onset of neurological deficit
- Associated mitral stenosis with atrial fibrillation

Left middle cerebral artery occlusion at the level of internal capsule is evidenced by

- Usual vascular territory involved in embolic CVA
- Presence of UMN facial palsy with hemiplegia with equal loss of power in the upper limb and lower limb (internal capsular lesion).

Features favouring the diagnosis of mitral stenosis with atrial fibrillation

- Mid diastolic murmur in the mitral area
- Irregularly irregular pulse (look other features of mitral stenosis and atrial fibrillation).

Note: Inability to speak (motor aphasia) or unable to understand (sensory aphasia) can occur in a patient of right sided hemiplegia due to involvement of speech centre on the left cerebral cortex.

Cardiovascular system examination in a patient of CVA may reveal the following features

- Evidence of valvular lesions like mitral stenosis
- Evidence of endocarditis
- Evidence of atrial fibrillation

In a patient of nervous system disease following observations are important

- Presence of nasogastric tube (in patient's of altered sensorium and dysphagia)
- Catheterisation of urinary bladder–for urinary retention/incontinence
- Pressure palsy, e.g. lateral popliteal nerve palsy causing foot drop
- Decubitus ulcers: Bed sores/pressure sores
- Aspiration pneumonia

Example 2: Thrombotic Cerebrovascular Accident

70-year-old male presented with weakness of right upper limb and progressed to involve the right lower limb with deviation of angle of mouth to the left side. There is previous history of TIA causing transient upper limb weakness. There was also history of minimal headache, hypertension and diabetes mellitus.

Possible Neurological Diagnosis

Cerebrovascular accident, right-sided hemiplegia right UMN facial palsy, lesion at the level of internal capsule, left middle cerebral artery occlusion due to thrombosis with hypertension with diabetes mellitus.

Evidence for Thrombotic Stroke

Slowly progressive neurological deficit.

Previous history of TIA, diabetes mellitus, hypertension favors the diagnosis of cerebral atherosclerosis and cerebral thrombosis. (other symptoms and signs are same as under embolic CVA).

Example 3: Intracerebral Hemorrhage

60 years old male presented with sudden onset of headache, vomiting and altered sensorium with weakness of right half of the body and deviation of angle of the mouth to the left side. He is a known case of hypertension.

Possible Neurological Diagnosis

Cerebrovascular accident with right-sided hemiplegia due to intracerebral hemorrhage.

Evidence for Intracerebral Hemorrhage

Sudden onset of headache, vomiting, altered sensorium associated with hypertension and neurological deficit (other symptoms and signs are same as for cerebral embolism).

Important Causes of Stroke in the Young (Less than 40 years of age)

Embolism of cardiac cause: Atrial fibrillation secondary to rheumatic heart disease.

CNS infections: Viral, tubercular and HIV infection

Collagen vascular disease

Vasculitic syndrome

Hematological disorders—bleeding/clotting disorder/hyperviscosity syndrome.

Cerebral Arterial occlusions of Clinical Significance

Middle Cerebral Artery Stem Occlusion

- *At its origin:* Deficit—contralateral hemiplegia, hemianaesthesia and hemianopia.
- Additional features (if occlusion is on the dominant side, usually left): Above features with global aphasia.
- Additional features (if occlusion is on the non dominant side (usually right side): Above features with hemineglect, anosognosia and constructional apraxia.

Occlusion of Middle Cerebral Artery Branches

Occlusion of superior division of middle cerebral artery

- It occlusion is on the dominant side (left side): Contralateral hemiplegia + hemi anesthesia and motor aphasia.
- It occlusion is on the non-dominant side (right side): Contralateral hemiplegia

Occlusion of the inferior division of middle cerebral artery

- It occlusion is on the dominant side (left side): Sensory aphasia without limb weakness.
- It occlusion is on the non-dominant side (right side): Contralateral hemineglect without limb weakness.
- Branch occlusion of middle cerebral artery can produce partial deficits like weakness only of one arm or one hand or face or only aphasia.
- Occlusion of lenticulostriate branches of middle cerebral artery causes lacunar strokes.

Clinically important lacunar syndromes

Lacunar syndrome	*Site of lesion*
• Pure motor stroke	Internal capsule
• Pure sensory stroke	Thalamus
• Ataxic hemiparesis	Internal capsule/ basis pontis Other possible sites: Corona radiata, thalamus
• Dysarthria clumsy hand syndrome	Internal capsule

Multiple lacunes (lacunar state) can present as pseudobulbar palsy

Occlusion of the anterior cerebral artery

Proximal part of the anterior cerebral artery (A1 segment) occlusion is well-tolerated because of collateral circulation.

Occlusion of A2 segment

(Distal to the origin of the anterior communicating artery)

Deficit on the opposite side of the occlusion

- Lower limb paralysis
- Minimal involvement of upper limb
- Bladder incontinence
- Cortical sensory loss of lower limb

Other features: Gait apraxia, abulia, presence of primitive reflexes (grasp reflex)

Occlusion of A2 segment (if both A2 segments arising from single anterior cerebral artery)

Neurological deficit

- There will be involvement of both hemispheres
- Bladder incontinence
- Severe abulia

Occlusion of anterior choroidal artery

Neurological deficit on the opposite side–hemiplegia, hemianaesthesia and hemianopia.

Occlusion of internal carotid artery

Causes occlusion of origin of both middle cerebral and anterior cerebral arteries; neurological deficit on the opposite side: Hemiplegia, hemianasthesia, hemianopia, aphasia and abulia can also occur.

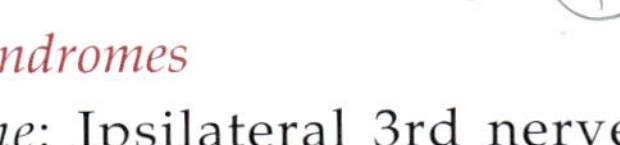

Occlusion of Posterior Cerebral Artery

Important clinical syndromes

- *Weber's syndrome*: Ipsilateral 3rd nerve palsy with contralateral hemiplegia (injury to cerebral peduncle)
- *Benedict's syndrome*: Ipsilateral 3rd nerve palsy with contralateral tremor and choreoathetosis (injury red nucleus)
- *Claude's syndrome*: Ipsilateral 3rd nerve palsy with contralateral tremor and ataxia

Table 5.3: Features of lateral medullary syndrome

Neurological deficit on the side of occlusion	*Structures involved*
• Nausea, vomiting, vertigo, nystagmus	Vestibular nucleus
• Cerebellar abnormality	Connection of restiform body and cerebellum
• Horner's syndrome	Descending sympathetic trunk
• Sensory loss over the half of face	Descending tract of trigeminal nerve
• Palate paralysis and absent gag reflex 9th and 10th nerve palsy	9th and 10th nerve nucleus
On the opposite side of the occlusion:	
Neurological deficit	*Structure involved*
• Pain and temperature loss in the opposite upper limb and lower limb	Spinothalamic tract

(injury to red nucleus and cerebellar peduncle)

- *Nothnagel's syndrome*: Ipsilateral 3rd nerve palsy with contralateral cerebellar ataxia (injury to superior cerebellar peduncle).

Thalamic Syndrome (Déjérine-Roussy)

Due to the occlusion of thalamogeniculate artery: Neurological deficit : Hemisensory loss on the opposite side with hyperpathia.

Occlusion of P2 Segment of Posterior Cerebral Artery

On the opposite side–there will be

- Macular sparing homonymous hemianopia
- Anton's syndrome:
  - Occurs due to bilateral occlusion of distal posterior cerebral artery.
  - There will be cortical blindness (patient will be unaware of blindness).
  - Normal pupillary light reflex.

Balint's syndrome

- Occurs due to infarction in the watershed area of posterior cerebral and middle cerebral arteries
- Involvement of bilateral visual association areas
- *Deficit*: Visual image persists in spite of looking at other objects
- *Asimultagnosia*: Difficulty in making out whole image of the surroundings

TOP OF BASILAR SYNDROME

Occurs due to the occlusion of the top of basilar artery by an embolus.

Features: Altered sensorium , bilateral ptosis, abnormality of pupil, bilateral UMN signs.

Medial Medullary Syndrome

Occurs due to the occlusion of vertebral artery or its branches.

Features

- On the side of occlusion: LMN 12th nerve palsy
- On the opposite side of occlusion: Hemiparesis due to involvement of pyramidal tract.

Lateral Medullary Syndrome (Table 5.3) (Wallenberg's syndrome)

- Occurs due to the occlusion of vertebral artery on the same side
- Can occur also due to the occlusion of PICA (posterior inferior cerebellar artery).

Disorders of Muscle and Peripheral Nerves

6

CHECKLIST FOR GENERAL PHYSICAL EXAMINATION

- Symptoms and signs of muscle disorder
- Peripheral neuropathy
- Diagnosis of peripheral neuropathy
- General examination in peripheral neuropathy
- Different types of peripheral neuropathy
- Ophthalmoplegias
- Ulnar and median nerve examination and claw hand
- Horner's syndrome

Muscular Atrophy

General term used for decrease of the muscle size (especially skeletal muscle) either due to muscle cell involvement or disease of the lower motor neuron.

Muscular Dystrophy

Group of hereditary disorders involving the skeletal muscle resulting in weakness and wasting of muscles.

Amyotrophy

Weakness and atrophy of muscle due to the disease of the motor neuron supplying the affected muscle.

Myopathy

Disease of the skeletal muscle not caused by neuronal disorders, e.g. endocrine myopathy.

Symptoms of Muscle Disease

Patient with disease of the muscle can present with any of the following symptoms.

- Muscle weakness
- Muscle fatigue
- Muscle pain
- Muscle wasting/enlargement
- Muscle cramps
- Muscle stiffness
- Myotonia
- Muscle contracture

Muscle Weakness

Enquire the following details about muscle weakness

- Acute/chronic
- Intermittent/persistent
- Proximal or distal weakness
- Painful or painless

Muscle disorders causing acute onset of muscle weakness

- Acute polymyositis
- Periodic paralysis
- Drug induced rhabdomyolysis

Causes of chronic muscle weakness due to muscle disorders

- Muscular dystrophies
- Chronic polymyositis
- Thyroid dysfunction

Causes of intermittent muscle weakness
- Myasthenia gravis
- Eaton Lambert's syndrome
- Periodic paralysis
- Myophosphorylase deficiency
- Mitochondrial myopathy

Causes of persistent muscle weakness due to muscle disorders, e.g.
- Muscular dystrophy
- Endocrine myopathy, e.g. thyroid disease diabetes mellitus.

Muscular disorders causing distal weakness: For example distal myopathies.

Causes of painful muscle weakness
- Polymyositis
- Osteomalacia
- Diabetic amyotrophy

Significance of Weakness of Different Groups of Muscles

Ocular Muscle Weakness
- Myasthenic disorders
- Ocular myasthenia
- Oculopharyngeal dystrophy

Weakness of Extensors of Neck (Causes head drop)
- For example: polymyositis
- Amyotrophic lateral sclerosis
- Myasthenia gravis

Muscle disorders causing predominant quadriceps weakness, e.g. inclusion body myositis, myotonic dystrophy.

Muscle Fatigue
- Difficulty in maintaining the force of contraction is a feature of muscle fatigue.
- Muscle fatigue should be differentiated from asthenia (general fatigability).

Features Suggestive of Asthenia (General fatigue)
- Person avoids physical activity
- There will be a general feeling of stress/depression
- Person feels drowsy during day time
- Tiredness with a feeling of loss of energy is indicative of asthenia.

Muscle disorders associated with muscle fatigue
- Myopathies
- Myasthenic syndromes
- Mitochondrial/glycogen storage disorders.

Muscle Pain

Causes of muscle pain: Localized muscle pain due to trauma.

Disorders associated with muscle pain, e.g.
- Polymyositis
- Polymyalgia rheumatica along with temporal arteritis
- Fibromyalgia
- Drug induced, e.g. zudovudine, statins, penicillamine.

Disorders associated with acute onset of generalized muscle pain
- Dengue fever
- Leptospirosis
- Influenza
- Acute polymyositis

Muscle Cramps (Spasms)

Muscle cramp is characterized by localised involuntary contraction of muscle which is associated with pain and hardening of muscle which is visible and palpable.

Disorders associated with muscle cramps, e.g.
- Polyneuropathy
- Pregnancy
- Amyotrophic lateral sclerosis

Muscle cramps are sudden in onset and usually of shorter duration. Muscle disorders are not usually associated with muscle cramps except in patients with Duchenne's muscular dystrophy.

Muscle Contracture
- Muscle contracture is characterized by difficulty in relaxing the muscle after active contraction the muscle

- Muscle contracture disorders are associated with energy failure as in glycogen disorders.
- Muscle contracture should not be confused with fixed contracture due to muscle fibrosis.

Muscle disorders associated with muscle contractures, e.g. Emery-Dreifuss muscular dystrophy, Bethlem myopathy.

Fibrous Contraction of the Muscle

In fibrous contraction of the muscle, stretching of the muscle to its proper length is not able to sustain.

Muscle Stiffness

- Muscle stiffness due to muscular disorders should be differentiated from inflammatory disorders of joints as they can also cause muscle stiffness.
- Affected muscle becomes rigid stiff but relax during sleep.
- Emotional upset, loud noise and sudden movement can precipitate muscle stiffness.

Disorders associated with muscle stiffness

Stiffman syndrome, neuromyotonia (Issac's syndrome).

Myotonia

Myotonia is characterized by prolonged muscle contraction with delayed relaxation of the muscle.

Action myotonia: Myotonia occurs after contraction of the muscle, e.g. person has got difficulty in releasing object after a firm grip.

Percussion myotonia: Myotonia occurs after mechanical stimulation of the muscle on the thenar eminence, over the tongue.

Disorders associated with myotonia

- Myotonic dystrophy
- Myotonia congenita

Paramyotonia congenita: Repeated activity of the muscle result in worsening of myotonia.

Muscle Enlargement and Atrophy

Causes of muscle enlargement

- Local infection, focal myositis, hematoma
- True or work hypertrophy
- Pseudohypertrophy
- Hypothyroidism

Localised muscle enlargement

Causes: Cysticercosis, sarcoid and amyloid deposit.

Pseudohypertrophy: Occurs in calf muscle, e.g. Duchenne's muscular dystrophy.

Atrophy or thinning of muscle

Cause: Long-standing muscle disease or lower motor neuron disease.

Clinical Features of Important Muscular Dystrophies

Duchenne's Muscular Dystrophy

Inheritance: X-linked recessive disorder.

Muscle weakness

- Recognized usually between 3 and 6 years of life.
- Starts as weakness of proximal muscle of lower limb resulting in difficulty in walking/climbing of stairs.
- Weakness of pretibial muscle: Person develops toe walking and foot drop.
- Progressive development of upper limb muscle weakness.
- Respiratory muscle weakness.
- Lordotic posture: Protuberant abdomen develop due to weakness of paravertebral and abdominal muscles.
- By the age of 12 years person are wheel chair bound and around 16–18 years of age develop serious respiratory infection and death.

Muscle Hypertrophy

Pseudohypertrophy of muscle is characteristic of Duchenne muscular dystrophy. Usual muscles which undergo pseudohypertrophy: Gastrocnemius, vastus lateralis and deltoid.

Important Clinical Signs of Duchenne Muscular Dystrophy

- Gower's sign
- Waddling gait

Systemic involvement

- Mild mental retardation
- Cardiomyopathy and cardiac arrhythmias.

Becker's Type of Muscular Dystrophy

Features

- X-linked recessive disease
- Milder from compared to Duchenne type
- Starts in 2nd decade of life (5–45 yeas of age)
- Muscle involvement is similar to Duchenne type
- Mentation is usually normal and cardiac abnormality is unusual.

Fascioscapulo humeral type

- Age group involved: 6 to 20 years of age
- Pattern of muscle weakness: Facial muscle weakness: Orbicularis oris and zygomaticus.
- Progressive involvement of latissimus dorsi. Rhomboids, erector spinae and later deltoid.

Important Clinical Signs Associated with Fascioscapulo Humeral Dystrophy

- Winging of scapula
- *Popeye effect:* Upper arm thinner than forearm
- Presence of Beevor's sign
- Congenital absence of muscles, e.g. pectoralis/brachioradialis.

Muscle biopsy: Inflammatory infiltration in the muscle.

Limb Girdle Muscular Dystrophy

Features

- Onset 1st to 4th decade
- Weakness of pelvic and shoulder girdle muscles
- Diaphragm weakness causing respiratory insufficiency
- Can be associated with cardiomyopathy

Myotonic dystrophy

- 2 types: Distal–type I
- Proximal–type 2

Pattern of muscle weakness

- Flexor muscle of neck
- Quadriceps weakness
- Distal limb muscle weakness

Facial characteristics

- Frontal baldness
- Hatchet face and facial muscle weakness and atrophy.

Myotonia

- When the person is asked to close the grip, he will be able to relax the grip only slowly
- Myotonia can also be demonstrated after percussion over the tongue or the thenar eminence (formation of dimple over the muscle groups).

Other Features of Myotonic Dystrophy

- Testicular atrophy
- Cataract
- Insulin resistance
- Complete heart block
- Hypersomnia
- Motility disorders of colon/oesophagus.

Inclusion Body Myositis Features

- Common after 50 years of age
- Quadriceps weakness occurs early
- Foot drop occurs due to foot extensor weakness and associated with weakness of deep finger flexors.
- Systemic connective tissue disorders may be associated
- Extramuscular manifestations including joint, cardiac and pulmonary dysfunction can coexist.

Polymyositis and Dermatomyositis

Polymyositis

- Painful weakness of predominantly proximal muscles
- Pharyngeal muscles and flexor muscles of neck are commonly involved
- Facial and ocular muscle are usually not involved

- Deep tendon reflexes are not affected till late
- In advanced cases muscles of respiration will be affected.
- Connective tissue disorders and extra-muscular involvement can coexist.

Dermatomyositis

Features

- Muscle weakness may cause quadriparesis
- Characteristic rash **heliotroph rash**
  - Usually precedes muscle weakness
  - Edema of upper eye with bluish purple colored rash

Gottron's sign: Scaly raised violaceous lesions over the knuckles

V-sign: Rash over the anterior chest

Shawl sign: Rash over the back and shoulders.

- Extra-muscular involvement occurs in the form of fever, joint involvement, cardiac and pulmonary disturbances
- Scleroderma and MCTD can overlap with dermatomyositis.

Neuromuscular Causes of Ocular Muscle Involvement (Ptosis/ophthalmoplegia)

Disorders of myoneural junction

- Myasthenia gravis
- Lambert-Eaton syndrome
- Botulism, snake bite (neurotoxic)

Disorders of peripheral neuropathy

- Diabetes mellitus
- Miller Fisher syndrome

Disorders of muscles

- Oculopharyngeal dystrophy
- Progressive external ophthalmoplegia

Ophthalmoplegia not associated with ptosis

Hyperthyroidism/Grave's disease

Different Types of Ophthalmoplegia

- Supranuclear–due to involvement of supranuclear control of gaze, e.g. progressive supranuclear palsy and encephalitis.
- *Nuclear:* Due to involvement of cranial nerve nuclei of 3rd, 4th and 6th cranial nerve.
- *Infranuclear:* Occurs due to the damage to the cranial nerves 3rd, 4th, 6th along their course.
- *Internuclear:* Occurs due to damage to the MLF and its connections.

Important Causes of Ophthalmoplegia

Painful Ophthalmoplegia

Causes

- Cavernous sinus thrombosis
- Diabetes mellitus and Graves' disease
- Posterior communicating artery aneurysm
- Tolosa hunt syndrome
- Herpes zoster

Painless Ophthalmoplegia

Causes

- Guillain-Barré syndrome
- Multiple sclerosis
- Brainstem infarction
- Wernicke's disease
- Progressive external ophthalmoplegia.

Important Clinical Points to be Remembered while Examining the 3rd, 4th and 6th Cranial Nerve Palsy

3rd (Oculomotor) Cranial Nerve Palsy

Total paralysis of the 3rd cranial nerve—position of the eye will be out and down.

Lesion of the oculomotor nucleus in the midbrain produces bilateral ptosis (levator palpabrae muscles on both sides is supplied by single oculomotor nucleus in the mid-brain).

Oculomotor nuclear palsy causes weakness of opposite superior rectus muscle.

4th (Trochlear) Cranial Nerve Palsy

4th cranial nerve fibers exit from the dorsal part of the brainstem. Fibers cross to the opposite side and supply contralateral superior oblique.

Patients with 4th nerve palsy tilt the head away from the side of the muscle palsy (head tilt) to avoid diplopia.

Trochlear nerve can be easily injured with the concussion injury of the brain.

6th (Abducens) Cranial Nerve Palsy

Nuclear lesion of the 6th nerve produces complete horizontal gaze palsy (paralysis of ipsilateral) lateral rectus and contralateral medial rectus. (6th nerve nucleus contains interneurons that connect medial rectus nucleus of opposite 3rd nerve nucleus via medial longitudinal fasciculus). 6th nerve lesion produces only unilateral abducens palsy.

PERIPHERAL NEUROPATHY

Features Favoring the Diagnosis of Peripheral Neuropathy

- Bilaterally symmetrical onset of symptoms.
- Lower limb is involved greater than upper limb
- Distal part of the limb is moral involved than proximal.
- Graded type of sensory loss.

Important General Physical Examination Signs in Peripheral Neuropathy

- *Pallor (anemia)*: B_{12} deficiency/folic acid deficiency
- *Pigmentation*: B_{12} deficiency/drug induced (antineoplastic)/paraneoplastic
- *Hypopigmented maculoanaesthetic patch*: Leprosy
- Blue line–on the gum: Lead neuropathy
- *Oral candidiasis*: HIV infection/diabetes mellitus

Key Points

- In patients with peripheral neuropathy sensory symptoms preceede motor symptoms.
- Motor symptoms begin later, can present as distal weakness, loss of ankle jerk and wasting of muscles.

- *Subcutaneous swelling*: Neurofibromatosis
- *Butterfly rash, polyarthritis*: Connective tissue disorder–SLE
- *Trophic ulcers*: Diabetes mellitus/leprosy
- *Mei's lines*: Chronic arsenic poisoning (multiple transverse ridges over the nails).

Importance of Peripheral Nerve Palpation in Patients with Peripheral Neuropathy

Look for

- Focal thickening
- Presence of neurofibromatosis
- Tenderness over the nerve

Conditions Associated with Peripheral Nerve Thickening

- *Leprous neuritis*: Fusiform nerve thickening
- *Amyloid neuropathy*: Bleeding of nerve trunks
- *Genetically determined neuropathy*: Uniform thickening of nerves.

Important Causes and Types of Peripheral Neuropathy

Pure motor neuropathy

Causes:

- Lead poisoning
- Acute intermittent porphyria
- Guillain-Barré syndrome

Predominant sensory neuropathy

Causes: 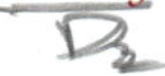

- Diabetes mellitus
- Drugs: INH, vincristine and alcohol

Acute Onset Neuropathy

Causes

- Guillain-Barré syndrome
- Diabetes mellitus
- Porphyria

Peripheral neuropathy with cranial nerve palsy

Causes: Diabetes mellitus (ophthalmoplegia, VII nerve palsy)

Guillain-Barré syndrome (ophthalmoplegia, VII nerve palsy)

Leprosy: VII nerve palsy

Mononeuropathy multiplex: (Asymmetrical involvement of multiple peripheral nerves)

Causes:
- Vasculitic syndrome
- Diabetes mellitus
- Leprosy

Peripheral neuropathy with thickened peripheral nerves

Causes:
- Leprosy
- Amyloidosis
- Hereditary neuropathies
- Déjérine-Sottas disease
- Refsum's disease

Polyneuropathy

Widespread and symmetrical distribution of peripheral neuropathy.

Plexopathy

Involvement of nerve plexus, e.g. brachial/lumbar plexopathies due to diabetes mellitus type 2.

Axonal Neuropathy

Features: Glove and stocking distribution of symptoms. Sensory symptoms are more dominant than motor symptoms.

Demyelinating Neuropathy

- Motor and sensory involvement may be equal.
- Larger fibers are more involved than smaller fibers.

Symptoms of peripheral neuropathy depending on the fiber involved:
- *Small fiber neuropathy:* Presents as burning feet, e.g. diabetes mellitus
- *Large fiber neuropathy:* Presents as sensory ataxia, e.g. paraneoplastic syndrome
- Sjögren's syndrome

Small Fiber Neuropathy

Mainly presents as burning sensation—cutting like pain and paraesthesia (tingling, pins and needles).

Large Fiber Neuropathy

Presents as gait disturbances, tingling numbness with loss of reflexes.

Note: Usually sensory disturbance starts in the toes and spreads upwards.
When sensory disturbance reaches the level of knee symptoms appear in the upper limb.
Paraesthesia developing in one hand may suggest entrapment neuropathy.

Leprosy Neuritis

- Peripheral nerves which are present in the cooler parts of the body are mainly affected.
- Anaesthetic parts can be present in any part of the body, less common in the scalp, axilla and groin (warmer pats).
- Mononeuropathy can occur near any leprosy patch.
- Cranial nerves 5th and 7th can be affected in leprosy.
- Foot drop, claw hand and inability to close the eye can occur in long-standing untreated case of leprosy.

Examination of Small Muscles of Hand, Median and Ulnar Nerves

Small Muscles of Hand

Thenar eminence
- Abductor pollicis brevis
- Flexor pollicis brevis
- Opponens pollicis

Hypothenar eminence
- Abductor digiti minimi
- Flexor digiti minimi
- Opponens digiti minimi

Action of lumbricals: Flexion of metacarpophalangeal joint and extension of both interphalangeal joints (writing muscles).

Supply of Median Nerve in the Hand

Motor supply: Abductor pollicis brevis, flexor pollicis brevis, opponens pollicis, 1st and 2nd lumbricals.

Sensory supply: Lateral 3½ digits and corresponding part of palm on the palmar aspect and index, middle and ring fingers on their dorsal aspect.

Deformities Produced by Median Nerve Lesions

Ape thumb: Due to the paralysis of opponens pollicis, thumb becomes in line with the other fingers.

Pointing index (finger): Index finger of the affected side remains straight when the other fingers flex due to intact flexor digitorum profundus (medial half) supplied by ulnar nerve.

Tests for Median Nerve Lesions

Abductor pollicis brevis

Action: Draws the thumb forwards at right angles to the plane of the palm of the hand.

Tests: Pen test: Keep the hand of the patient flat with the palm facing upwards.

Patients is asked to touch the pen with the thumb which is held infront of it.

Opponens pollicis

Test: There will be difficulty in touching the ends of fingertips with the tip of the thumb.

Flexor digitorum superficialis and profundus

Tests: Clasping test: Person is asked to clasp the hands there will be failure of flexion of index finger-produces "pointing index".

Flexor pollicis longus: Person is not able to flex the terminal phalanx of the thumb (examiner should hold the proximal phalanx firmly to avoid the action of short flexors).

Ulnar Nerve

Supply of ulnar nerve in the hand

Motor supply: Abductor digiti minimi, opponens digiti minimi, flexor digiti minimi, 3rd and 4th lumbricals, 4 palmar interossei, 4 dorsal interossei, 2 parts of adductor pollicis.

Sensory supply: Supplies 5th digit and medial half of 4th digit and corresponding part of palm on the palmar aspect and corresponding digits on the dorsal aspect of nails.

Action of interossei

Palmar interossei–adduction of fingers

Dorsal interossei–abduction of fingers.

Interossei also extend middle and terminal phalanx.

Tests for Ulnar Nerve Lesion

For interossei: Person is asked to bring the fingers close (adduct) and spread out (abduct) against resistance.

Card test: Person is asked to keep the finger straight. He is asked to grip a piece of paper or card which is held in between the fingers (examiner tries to withdraw the paper).

In ulnar nerve lesion: Person is not able to grip the paper and offer poor resistance to withdrawl.

Book test (Froment's sign): This is the test for 1st palmar interosseus and adductor pollices.

Test: Person is asked to grasp the book between the thumb and other fingers.

In normal person: Thumb remains straight (due to the action of intact adductor pollicis, Ist palmar interosseus and flexor pollicis longus).

In ulnar nerve lesion: Immediate flexion of the thumb on the affected side (due to action to of intact flexor pollicis longus alone).

Note: Flexor pollicis brevis is supplied by both median and ulnar nerve.

Claw Hand

Characteristics

- Metacarpophalangeal joint is extended and proximal and distal phalangeal joints are flexed.
- Classically seen in ulnar nerve lesion or combined lesion of ulnar and median nerves.
- *Extension of metacarpophalangeal joint occurs due to:* Paralysis of lumbricals with unopposed action of long flexors and extensors of forearm.

Appearance of hand in claw hand deformity: 1st phalanges of fingers are extended and 2nd and 3rd phalanges are flexed.

Ulnar paradox: In person with ulnar nerve palsy if the lesion is more proximal clawing of the hand is less severe because of the loss of innervations of more number of muscles.

Pathogenesis of ulnar paradox: Proximal lesion of the ulnar nerve (at elbow). There will be loss of function of both intrinsic muscles of hand and long flexors of forearm resulting in less flexion of 4th and 5th digits resulting in less clawing.

Distal lesion of ulnar nerve (at hand): There will be loss of function of intrinsic muscles of the hand with normal action of long flexors of forearm resulting in more flexion of 4th and 5th digits with significant clawing.

Causes of Wasting of Small Muscles of Hand

Spinal cord lesions: Compressive: Cervical spondylosis, syringomyelia, non-compressive.

Anterior horn cell disease

- Motor neurone disease
- Poliomyelitis
- Spinal muscular atrophy

Lesion of brachial plexus

Nerve roots (C_8–T_1): Carcinoma lung (Pancoast's tumor)

Lesion of peripheral nerves (medial ulnar nerves): Leprosy, vasculitis, diabetes and CIDP

Disease of muscles: Distal myopathy and myotonic dystrophy

Causes of wasting of small muscles of hand (predominantly unilateral)

- Cervical rib
- Pancoast's tumor
- Leprosy
- Vasculitis
- Carpal tunnel syndrome
- Diabetes mellitus.

Horner's Syndrome

Clinical significance of different sites of lesions in Horner's syndrome.

Site of lesion: Central lesion (1st order neuron is involved).

Produces: Absence of sweating on one side of the body.

Lesion of sympathetic chain (2nd order neuron is involved): Absence of sweating on one side of the face.

If the lesion is distal to the bifurcation of common carotid: Loss of sweating at medial side of forehead and side of nose.

7 Hematological Disorders

CHECKLIST FOR GENERAL PHYSICAL EXAMINATION

- Symptoms due to manifestation of anemia
- Symptoms attributing to the cause of anemia
- Past history
- Personal history
- Family history
- Menstrual history
- General physical examination
- Examination of face, oral cavity, skin, nails, leg ulcers, bone tenderness and bleeding spots.
- Vital signs

APPROACH TO A PATIENT OF ANEMIA AND OTHER HEMATOLOGICAL DISORDERS

Physiological Adaptation to the Development of Anemia

1. Symptoms of anemia depend on the rate of development of anemia and person's cardiovascular status.
2. Younger age and slower development of anemia are better tolerated.
3. Decrease in the oxygen carrying capacity of blood and tissue hypoxia (Hb% < 5 gm) leads to increase in the level of circulating 2–3 diphosphoglycerate (2–3 DPG) resulting in increased release of oxygen from the RBCs.
4. There will be increase in the circulating plasma volume with redistribution of blood flow to the vital organs.
5. Increased flow of blood and increase in the stroke volume occurs as a result of compensatory mechanisms.

History Taking of Anemia and other Haematological Disorders

Symptoms due to the Manifestations of Anemia

- Fatigue
- Dizziness
- Syncope
- Headache
- Blurring of vision

Cardiovascular Symptoms

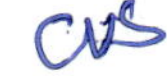

- Chest pain
- Palpitation
- Dyspnea
- Pedal edema

Gastrointestinal Symptoms

- Appetite loss
- Abdominal pain
- Jaundice
- Diarrhea
- Dysphagia
- Constipation

Neurological Symptoms

- Tingling and numbness
- Swaying while walking, weakness of limbs
- Altered sensorium

Miscellaneous Symptoms

- Fever
- Bleeding tendencies
- Bony pain

Symptoms Attributable to the Cause of Anemia

- History of blood loss
- Nutritional intake
- History suggestive of malabsorption
- History suggestive of worm infestations.

Past History

- Drug intake
- Exposure to chemicals and radiation
- Anemia since childhood, recurrent jaundice and recurrent blood transfusions.

Personal History

- Appetite loss, weight loss
- Alcohol intake
- Smoking
- Urine output
- Bowel habits

Family History

Anemia in the family members.

Menstrual History

Details of menstrual blood loss.

SYMPTOM ANALYSIS OF AN ANAEMIC DISORDER

Non-specific Symptoms

Fatigue, dizziness, headache and syncope may be due to severe anemia causing tissue hypoxia.

Cardiovascular symptoms

- Symptoms like chest pain, dyspnea and palpitation are due to hypoxia of the myocardium.
- Anemia can cause aggravation of pre-existing heart disease (due to high cardiac output state).
- Adult without any coexisting illness may develop exertional dyspnea when Hb% reaches 7 gm/dl. Dyspnea can also occur at rest especially in individuals with severe anemia (when Hb% < 3 gm/dl) and anemia causing cardiac failure.
- *Chest pain:* Elderly persons with pre-existing coronary heart disease will have aggravation of chest pain with development of significant anemia.

Gastrointestinal Symptoms

- *Loss of appetite:* Severe anemia can cause appetite loss. Appetite loss may also be a manifestation of systemic disease causing anemia, iron deficiency anemia can be associated with pica (*see* below).
- *Jaundice:* Jaundice may be the manifestation of the hepatobiliary disease causing anemia or may be due to hemolytic anemia.
- *Dysphagia:* Chronic severe iron deficiency can cause dysphagia due to postcricoid web, e.g. Plummer-Vinson syndrome—combination of iron deficiency, glossitis and dysphagia due to postcricoid web.
- *Abdominal pain:* Abdominal pain with anemia may due to peptic ulcer disease, GI malignancy or due to ancylostoma infestation.
- *Diarrhea:* Diarrhea may be a manifestation of malabsorption syndrome. Megaloblastic anemia itself can be associated with diarrhea.
- *Pica:* Person eats persistently non-nutritive substances like soil, leaves, pastes, etc. Pica is usually associated with iron deficiency anemia.

Neurological Symptoms

- *Paresthesia:* Folic acid and vitamin B_{12} deficiency leads onto peripheral neuropathy causing tingling and numbness of hands and feet.
- *Weakness of limbs*
  - Vitamin B_{12} deficiency can also result in sub acute combined degeneration of the spinal cord.
  - This causes pyramidal disturbance with weakness of lower limbs and also swaying while walking in the dark due to posterior column disturbance.
  - Severe anemia can also cause altered sensorium due to hypoxic encephalopathy.

Miscellaneous Symptoms

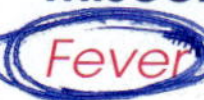

Fever

- Severe anemia itself may be associated with mild fever.
- Pyrexia in a patient of anemia may be due to associated systemic disease like:
  - Infections, e.g. malaria
  - Lymphoma
  - Leukemia
  - Endocarditis
  - Collagen vascular disease

Note: Pancytopenia conditions are associated with fever due to sepsis.

Bleeding Tendencies and Bony Pain

- Hematological malignancies like leukemia, myeloma or lymphoma can cause bony pain and bleeding tendencies.
- Bleeding tendencies may also be due to platelet/clotting disorder.

Symptoms due to Systemic Illness

- Chronic renal, hepatic, musculoskeletal and other systemic disorders can cause severe anemia.
- All persons with severe anemia should be evaluated for associated systemic illness.

SYMPTOMS ATTRIBUTABLE TO THE CAUSES LEADING ONTO ANEMIA

History of Blood Loss

- Enquire the history of haematemesis, malaena, haemoptysis and menstrual blood loss in all patient with anemia.
- Recurrent small amount of blood loss can cause severe anemia (occult bleeding from GIT).
- Enquire also symptoms like heartburn, altered bowel habit and abdominal pain for ruling out chronic occult GIT blood loss.

Nutritional Intake

1. Details of nutritional intake should be enquired. Inadequate dietary intake causes iron, folic acid and vit B_{12} deficiency. Strict vegetarians have more chance of developing vit B_{12} deficiency.
2. Symptoms of malabsorption like diarrhea, steatorrhoea should be enquired in all patients with unexplained anemia.

Worm Infestation

- Hookworm infestation is an important cause of iron deficiency.
- *Ancylostoma duodenale* can cause 0.2 ml blood loss/worm/day.
- *Nicator americanus* can cause 0.03 ml blood loss/worm/day.

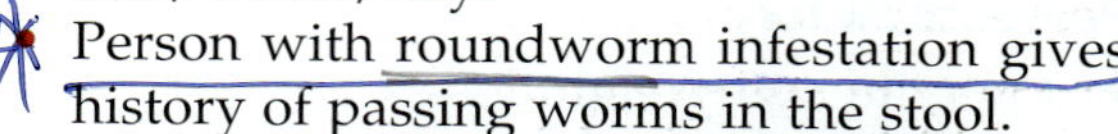

- Person with roundworm infestation gives history of passing worms in the stool.
- Poor hygiene and poor toilet facilities give an indirect indication of worm infestation.
- Persons with hookworm infestation may have epigastric pain and inflammatory diarrhea.

Past History

- Anemia since childhood with recurrent history of blood transfusion is a feature of congenital hemolytic anemia or a bleeding/clotting disorder since childhood.
- Intrauterine and childhood death can be due to thalassemia disorders.
- Exposure to chemicals like benzene and exposure to radiation may be responsible for the development of aplastic anemia.

Importance of Drug History in a Patient of Anemia

- Long-term intake of NSAIDs and corticosteroids cause erosive gastritis and chronic blood loss.
- Chloramphenicol, cytotoxics, oxyphenbutazones, gold salts can cause bone marrow suppression and aplastic anemia.
- Primaquine intake causes hemolysis in patients with G6PD deficiency.

Note: Previous history of jaundice due to viral hepatitis may be responsible for the development of aplastic anemia.

Personal History

- *Appetite loss:* Due to anemia itself or systemic disease causing anemia.
- *Weight loss:* Suggests systemic disease and decreased nutritional intake.
- *Alcohol:* Can cause erosive gastritis, bleeding due esophageal varices. Alcoholics can have associated nutritional deficiency.
- *Smoking*: Causes peptic ulcer and reflux esophagitis causing blood loss.

Family History

- Congenital hemolytic anemia can involve several members of a family.
- History of consanguinity between parents should be enquired in all patients with hereditary disorders of haemoglobin and also disorders like haemophilia.
- Worm infestation can affect several family members causing anemia.
- People of low socioeconomic groups will have decreased nutritional intake causing anemia affecting several family members.

Menstrual history

- Excessive menstrual loss of blood is an important cause of anemia in females.
- Repeated childbirth is also a contributory factory for the development of anemia.

EXAMINATION

Scheme of Examination

General Physical Examination

- Pallor
- Clubbing
- Jaundice
- Lymphadenopathy
- Cyanosis Edema

Vital signs: Pulse, blood pressure, respiratory rate and temperature.

Other Specific Examination Related to Anemia

Examination of face/oral cavity/skin/nails/leg ulcers/bone tenderness/bleeding spots.

Systemic Examination

- *Cardiovascular system:* Cardiomegaly/murmurs/cardiac failure/venous hum
- *Respiratory system:* Evidence of pulmonary disease.
- *Gastrointestinal tract:* Mass lesion/hepatomegaly/splenomegaly/ascites.
- *Central nervous system:* Motor, sensory and cranial nerve deficits.
- Urogenital, musculoskeletal, hepatobiliary system and other systemic examination wherever necessary.

General Physical Examination

Build and Nourishment

1. Chronic anemic disorders are associated with stunted skeletal growth, e.g. hemolytic anemias.
2. Persons with deficiency anemias like iron, folic acid are usually poorly nourished with decreased muscle bulk and subcutaneous fat due to associated calorie deficiency.

Pallor

Conjunctival pallor may be mild or severe. Iron deficiency may be associated with pearly white sclera (*see* Chapter 1, general physical examination).

Icterus

- Hemolytic anemias are associated with mild icterus (lemon yellow tinge to the sclera).
- Hemolytic anemias with pigmented gallstones can have' severe icterus.

Cyanosis

- Severe anemia (Hb% < 5 gm/dl) is usually not associated with cyanosis.
- Cyanotic patients will be polycythemic with suffused conjunctiva.

Clubbing

Presence of clubbing may suggest associated systemic disease in an anemic patient.

Lymphadenopathy

Causes of lymphadenopathy with severe anemia

a. Supraclavicular lymphadenopathy: GIT malignancy (left supraclavicular)/bronchogenic carcinoma.

b. Generalised lymphadenopathy:
   - Acute and chronic leukemia/lymphomas/systemic causes of generalised lymphadenopathy.
   - See also general examination for details on lymphadenopathy.

Edema

Pedal edema in an anemic patient may be due to

- Severe anemia itself (due to renal retention of salt, water and also may be due altered capillary permeability)
- Congestive cardiac failure
- Systemic causes like renal and hepatic diseases
- Associated hypoalbuminemia

Non-pitting edema–myxedema can be associated with severe anemia.

Examination of Face and Oral Cavity

- *Facial abnormality:* Look for pallor/puffiness of face.
- *Chip-monk facies:* Frontal bossing, malar prominence with protuberant teeth. Seen in patients with thalassemia major.

Note: Agranulocytosis will result in ulcers in the oral cavity and pharynx.

Bony Tenderness

- Bony tenderness is detected by applying pressure on the body of the sternum (often-lower end)/part of the sternum corresponding to the 5th intercostal space.
- Common sites for bony tenderness–body of sternum, ribs, clavicles, pelvic bones and skull.

Causes of bony tenderness

- *Common causes:* Acute leukemias, multiple myeloma, chronic leukemia
- *Rare causes:* Severe anemia, osteomalacia and osteoporosis.

Note: Bony pain and tenderness is usually due to the expansion of the marrow and sub-periosteal leukemic infiltration.

Focal bone tenderness is due to secondary deposits in the bone.

Bleeding Spots

- *Common sites*
  - Oral cavity, conjunctiva, gum (gum hypertrophy and bleeding is common in case of AML), limbs.
- *Associated conditions*
  - Bleeding and clotting disorders
  - Systemic causes like vasculitis
  - Leukemic disorders
  - Aplastic anemia

Skin Examination

For pallor, bleeding spots, pigmentation (megaloblastic anemia, Addison's disease).

Table 7.1: Oral cavity examination: Check for the following abnormalities

Site	*Abnormality*
1. Oral mucosa	Pallor
2. Tongue	
• Pale and bald (atrophy of papillae)	• Iron deficiency
• Beefy red appearance	• Niacin deficiency
• Magenta colored	• Riboflavin deficiency
3. Palate and gum	Bleeding spots (bleeding and clotting disorder) Gum hypertrophy and bleed—acute myeloid leukemia (acute monocytic)

Nails

- Platynychia (flat nails)
- Koilonychia (spoon shaped)

} Iron deficiency anemia

- Brittle nails and
- Longitudinal ridges

} Severe chronic anemia

Leg Ulcers

Site: Medial aspect of tibia above the ankle.

Characteristics

- Chronic ulcers
- Single or multiple
- Unilateral or bilateral
- Only scarring of healed ulcers may be present.

Significance: Commonly associated with sickle cell anemias and hereditary spherocytosis.

Mechanism of leg ulcers: Leg ulcers are due to ischemia and super-added infection in the distal circulation.

Retinal Examination

- Pallor (severe anemia)
- Hemorrhages (severe anemia, bleeding disorder)
- Roth spots (infective endocarditis)
- Hypertensive and chronic renal failure changes
- Papilledema (severe anemia can cause papilledema).

Vital Signs

Vital sign changes ill anemic disorders

- *Pulse:* Severe anemia causes tachycardia and high volume pulse.
- *Blood pressure:* Wide pulse pressure occurs due to anemia.
- *Temperature:* Minimal raise of temperature—due to severe anemia itself.

  Severe rise of temperature–suggestive of systemic illness.

SYSTEMIC EXAMINATION

Clinical Findings on Systemic Examination

Cardiovascular System

a. Cardiomegaly with hyperdynamic apex.

b. *Murmurs*

- Ejection systolic murmur at the left sternal border (pulmonary area), murmur occurs due to the increased velocity of blood flow with decrease in the viscosity of blood.
- Murmurs may also be due to underlying heart disease.

c. Congestive cardiac failure

d. Venous hum in the neck

Note: In Patients with chronic anemia, who are adjusted to very low Hb concentration, sudden transfusion of blood can expand the intravascular volume and increase in the LV filling pressure can precipitate cardiac failure.

Respiratory System

Check for evidence of tuberculosis, malignancy, chronic suppurative lung disease which can cause significant anemia.

Central Nervous System

Severe anemia may be associated with

- Altered sensorium (severe anemia with encephalopathy).
- *Peripheral neuropathy:* Loss of sensation (glove and stocking type), loss of deep reflexes (ankle jerks).
- Subacute combined degeneration of spinal cord (patients with chronic vitamin B_{12} deficiency)–pyramidal tract abnormality and posterior column disturbance.

Examination of other Systems

- Systemic examination should also include examination of hepatobiliary, musculoskeletal and other systems in relevant cases.
- Patients of anemia should undergo per rectal examination.

- Per rectal examination may reveal—haemorrhoids, rectal bleeding, occult blood loss.
- Per vaginal examination is helpful to find the etiology of anemia in female patients.

Differential Diagnosis and Investigations of Hematological Disorders

Iron deficiency anemia

Features

- History of blood loss
- Dietary lack of iron
- Occasionally dysphagia and pica.

Signs

- Severe anemia
- Pale and bald tongue
- Koilonychia and platynychia

Investigations

- For evidence of iron deficiency
- Microcytic hypochromic anemia
- Serum iron decrease with increase in the iron binding capacity.
- Bone marrow iron stores depleted (stained by Prussian blue).

For the cause of iron deficiency

- Stool for ova, cyst and occult blood.
- Upper and lower GIT endoscopy and Barium studies—for evidence of blood loss.
- Gynecological evaluation—for evidence of blood loss.

Folic Acid Deficiency

Clinical features

- Poor dietary intake, symptoms of malabsorption
- Anemia, red bald tongue
- Peripheral neuropathy—rare

Investigations

- Macrocytic anemia, hypersegmented neutrophils
- Megaloblastic marrow and low serum folate level.

Vitamin B_{12} Deficiency

Clinical features

- Strict vegetarians, diarrhea may be present
- Disease of terminal ileum, previous gastrectomy

Gastrointestinal tract

Oral cavity (*see* above)

Abdomen: *Check for*

Epigastric tenderness	• May suggest peptic ulcer
Epigastric mass	• May suggest carcinoma stomach
Right iliac fossa mass	• May suggest carcinoma caecum
Retroperitoneal mass with severe anemia	• Secondary carcinoma Chronic lymphatic leukemia Lymphoma
Hepatomegaly due to	• Anemia itself Anemia with CCF Systemic disease involving the liver; leukemia, lymphoma, cirrhosis, etc.
Splenomegaly due to	• Anemia itself, e.g. hemolytic anemia Systemic conditions like leukemia, lymphoma, etc.
Ascites due to	• Anemia with congestive cardiac failure Anemia with hypoalbuminemic states Exudative causes of ascites associated with anemia

- Pallor, mild icterus (lemon yellow)
- Peripheral neuropathy, subacute combined degeneration of spinal cord.

Investigations

- Macrocytic anemia, megaloblastic marrow
- Serum B_{12} level very low
- Abnormal B_{12} absorption test (Schilling's test).

Aplastic Anemia (Primary)

Clinical features

- Infection, pharyngeal ulcers
- Bleeding tendencies, anemia, no organomegaly.

Investigations

- Pancytopenia, hypoplastic/aplastic bone marrow (dry tap).

Hemolytic Anemia

Features

- Anemia, jaundice—since childhood
- Positive family history
- Severe anemia, mild jaundice and splenomegaly.

Evidence of hemolysis

- Reticulocyte count
- RBC enzyme LDH
- Urine urobilinogen increased
- Marrow—erythroid hyperplasia
- Reduced serum haptoglobin level

Hereditary Spherocytosis

Features

- Anemia, jaundice, splenomegaly, leg ulcers.
- Evidence of hemolysis, osmotic fragility ↑
- ^{51}CR labeled RBCs—destroyed in the spleen.

Sickle Cell Anemia

Features

- Anemia, aplastic and infarction crises
- Splenomegaly and later autosplenectomy
- Leg ulcers

Investigations

- Sickle cells in the smear
- Sickling phenomenon—demonstrated by adding sodium metabisulphite
- Hb electrophoresis—HbS (beta chain of Hb at 6th position—valine is replaced by glutamic acid.

Thalassemia Major

Features

- Anemia since childhood
- Incompatible without recurrent transfusion or marrow transplant
- Splenomegaly

Investigations

- Microcytic hypochromic anemia.
- *Hb electrophoresis:* Hb-A_1 (α_2 and β_2) is decreased and HbF (α_2 and γ_2) is increased.

Thalassemia Minor (β)

Features

- Anemia and splenomegaly
- Not responding to iron therapy

Investigations

- Microcytic and hypochromic anemia
- Osmotic fragility of RBCs is ↓ HbA_2 (α_2 and δ_2) is ↑↑.

Autoimmune Hemolysis

Features

- Anemia at any age
- Hepatosplenomegaly
- Microspherocytes and polychromasia in the peripheral smear
- Positive Coombs' test.

Polycythemia Vera

Features

- Suffused conjunctiva with plethoric appearance
- Splenomegaly
- Hb% ↑↑ and RBC mass ↑↑

Marrow

- Hypercellularity of all marrow elements
- ↑↑ Neutrophil ALP increased
- ↑↑ Serum B_{12} level increased

Decrease in the serum erythropoietin level.

Agranulocytosis

Features

- Severe opportunistic infection
- Mouth and pharyngeal ulcers
- Sepsis syndrome
- Granulocytes decreased, marrow granulocyte precursors decreased.

Acute Lymphoblastic Leukemia (ALL)

Features

- Younger age
- Acute onset–anemia, bleeding and infection
- Bone tenderness
- Generalised lymphadenopathy and hepato splenomegaly.

Investigations

- Severe anemia
- Peripheral smear–very high WBC count (>5000 cells/cu) with blast cells
- Bone marrow ≥ 20% lymphoblasts.

Acute Myeloblastic Leukemia (AML)

Features

- Acute onset anemia, bleeding and infection.
- Lymphadenopathy less common compared to ALL
- Hepatosplenomegaly
- Bleeding due to DIC common with M_3 (promyelocytic)
- Gum hypertrophy common with M_5 (monocytic)

Investigations

- Very high WBC count (>50000 cells/cu)
- Marrow—myeloblasts 20%, myeloblasts—auerrods +ve, myeloperoxidase stain +ve.

Chronic Myeloid Leukemia (CML)

Features

- Third to fifth decade
- Anemia with massive splenomegaly

Investigations

- WBC count >50000 cells/cu, platelet count is increased.
- Peripheral smear—myelocytes, metamyelocytes with matured neutrophils. *Marrow* ↑↑ cellularity of myeloid series, blasts-normal or mild (5%)
- Philadelphia chromosome +ve.
- Serum B_{12} is increased and leukocyte alkaline phosphatase is decreased.

Chronic Lymphocytic Leukemia (CLL)

Features

- Age: 45 to 65 years, slowly progressive anemia
- Generalised lymphadenopathy, hepatosplenomegaly.

Investigations

- WBC counts 50000/cu, ↑ small lymphocytes
- Marrow ↑ cellularity of lymphoid series

Multiple Myeloma

Features

- Elderly age group
- Bone pain and pathological fracture
- Anemia and renal failure

Investigations

- Urine—presence of Bence Jones protein
- Serum protein electrophoresis—presence of 'M' band
- Marrow—malignant plasma cells.

Table 7.2: Differences between bleeding disorders and clotting disorders

	Bleeding disorder (defect of primary hemostasis)	*Defects of secondary hemostasis (clotting defect)*
a. Site of bleed	Superficial–skin and mucosa	Deep–muscle, joint, etc.
b. Family history	May not be present	Usually present
c. Sex involved	Females/males occasionally	Males
d. Bleeding	Immediate	Delayed (hours to days) after trauma
e. Findings	Petechiae and ecchymoses	Muscle hematomas, hemarthrosis
f. Treatment	Local measures effective	Requires systemic treatment

Hodgkin's Lymphoma

Features

- Early adolescence and later age group
- Lymphadenopathy with hepatosplenomegaly
- B symptoms—fever (>38°C), weight loss, itching.

Investigations

ESR, lymph node biopsy–Reed-Sternberg cells.

Non-Hodgkin's Lymphoma

Features

- At any age usually at later ages
- More common with HIV positives
- Waldeyer's ring and epitrochlear nodes—commonly involved
- Abdomen and tissue involvement—more common
- Lymph node biopsy—abnormal lymphocytes depending on the histological type.

8 Renal and Urogenital System

CHECKLIST FOR GENERAL PHYSICAL EXAMINATION

- Symptoms and history of present illness
- Past history
- Family history
- Personal history
- Obstetrics and socioeconomic history
- General physical examination
- Vital signs
- Specific examination related to renal and urogenital disorders
- Systemic examination

Diagnosis of renal and urogenital diseases which are encountered in clinical practice is made in the following circumstances:

a. On routine clinical and laboratory investigation of an asymptomatic patient.
b. Persons with symptoms of renal disease and diagnosed on clinical/laboratory examination.
c. Positive family history of inherited kidney disease.
d. Systemic disease with secondary renal involvement.

APPROACH TO A PATIENT OF RENAL AND UROGENITAL DISEASE

SCHEME OF HISTORY TAKING

Symptoms and History of Present Illness

- Pain during the act of micturition.
- Symptoms due to the disturbance during the act of voiding the urine:
  - Increased frequency
  - Dysuria
  - Precipitancy
  - Incontinence
  - Retention
- Change in the colour and appearance of urine.
- Change in the urinary volume.
- General symptoms due to renal dysfunction.

Past History

- Previous history of urinary infection
- Recurrent febrile episodes in childhood
- Previous history of sore throat, pyoderma
- Long-standing sepsis
- H/o recurrent joint pain
- History of hypertension, diabetes mellitus and hypercalcemia
- Drug intake
- Recurrent puffiness of face, edema and steroid therapy.

Family History

- History of renal disease
- Consanguinity between parents.

Personal, Obstetric and Socioeconomic History

SYMPTOM ANALYSIS

Pain during the Act of Voiding the Urine

Pain during the act of micturition may be indicative of pathology in the kidney, ureter, prostate, and urethra.

I. Pain of different Renal and Urogenital Disorders

Characteristic features

a. *Acute glomerulonephritis:* Dull aching pain in the lumbar region.

b. *Acute pyelonephritis*: Renal angle pain on the affected side.

c. *Prostatitis:* Perineal or rectal pain.

d. *Cystitis/urethritis:* Person feels burning or scalding discomfort during or at the end of micturition.

e. *Perinephric abscess:* Causes severe back pain.
   - Tracking of perinephric abscess towards diaphragm: Shoulder pain due to diaphragm irritation.
   - Tracking of perinephric abscess towards the Psoas: Extension of hip causes pain.

f. *Loin pain hematuria syndrome*: Intermittent dull aching loin pain associated with hematuria.

g. *Obstruction to the urine flow:* Obstruction to the urine flow may be due to calculus, pus, blood clots, infection.

> *Note:* Acute urinary obstruction causes colicky pain, chronic obstruction may be painless.

h. *Ureteric colic*
   - Severe spasmodic pain.
   - Starts from the renal angle and radiates up to the groin (testes or medial thigh).
   - Patient: Restless associated with vomiting and sweating.
   - Pain increases by jolting or movement and may last up to few hours (common with calculus disease).
   - Dull aching pain may persist in the loin in between the attacks.

i. Bladder and urethral obstruction pain: Referred to lower abdomen, perineum and glans penis in the male.

j. *Strangury:* Painful passing of urine drop by drop.

l. *Dysuria:* Difficulty in passing urine may be associated with pain or discomfort.

> *Note:* Grossly enlarged or scarred kidneys may occasionally cause dull aching flank pain.
>
> "Progressive and advanced renal disease may be without discomfort".

II. Symptoms due to Disturbance during the Act of Voiding the Urine

Increased frequency of micturition

Causes

1. Due to increased urinary volume—all causes of polyuria.
2. Frequency with normal urinary volume:
   - Due to irritation of bladder, e.g. calculus, growth, infection or blood clot.
   - Due to decreased bladder capacity, e.g. extrinsic compression of the bladder from a pelvic mass, fibrosis of the bladder.
3. Neurological disorder affecting the bladder.

Nocturia (Frequency of urine more at night)

Frequency of urine is more easily recognised at night than the day.

> *Note:*
> - Disturbed sleep leads to decreased ADH level
> - During recumbency renal blood flow increases
> - Above mechanisms result in increased urine formation at night
> - All causes of increased frequency can have nocturia
> - Specific causes of nocturia: Renal failure, early CCF.

Precipitancy

Person passes urine suddenly without prior warning symptoms, e.g. Neurological disorders of bladder, occasionally gynecological causes.

Incontinence

Person has difficulty in holding the urine.

Causes

Overflow incontinence:
- Spinal cord damage due to multiple sclerosis/trauma

- Stress incontinence: Due to increased abdominal pressure causes incontinence.
  - For example, uterine prolapse with cystocoele
  - Weakness of pelvic floor
  - Vesico-vaginal fistula.
- Frontal lobe disease: Due to cerebro-vascular disease can also cause incontinence.

Urinary Retention

Person has difficulty in passing urine.

Causes

1. Obstruction to urine outflow:
   - Vesical calculus
   - Stricture urethra
   - Prostatic enlargement. BPH
2. *Neurological*: Spinal cord or sacral nerve root disease.
   - Preceding to total obstruction of urine flow there may be poor stream of urine
   - Person has difficulty in initiating the act of micturition (hesitancy) and terminal dribbling of urine.

Acute retention of urine in females

Causes

- Retroverted gravid uterus
- Ovarian cyst
- Ectopic pregnancy/rupture of ectopic pregnancy.

III. Alteration in the Colour (Appearance) of Urine

Hematuria (Table 8.1)

- Passing of blood in the urine.
- Hematuria may be macroscopic or microscopic (centrifuged urine).

Causes

- Cystitis and urethritis
- Glomerulonephritis
- Carcinoma kidney
- Renal tuberculosis
- Papillary necrosis
- Bleeding into the urinary tract.

Causes of Brownish/Reddish Colored Urine

a. *Drugs:* Rifampicin, metronidazole, phenacetin, phenytoin
b. *Vegetables:* Beetroot and food coloring materials
c. Haematuria
d. Haemoglobinuria
e. Alkaptonuria
f. Porphyria.

Clinical Significance of Different Types of Urine Discoloration

- Frothy urine–proteinuria
- Blue coloured urine–methylene blue intake
- Orange coloured–rifampicin intake
- Dark yellow–conjugated bilirubin excess
- Pus in the urine–urinary infection
- Cloudy urine with offensive smell–infected urine
- White urine–phosphaturia, chyluria
- Appearance of small tissue pieces in urine–papillary necrosis.

IV. Change in the Urinary Volume

Normal individual requires to pass minimal 400 ml/day for clearing the metabolic waste products.

Table 8.1: Approach to a patient of haematuria

Types of hematuria	*Associated disorder*
1. Transient hematuria	• Severe exercise
2. Intermittent hematuria	• IgA nephropathy
3. Passing blood during initial part of micturition	• Urethral bleed
4. Hematuria at mid and later part of micturition	• Bladder and prostate bleed
5. Smoky or tea colored (red brown) urine	• Glomerular bleed

Oliguria: Urine output less than 400 ml/day.

Causes

Pre-renal:

- Due to decreased renal blood flow
- Hypovolemic shock
- Dehydration
- Congestive cardiac failure

Renal: Acute glomerulonephritis.

Anuria: No urine output within 24 hours.

Commonest cause: Obstruction to the urine flow

Other causes

- Renal infarction: Massive embolisation, renal artery occlusion
- Dissecting aneurysm of aorta.
- Bilateral cortical necrosis: Postpartum hemorrhage
- Bilateral calculus disease
- *Rarer causes*: Retroperitoneal fibrosis.

Polyuria: Passing urine volume greater than 3 liters/day

Causes (common)

- Diabetes insipidus
- Hypercalcemia
- Diabetes mellitus
- Diuretic therapy

Other causes

- Consumption of alcohol, coffee and tea
- Anxiety
- CRF
- Diuretic phase of ARF

V. General Symptoms of Renal Disease

Pedal edema

Causes:

- Acute glomerulonephritis
- Nephrotic syndrome
- Chronic renal failure

Puffiness of Face

Fluid collection in the loose areolar tissue around the eyes causes periorbital edema more common in the early morning hours.

Causes

- Acute glomerulonephritis
- Nephrotic syndrome

Generalised Edema

Nephrotic syndrome causes generalised edema.

Late stages of CRF with GFR <5 ml/min and 95% nephron loss will have edema of face and feet.

Symptoms due to High Blood Pressure

Acute glomerulonephritis causes sudden raise in the blood pressure causing headache, vomiting, convulsions (due to hypertensive encephalopathy) and dyspnea due to congestive cardiac failure.

Uremia

Clinical syndrome which develops in a patient with severe renal failure. Uremia develops with 95% loss of renal function.

Nonspecific Symptoms of Uremia

- Tiredness
- Nausea
- Vomiting
- Pruritis
- Irritability
- Confusion
- Convulsions
- Stupor

Systemic Symptoms

- *Hematological*
  - Severe anemia
  - Platelet and coagulation defect
- *Cardiovascular*
  - Pericarditis pain
  - Angina
  - Dyspnea
- *Respiratory*
  - Haemoptysis
  - Pleuritic pain
  - Dyspnea
  - Hyperventilation due to metabolic acidosis
- *Musculoskeletal*
  - Muscular weakness
  - Bony pain
- *Nervous system*
  - Convulsions
  - Coma

- CVA
- Peripheral neuropathy symptoms

- *Eye disturbance*
  - Blurring of vision due to retinal damage and retinal vascular disease
- *Urogenital*
  - Polyuria, nocturia
  - Impotence and loss of libido
  - Secondary amenorrhea
- *Gastrointestinal*
  - Anorexia, nausea and vomiting
  - Loss of weight
  - Ammoniacal odour of breath

Bronchiectasis: Can cause nephrotic syndrome due to amyloid deposition in the kidney.

> *Note:* Chronic renal failure can cause hypertension. Long-standing hypertension itself can result in renal failure.

Family History

Following urogenital disorders can have positive family history:

- Cystic disease of the kidney
- Alport syndrome
- Nail patella syndrome
- IgA nephropathy
- Vesicoureteric reflux disease

Enquire parental consanguinity in suspected familial renal disorders.

Importance of Socioeconomic, Occupational, Dietary and Gynecological History in Renal and Urogenital Disease

Socioeconomic History

- Overcrowding and poor hygienic conditions predispose to streptococcal infection and glomerulonephritis.
- Multiparous and lower socioeconomic patients are more prone to develop bacteriuria.
- Drug addiction may be a predisposing factor for HIV nephropathy.

Occupational History

Examples of occupation related renal and urogenital disorders:

- Sewage workers–leptospirosis with renal involvement.
- Aniline dye exposure–uroepithelial tumours.
- Hot atmospheric conditions with increased sweating–increased incidence of calculus disease

Diet History

Renal disorders in relation to the dietary intake:

Past history

Significance of previous illness in a patient of renal disease:

Previous illness	*Associated disorders*
• Previous recurrent UTI	Leads to chronic UTI, may be associated with obstructive uropathy–causing pyelonephritis
• Previous sore throat and pyoderma (2–3 weeks before)	Acute glomerulonephritis
• History of long-standing hypertension	Chronic renal failure
• History of recurrent joint pain (connective tissue disorder)	Chronic renal failure
• History of diabetes mellitus and hypercalcemia	Nephropathy
• History of febrile episodes in childhood	Recurrent UTI and vesicoureteric reflux
• History of long-term intake of:	
NSAIDs	Nephropathy
ACE inhibitors	Aggravate renal failure
Penicillamine and gold	Nephropathy
Aminoglycoside intake	Acute renal failure

- Excess salt intake—hypertension and hypertension induced renal disease
- Nonvegetarian diet—calculus disease (calcium oxalate and uric acid stones)
- Food hypersensitivity—nephrotic syndrome

EXAMINATION OF RENAL AND UROGENITAL SYSTEM

GENERAL PHYSICAL EXAMINATION

- Build and nourishment
- Pallor
- Icterus
- Cyanosis
- Clubbing
- Lymphadenopathy
- Edema

Vital signs

- Pulse
- Blood pressure
- Temperature
- Respiratory rate
- Examination of skin/face/eye/hands and feet

Systemic Examination

- Urogenital system
- Cardiovascular system
- Respiratory system
- Gastrointestinal system
- Nervous system
- Musculoskeletal system

Height and Nourishment

Chronic renal disease in a child causes growth retardation and decreased height.

Renal osteodystrophy in a chronic renal disease can result in bony abnormalities.

Pallor: Chronic renal failure will be associated with severe anemia and pallor.

Edema

1. *Sites*: Periorbital edema:
    - Ankle edema
    - Genital edema
    - Generalised edema
2. *Renal disorders associated with edema*
    - Acute glomerulonephritis
    - Chronic renal failure
    - Nephrotic syndrome (associated with anasarca).

Spine

Soft vertebrae with loss of spinal curvature–chronic renal disease with abnormal vitamin D metabolism

Vital signs

Pulse: Rate, rhythm, volume, character and vessel wall thickening (check for abnormalities).

Blood pressure: Hypertension is common in patients with:

- Acute glomerulonephritis
- Chronic parenchymal renal disease
- Polycystic kidney
- Renal artery stenosis

Respiratory rate: Metabolic acidosis (acute and chronic renal failure) is associated with hyperventilation.

SYSTEMIC EXAMINATION

Check for the following abnormalities.

Cardiovascular System

- Changes due to hypertension—cardiomegaly with heaving apex/murmurs
- Due to hypertension and volume overload—CCF
- Due to renal failure—pericarditis with rub
- Connective tissue disease—pericardial effusion.

Respiratory System

- Changes due to fluid retention–pleural effusion
- Due to renal failure–uremic lung
- Due to volume overload–crepitations at lung bases
- Kussmaul's breathing–renal disease with metabolic acidosis.

Examination of skin in a renal disorder

Dermatological abnormalities in renal disease

Salmon yellow appearance of skin	Due to retention of urinary pigment in CRF.
Purpuric spots	CRF with platelet abnormalities, Henoch-Schönlein purpura with renal involvement
Scratch marks	CRF
Uremic frost	Manifestation of terminal uremia—due to deposition of crystals of urea from sweat
Decreased skin turgor	Volume depleted lax skin in patients with—hypovolemia and renal failure
Pyoderma	Post-streptococcal glomerulo nephritis (PSGN)

Examination of face

Abnormalities	*Associated disorders*
Edema and puffiness	Nephritic/nephrotic syndrome
Oral candidiasis	Steroid and cytotoxic drugs (nephrotic syndrome/after renal transplantation)
Butterfly rash	SLE with renal involvement
Nose: Destruction of nasal septum	Wegener's Granulomatosis with renal disease
Deafness	Aminoglycoside therapy Alport's syndrome
Thick and tight skin	Systemic sclerosis
Steroid face	Steroid therapy for nephrotic syndrome
Pharyngitis	Post streptococcal glomerulo nephritis

Examination of eye

Abnormalities associated disorders

Periorbital edema	Glomerular disease (nephritis/nephrosis)
Sub-conjunctival hemorrhage	Renal involvement with leptospirosis and vasculitis
Cataract	Hypercalcemia with renal failure), steroid therapy for nephrotic syndrome

Ophthalmic fundus

Exudates	Diabetes mellitus and vasculitis
Hemorrhages	CRF and hypertension
Macular star	CRF

Examination of hands, lower limbs and spine

Hands: *Check for:*

Beau's line	Transverse ridges (recurrent severe illness)
White nail	Hypoalbuminemia (nephrotic syndrome)
Short fingers	Terminal phalanx resorption due to secondary hyperparathyroidism with renal failure
AV anastamoses (constructed over the forearm)	In patients undergoing chronic hemodialysis
Lower limbs: check for—pedal edema	Acute glomerulonephritis, nephrotic syndrome and CRF
Knock knees/Bow legs	Renal rickets
Peripheral neuropathy	CRF
Absence of patella	Nail patella syndrome

Gastrointestinal Tract and Abdomen

Check for:

- Ammoniacal odour of breath due to uremia
- Bloody diarrhea due to renal failure.

Abdomen

Inspection and palpation: Check for:

1. Renal mass is associated with:
   - Polycystic kidney
   - Hydronephrosis
   - Renal tumors
2. Distended bladder: Forms a pyriform swelling arising from the pelvis may be up to the umbilicus, e.g. obstruction to the bladder neck.
3. Palpate for the renal angle tenderness (renal angle: Angle made by last rib with erector spinae).

   Causes of renal angle tenderness: Acute pyelonephritis and perinephric abscess. Occasionally acute glomerulonephritis.
4. Fullness at the renal angle: Perinephric abscess.

Percussion

Percuss for the evidence of free fluid (ascites).

Renal disorders associated with ascites

- Nephrotic syndrome
- Acute glomerulonephritis
- Chronic renal failure
- Malignant disorders of the kidney.

Percuss also for distension of the urinary bladder.

Auscultation: For renal artery bruit—in renal artery stenosis.

> *Note:* P/R examination for prostatomegaly should be done in all patients with suspected obstructive uropathy.

Nervous system: Check for the following manifestations due to renal failure:

- Twitching of limbs (myoclonus)
- Peripheral neuropathy
- Cerebrovascular accident (associated with hypertension)
- Flapping tremor
- Altered consciousness
- Proximal muscle weakness (usually due to steroid therapy).

Patients with suspected collagen disease with renal involvement should undergo detailed musculoskeletal examination.

EXAMINATION OF INGUINAL REGION AND GENITALIA

MALE GENITAL EXAMINATION

Check for:

- Inguinal and femoral herniae
- Inguinal lymphadenopathy

Examination of Penis

Look for:

a. *Purulent discharge:* It may suggest urethritis, e.g. *E.coli*/gonococcal infection
b. *Meatal ulcer:* Causes painful micturition and hematuria.
c. *Balanoposthitis:* Inflammation of glans and prepuce, e.g. diabetes mellitus.
d. *Urethral stricture:* Palpate the penile part of urethra, e.g. post-traumatic, post-gonococcal urethritis.
e. *Hypospadiasis*: Urethral orifice is present on the ventral surface of the penis due to incomplete development.
f. *Phimosis:* Foreskin of the penis is tight and cannot be retracted.

> *Note:* Priapism is a condition characterised by erection of the penis which will be prolonged and painful, e.g. leukemia, sickle cell anemia and may be idiopathic.

Inguinoscrotal Swellings

Testicular swellings

- *Hydrocoele:* Due to accumulation of fluid in the tunica vaginalis.
- *Varicocoele*: Pampiniform plexus of veins within the spermatic cord become abnormally tortuous and dilated.

- Left-sided varicocoele is common in young men and boys producing dragging pain and felt as bag of worms.
- Infertility can occur due to varicocoele as a result of increased venous pressure and increase of temperature.

- *Orchitis:* Inflammatory swellings, e.g. mumps/bacterial
- *Testicular neoplasms:* Seminoma/teratoma/secondaries.
- *Epididymis:* Felt on the posterolateral aspect of the testis.
- *Epididymitis*: Filarial: Acute–presence of tenderness
  - Chronic–thickening of epididymis.
  - Tuberculosis–tenderness with modularity.
- *Vas deferens:* Felt as a smooth and discrete structure starting from the testis to the inguinal ring.
- Tuberculosis of vas deferens–thickening with beaded feeling.

Examination of Anus and Rectum

See gastrointestinal tract.

FEMALE GENITAL EXAMINATION

Check for

a. *Pruritis vulvae*
   - Causes vulval itching.
   - May be an early symptom of diabetes mellitus.
   - Vulva should be inspected for: Discharge/prolapsed uterus.

b. *Vulvovaginitis*

   Causes
   - Trichomonal infection
   - Gonococcal infection
   - Candidiasis

c. *Cystocoele*
   - Small cystocoele: Causes stress incontinence
   - Large cystocoele: Appears as projecting out from vulva can cause urinary retention.

Speculum Examination

a. Inspect vagina and cervix for vulvovaginitis.

   Swabs from the vagina, cervix and urethra should be taken for bacteriological examination.

b. Observe for–cystocoele
   - Cervical malignancy
   - Vesical fistula and
   - Paraurethral abscess.

Vaginal examination in the dorsal position

- Uterus and the uterine adnexa can be better assessed bi-manually in the dorsal position.
- Dorsal position also allows the palpation of ureteric calculus in its terminal position.

Different Clinical Syndromes Associated with Renal Disease

Acute Nephritic Syndrome

Features

- Oliguria
- Hematuria
- Hypertension
- Edema

Causes

- Acute post streptococcal glomerulonephritis
- Acute and sub-acute bacterial endocarditis
- Shunt nephritis (infection of ventriculo-atrial shunt)
- Viral, fungal and parasitic infection.

Nephrotic Syndrome

Features

- Anasarca
- Massive proteinuria (>3.5 gm/1.73 m^2/24 hours)
- Hypoalbuminemia
- Hyperlipidemia

Causes

Primary

- Idiopathic glomerulonephritis (GN)
- Minimal lesion GN
- Membranous GN

- Proliferative GN
- Focal and segmental glomerulosclerosis

Secondary

- *Infective:* Hepatitis B, HIV infection, malariae malaria
- *Metabolic:* Diabetes mellitus, amyloidosis
- *Drug induced:* Penicillamine, gold
- *Multi-system disease:* SLE.

Acute Renal Failure

Features

- Rapid decrease in GFR
- Usually reversible (persists days to weeks)
- Results in clinical syndrome of uremia.

Causes

- *Pre-renal*
  - Hypovolemic states
  - Low cardiac output
  - Intravascular hemolysis.
- *Renal*
  - Renovascular obstruction
  - Glomerular disease
  - Acute tubular necrosis
- *Post-renal*: Obstructive uropathy.

Chronic Renal Failure

Features

Irreversible destruction of glomeruli and renal function resulting in uremia.

Causes

a. Congenital disorders—polycystic kidneys
b. Vascular—vasculitis/arteriosclerosis
c. Glomerular disease—primary and secondary glomerulonephritis
d. Interstitial—chronic pyelonephritis, analgesic abuse
e. Obstructive uropathy.

Proteinuria

Causes

- Glomerulonephritis
- Bence-Jones proteinuria
- Diabetic nephropathy
- Amyloid kidney

Benign causes

- Orthostatic proteinuria
- Post-exercise

Micro-albuminuria

24 hours urinary albumin excretion >30–300 mg/day (>30 microgms/min), e.g. diabetic nephropathy.

9 Locomotor System

CHECKLIST FOR GENERAL PHYSICAL EXAMINATION

- Symptoms and history of present illness
- Association of age, sex and race with rheumatic disorders
- Family, socioeconomic and drug history
- General physical examination
- Vital signs
- Extra-articular manifestation
- Examination of individual joint
- Examination of other systems

APPROACH TO A PATIENT OF BONE AND JOINT DISEASE

Scheme of History Taking

1. *Symptoms and history of present illness*
   - Mode of onset and duration of symptoms
   - Pain and swelling
   - Pattern of joint involvement
   - Stiffness
   - Deformity
   - Impairment of movement
   - Constitutional and extra-articular symptoms
2. Association of age, sex and race with rheumatic disorders
3. Family, socioeconomic and drug history.

History of Present Illness

Mode of onset of Symptoms and Duration of Symptoms

Acute onset (duration less than 6 weeks)

Causes

- Gouty arthritis
- Septic arthritis
- Rheumatic arthritis

Gradual onset (duration more than 6 weeks)

- For example, rheumatoid arthritis
- Osteoarthritis
- Seronegative arthritis

Intermittent attacks of arthritis, e.g. gouty arthritis

Migratory attacks of arthritis, e.g. rheumatic fever

- Gonococcal arthritis
- Viral arthritis

Palindromic onset

Features

- Individual joints are affected.
- Pain and stiffness persists for few hours to days occurring in recurrent acute episodes.
- Usually progresses to typical rheumatoid arthritis.

Pain

Pain is an important symptom of bone and joint disease.

Bony pain: Continuous aching pain disturbing sleep.

Joint pain: Sharp pain related to posture or movement associated with stiffness.

Pain is usually well localised except pain originating from the hip joint which may be referred to the knee joint.

Assessment of Joint Pain

Mode of onset

1. Acute onset:
   - Septic arthritis
   - Rheumatic fever
   - Gouty arthritis
2. Gradual onset:
   - Rheumatoid arthritis
   - Osteoarthritis
3. Episodic and intermittent attacks:
   - Gouty arthritis
   - Palindromic rheumatism—see above.
4. Fleeting (migratory) type of joint pain:
   - Pain begins in one joint at a time and then involves the other joints.
   - Involvement of the other joints occurs after about 3–5 days, e.g. rheumatic fever Gonococcal arthritis.
5. Pain severe disturbing sleep:
   - Septic arthritis
   - Gout
6. *Effect of activity:* Pain appears after activity and decreases with rest, e.g. degenerative arthritis

Sites of Somatic Reference of Different Joint Pains

Joint pain	*Site of referred pain*
• Cervical spine	Head/over the shoulder
• Lumbar spine	Buttocks/posterior thigh
• Shoulder	Lateral aspect of upper arm
• Elbow	Forearm
• Hip	Outer aspect of thigh or knee or both

Referred pain of cervical and lumbar spine disorders increases on coughing, sneezing and straining at stool due to increase in the intraspinal pressure, e.g. sciatic pain is due to pressure on nerve roots.

Joint Swelling

Joint swelling is a predominant manifestation of inflammatory arthritis.

Swelling may be due to synovitis or excess accumulation of intra-articular fluid.

Swelling can also occur in degenerative arthritis due to bony hypertrophy.

Pattern of Joint Involvement

1. *Number of joints involved:*
   - *Monoarticular*: Single joint involved
   - *Acute onset*, e.g. gout, pseudogout, infective arthritis and trauma to the joint
   - *Gradual onset*, e.g. rheumatoid arthritis, ankylosing spondylitis, psoriatic arthritis and tubercular arthritis
   - *Oligo (pauci) articular:* 2 or 3 joints are involved, e.g. reactive arthritis and sero-negative arthritis
   - *Polyarticular:* More than three joints, e.g. rheumatoid arthritis and SLE
2. *Symmetrical arthritis*, e.g. rheumatoid arthritis
3. *Asymmetrical arthritis*: e.g. gout, rheumatic fever and seronegative arthritis.
4. *Site of joint involvement*
   - Upper extremities: Rheumatoid arthritis
   - Lower extremities: Reiter's disease gout
   - Axial skeleton: Osteoarthritis and ankylosing spondylitis.

Stiffness of Joints

Inflammatory arthritis

- Early morning stiffness persisting for more than 30 minutes occurs in inflammatory arthritis.
- Morning stiffness persisting for more than 1 hour is characteristic of rheumatoid arthritis.
- Stiffness is precipitated by prolonged rest and lasts several hours.
- Stiffness improves with activity and anti-inflammatory drugs.

Non-inflammatory arthritis

- Intermittent stiffness
- Stiffness may increase by activity
- Lasts less than one hour
- Stiffness is accompanied only by pain without other inflammatory symptoms.
- Stiffness may be due to pain or deformity.

Note: Early morning stiffness of pelvic and shoulder girdle is a characteristic feature of Polymyalgia rheumatica.

Deformities

Deformity occurs in both inflammatory and degenerative arthritis.

Alteration in the skull and spine: Paget's disease and acromegaly

Hands and legs deformities: Rheumatoid arthritis

Jaccoud's arthritis: Rheumatic fever

Deformity due to Heberden's nodes: Osteoarthritis. Deformity of spine can cause gradual loss of height and spinal curvature.

Impairment of Movement

Joint and bone disorders result in impairment of movement due to the following factors:

- Joint stiffness
- Joint pain
- Tendon damage
- Muscle weakness
- Neurological deficit

Crackling sensation of joint

- Crackling sensation on joint movement is a feature of degenerative arthritis.
- Osteoarthritis of knee joint characteristically produces crackling sensation on joint movement.
- Crackling sound is due to the badly damaged articular cartilage (due to loose bodies—fragments of cartilage).

Note: It is normal to hear minor clicks on joint movement.

Locking of joint

Locking: Jamming of the joint occurs at some point after certain range of movement (pain and sweating may be associated with locking).

Mechanism of locking: Part of menisci or cartilage (loose body within the joint) interferes with the movement at articular surfaces.

Constitutional and Extra-articular Symptoms in Relation to Rheumatic Diseases

Symptoms	*Associated rheumatic disorders*
Fever and sweating	Septic arthritis and rheumatic fever
Skin rash	Psoriatic arthritis, Reiter's disease, SLE and rheumatic fever
Dyspnea and chest pain (Pericardial and pleural disease)	Rheumatic fever, rheumatoid arthritis and SLE
Eyes	
Conjunctivitis	Reiter's disease
Dry eye	Sjögren's syndrome
Painful iritis	Ankylosing spondylitis
Blue sclera with multiple fractures	Osteogenesis imperfecta
Disturbance of vision and blindness	Giant cell arteritis
Blindness and deafness	Paget's disease
GIT disturbance (Altered bowel habits)	Scleroderma Inflammatory bowel disease. Malabsorption syndromes
Transient diarrhoea	Reactive arthritis
Recurrent mouth ulcers	Behcet's syndrome
Genitourinary symptoms	
Urethritis Asymptomatic urethral discharge	Reiter's disease
Second trimester abortion	APLA syndrome
Female vaginal ulcers	Behcet's syndrome
Neurovascular symptoms	
Entrapment neuropathies	Rheumatoid arthritis
Vascular headache Psychosis Dementia Stroke	SLE
Headache, jaw claudication	Giant cell arteritis SLE, systemic sclerosis and rheumatoid arthritis
Respiratory symptoms	
Symptoms of bronchial asthma	Churg-Strauss disease
Chronic nasal, sinus and middle ear discharge	Wegener's granulomatosis

Association of Age, Sex and Race with Rheumatic Disorders

Rheumatic Disorders Affecting Different Age Groups

- *Younger age*
  - Rheumatic fever
  - SLE
  - Reiter's disease
- *Middle age*
  - Rheumatoid arthritis
  - Fibromyalgia
- *Elderly age*
  - Osteoarthritis
  - Polymyalgia rheumatica

Rheumatic Disorders Affecting Different Sexes

- *Predominantly males*
  - Ankylosing spondylitis
  - Gout
- *Predominantly females*
  - Rheumatoid arthritis
  - SLE, fibromyalgia

Significance of Race in Rheumatic Diseases

- *Disorders predominantly affecting blacks*: Sarcoidosis, SLE
- *Disorders predominantly affecting whites*
  - Giant cell arteritis
  - Wegener's granulomatosis
  - Polymyalgia rheumatica

Drugs and Rheumatic Disease

Certain drugs can induce Rheumatic disease as given below.

Name of the drug	*Disorder produced*
Statins	Arthralgia, drug induced lupus and myopathy
Steroids	Myopathy and osteoporosis
Hydralazine and pencillamine	Drug induced lupus
Salicylates, alcohol	Gout
diuretics and quinidine	Athralgia and drug induced lupus

Psychogenic Symptoms

Functional disorders may present with chronic musculoskeletal symptoms. Objective evidence of organic disease will be absent.

Family History

Examples of musculoskeletal disorders with familial association:

- Rheumatoid arthritis
- Gout
- Psoriatic arthritis
- Ehlers Danlos syndrome
- Marfan's syndrome
- Ankylosing spondylitis
- Osteoarthritis with Heberdon's nodes.

EXAMINATION OF LOCOMOTOR SYSTEM

GENERAL PHYSICAL EXAMINATION—AS FOR OTHER SYSTEMS

(*See* extra-articular manifestations)

Vital Signs–Record the Vital Signs as for Other Systems

1. *Examination of Bony Structures*

- *Alteration of the bony structures may be due to*
  - Alteration in the bony outline
  - Alteration in the shape
  - Swelling over the bones
- *Localised swelling of bones occurs with*
  - Fractures
  - Tumors
  - Infections
  - Cysts

Rickets and Paget's disease of bones can have altered bone shapes.

2. *Palpation of Bones*

a. *Bony tenderness:* Bone tenderness can occur due to destruction of bones or periosteal stretching.

Causes of bony tenderness
- Multiple myeloma
- Infections
- Acute leukemias
- Carcinoma
- Osteitis fibrosa cystica

b. *Fractures*

Causes
- Trauma
- Spontaneous fracture (pathological)

Closed fracture

Fracture with intact surrounding tissue

Open fracture

Fractures associated with bony structures communicating with surface of the skin.

Causes of spontaneous (pathological) fractures
- Multiple myeloma
- Secondary carcinoma
- Osteogenesis imperfecta
- Osteoporosis

Check for the following points in a patient of fracture
- Deformity
- Pain and tenderness
- Hemorrhage
- Crepitus
- Restriction of movements.

EXAMINATION OF JOINTS

SCHEMATIC APPROACH TO THE JOINT EXAMINATION

Checklist for joint examination
- Swelling
- Redness
- Tenderness
- Effusion
- Synovial thickening
- Deformity
- Movements
- Muscle wasting
- Extra-articular features

Examination of joints also includes

a. Anatomical structures
- Articular structures
- Ligaments
- Bony structures
- Muscular and neurological structures

b. Signs of inflammation
- Tenderness
- Erythema
- Rise of temperature
- Synovial effusion.

c. Movements

d. Complications of joint disease
- Deformity
- Muscle wasting
- Instability
- Extra-articular features

Joint Swelling

Causes of joint swelling
- Effusion into the joints
- Thickening of the synovial tissues
- Bony enlargements or osteophytes (Heberden's nodes)

Joint Tenderness

Causes of extreme joint tenderness
- Septic arthritis
- Gouty arthritis
- Rheumatic arthritis

Joint tenderness may occasionally be due to tenosynovitis (inflammation of tendon sheaths).

Note: Enthesitis suggests inflammation of tendons or ligaments at their attachments. Tenderness over the joint may be minimal (patient says or winces on joint palpation) or severe (person does not allow to touch or may take away the joint before palpation).

Joint (Synovial) Effusion

Joint effusion leads to fluctuant swelling in the joint with sharply defined borders, e.g. effusion into the knee joint.

Synovial thickening: Palpate on either side of the joint for the feeling of the thickening.

Deformities and Contractures

Deformities suggest change in the size or shape of involved structures.

Deformities can occur as a result of

- Hypertrophy of bony parts
- Defective alignment of articular structures
- Damage to supportive structures around the joint.

Contractures: Muscle spasm or fibrosis of structures around the joint resulting in loss of full range of movement.

Common Types of Deformities Associated with Different Joint Diseases

Rheumatoid Arthritis

Deformities of hand and wrist

- *Spindling*: Due to swelling of proximal interphalangeal joint.
- *Ulnar deviation of fingers:* Due to anterior subluxation of metacarpophalangeal joints.
- *Swan neck deformity:* Hyperextension of proximal interphalangeal joint with fixed flexion at distal interphalangeal joint.
- *Button hole (Boutonniere's) deformity:* Fixed flexion of proximal interphalangeal joint with extension of terminal IP joint.
- *Z deformity:* Ulnar deviation of the digits with radial deviation of the wrist.

Deformities of feet

- Subluxation of metatarsophalangeal joints and clawing of toes.
- Calcaneal erosion at the insertion of achilles tendon.
- Valgus deformity can occur.

Osteoarthritis

- *Heberdens nodes*
  - Bony outgrowths or gelatinous cysts on the extensor aspect of terminal interphalangeal joints.
  - Associated with inflammation.
- *Bouchard's nodes*
  - Bony outgrowths at the proximal IP joints on the extensor aspect.

Jaccoud's Arthritis

- Deformity is supposed to occur due to chronic rheumatic polyarthritis.
- It is not a true synovitis but associated with periarticular fibrosis of metacarpophalangeal joint.

Ankylosing Spondylitis

Advanced disease

- Exaggerated thoracic kyphosis
- Obliteration of lumbar lordosis
- Forward stooping of neck

Joint Crepitus

Move the joint with one hand and palpate the joint with the other hand for crepitus, e.g. of joint crepitus: Osteoarthritis

Loose bodies (cartilaginous fragments in joint space).

Tendon crepitus can sometimes be felt predominantly in tendons of hand muscles.

Joint Movements, Stability and Gait

Check for both active and passive movement and note the direction and degree of movement.

Goniometer is used to measure the actual movements.

Movements are recorded from neutral position.

Hyperextensibility of the joint occurs due to lax ligaments, e.g. Ehlers Danlos syndrome, Charcot's joints.

Lack of joint movements due to pain

Causes: Trauma/inflammation

Lack of joint movement without pain

Causes:

- Spontaneous fusion (bony ankylosis)
- Surgical fusion (arthrodesis)

Joint subluxation

- Incomplete approximation of articular surfaces.
- There will be alteration of joint alignment.

Joint dislocation

Articular surfaces are not in contact due to their displacement.

Charcot's Joint

Enlarged painless and severely disorganised joints.

Usually associated with excess mobility of joints.

Causes

- Tabes dorsalis
- Peripheral neuropathy
- Syringomyelia

Pattern of joint involvement (Charcot's joint)

- Syringomyelia–shoulder and elbow
- Peripheral neuropathy–joints of the feet
- Tabes dorsalis–hip and knee joints

Loss of pain and position sense results in overstretching and degenerative changes in the joint which predominantly occurs when subjected to repeated trauma.

Stability of the Joint

Stability of the joint is assessed by application of manual stress in different directions and check for displacement.

Gait

Gait abnormality may be due to pain and stiffness or painless conditions like short limb/deformity/stiffness/muscle weakness.

Check the gait with feet fully exposed (without footwears): While the person is walking away/towards and while turning.

Extra-articular Features Associated with Joint Disease

Subcutaneous Nodules

Causes

- Rheumatic fever
- Rheumatoid nodules
- Nodules in SLE and polyarteritis nodules

Rheumatic Fever Nodules

- Non-tender, firm and round nodules of 0.5–2 cm size.
- Signifies severe disease associated with carditis.
- *Site:* Extensor aspects and tendons-elbow, wrist, occiput, etc.
- Spontaneous disappearance can occur.

Rheumatoid Arthritis Nodules

- Firm and non-tender nodules
- Found over the proximal ulna and pressure and friction sites
- Ulceration and infection can occur
- Associated with rheumatoid factor positivity.

Tophi

- Characteristic feature of gouty arthritis
- Palpate the helix of the ear for tophi
- Deposits of urate can be found over the joints and fingertips.

Cutaneous Vasculitis Lesions

Causes: SLE, rheumatoid arthritis, etc.

Due to vasculitic lesions there will be necrosis of the skin with gangrenous changes in the digits (malignant rheumatoid disease).

Skin Rash of SLE

- Erythematous and photosensitive.
- Involves cheek and bridge of the nose (butterfly rash).
- Sensitive to the UV light, may be flat or raised above the skin.

Skin Rash of Dermatomyositis

- Heliotroph rash
- Characteristics of heliotroph rash:
  - Upper eyelids are swollen with purplish discoloration.
  - Usually associated with periorbital edema.

Upper part of the body and face can also have rashes which are erythematous and not raised above the skin in a patient of dermatomyositis.

Skin Changes in Behçet's Syndrome

- *Oral lesions:* Recurrent, multiple painful ulcers (apthous ulcers)
- *Skin lesions:* Pustules/acne lesions, erythematous rash/erythema nodosum and other vasculitic lesions.

Lymphadenopathy

- Localised lymphadenopathy–septic arthritis
- Generalised lymphadenopathy–SLE, rheumatoid arthritis and polyarteritis nodosa.

Local edema: Localised edema occurs over the inflamed joints.

EXAMINATION OF INDIVIDUAL JOINTS

Shoulder Joint

Causes of shoulder pain:

- Synovitis 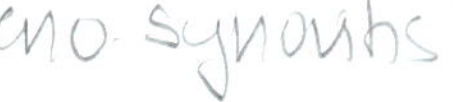
- Osteoarthritis
- Fractures
- Tumors
- Tendinitis

Movement of shoulders

- Abduction: 180°
- Adduction: 45°–50°
- Flexion: 180°
- Extension: 50°–60°
- Rotation: External rotation and internal rotation is 90°.

Supraspinatus Tendinitis
(Painful arc syndrome)

Characteristics

- Pain on abduction of arms and decreases by external rotation.
- Tenderness is present over the greater tuberosity of humerus.

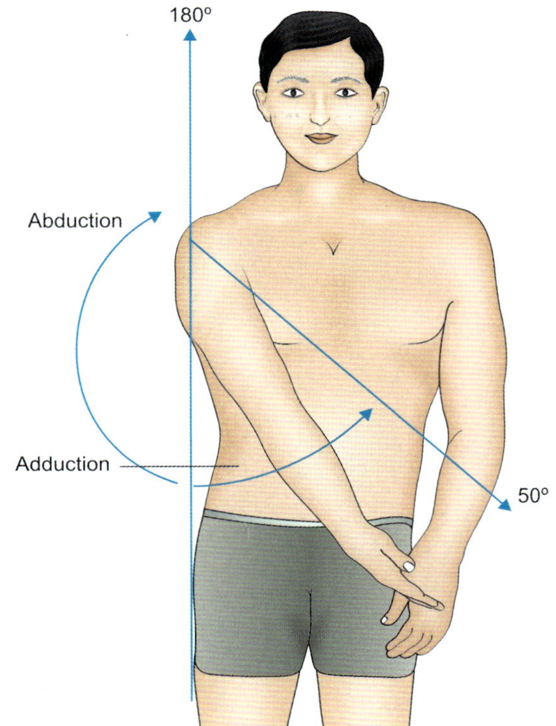

Shoulder movements

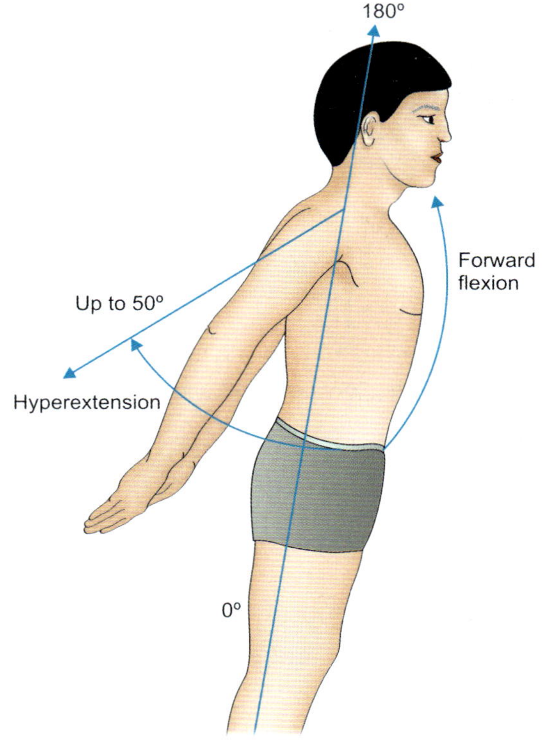

Shoulder movements

- Impingement of the supraspinatus tendon on the acromion causes painful arc syndrome.

Wrist Joint

Common abnormalities

- Arthritis
- Fractures
- Thickening of lower end of radius and ulna—hypertrophic osteoarthropathy.

Movements

- Dorsiflexion (extension)—around 10°
- Palmar flexion—around 70°
- Ulnar and radial deviation—around 20° to 30°
- Supination and pronation—around 80°.

Elbow

Movements

- Flexion—160°/hyperextension—180°
- Pronation and supination—90°

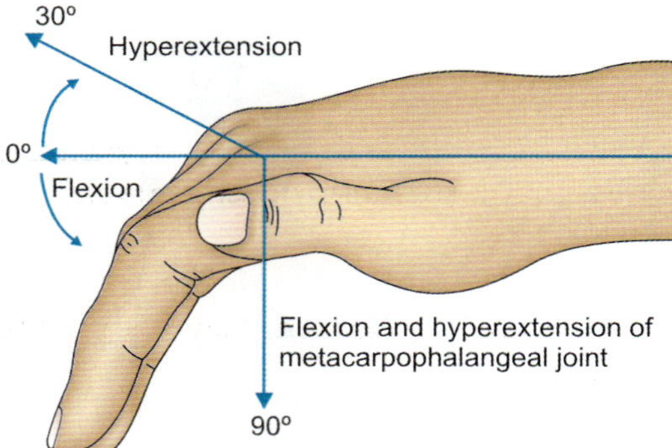

Movements of hand and wrist

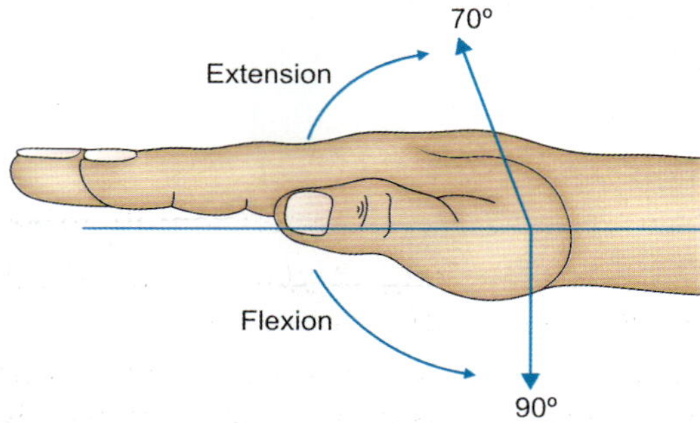

Movements of hand and wrist

- *Golfer's elbow*: Due to medial epicondylitis—may have nocturnal pain if severe.
- *Tennis elbow*: Due to lateral epicondylitis—may have pain on active movement.

Person will have night pain and painful movements.

Forearm

Movements

- Flexion and extension—70°
- Ulnar deviation—30°
- Radial deviation—20°
- Pronation and supination—80°

Hand Examination

Check the hand (power) grip and pinch grip (between index finger and thumb).

Hand Involvement in Ulnar and Medial Nerve Lesions

Ulnar Nerve Lesions

Characteristics

Sensory loss: Loss of sensation of little finger and ulnar half of ring finger.

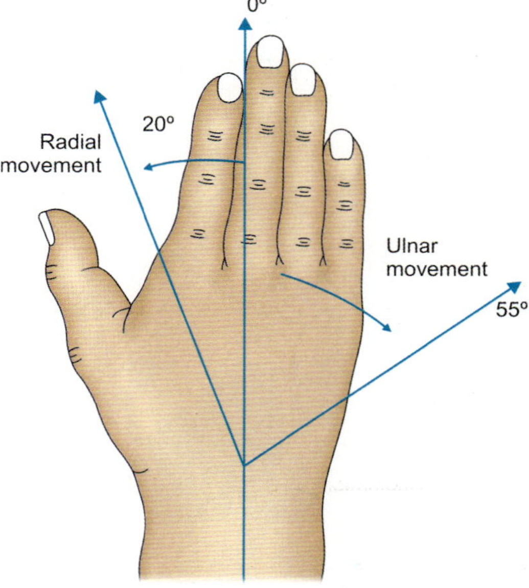

Movements of hand and wrist

Motor loss:

- Wasting of hypothenar eminence.
- Hyperextension of medial metacarpophalangeal joints–(little and ring fingers) due to paralysis of lumbricals and unopposed action of extensor digitorum.
- Flexion of middle and terminal phalanx–due to paralysis of interossei and unopposed action of long flexors.

Medial Nerve Lesions

Sensory loss: Loss of sensation of palmar aspect of thumb, index, middle and lateral half of ring fingers.

Motor loss: Wasting of thenar eminence.

True Claw Hand

Combined lesion of ulnar and medial nerves.

Features

- Hyperextended wrist and metatarsophalangeal joints.
- Flexion of interphalangeal joints.
- Due to paralysis of interossei and lumbricals.

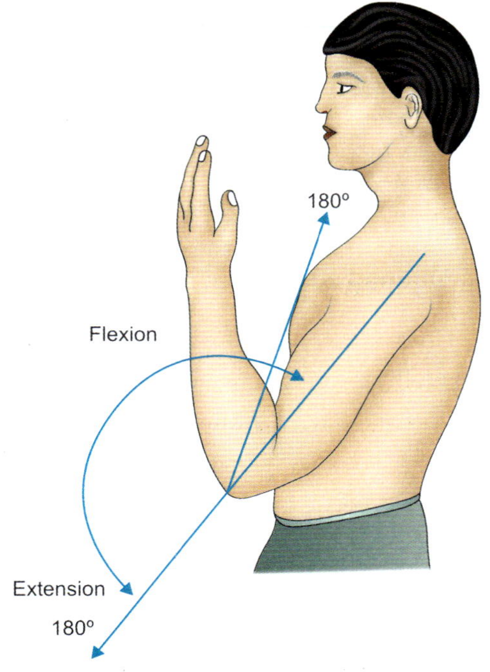

Range of elbow movement

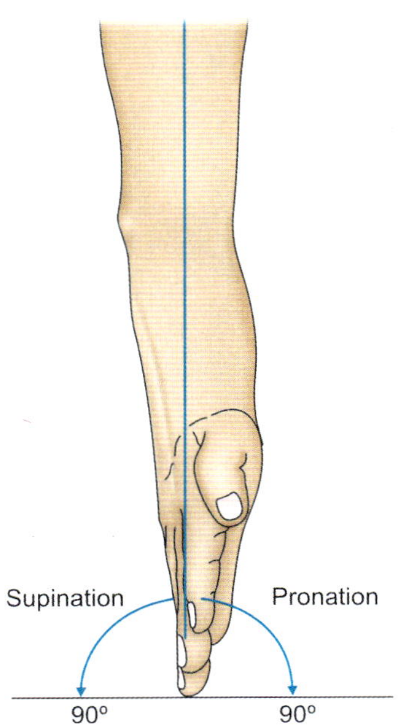

Range of elbow movement

Fingers

Test flexion at: Metacarpophalangeal joint and proximal and distal interphalangeal joint.

Thumb

Test for extension, flexion, opposition and adduction.

Hip joint

Movements

- Flexion—90°–120°
- Abduction—45°
- Adduction—30°
- Extension—30°
- Rotation inflexion and extension: 40° to 50°.

Look for wasting of gluteal and thigh muscles while examining the hip.

Prevent the tilt of pelvis by placing one hand over the pelvis while examining the hip with the other hand.

Knee Joint

Movements

- Flexion (around 135°–140°) and extension–hyperextension (up to 15°).
- Loss of flexion: Inability to flex results in loss of angle of flexion.
- Loss of extension: Person will have difficulty in keeping the knee flat onto the examining bed.

Abnormalities of Knee Joint

Joint swelling due to effusion into the joint.

Demonstration of Effusion into the Knee Joint

a. *Bulge test:* Medial parapatellar fossa appears to refill after the flat of the hand empties it.

b. *Patellar tap*
   - Extend the knee
   - Empty the suprapatellar fossa by application of downward pressure with one hand (to empty the fluid into the retropatellar space) and simultaneously.

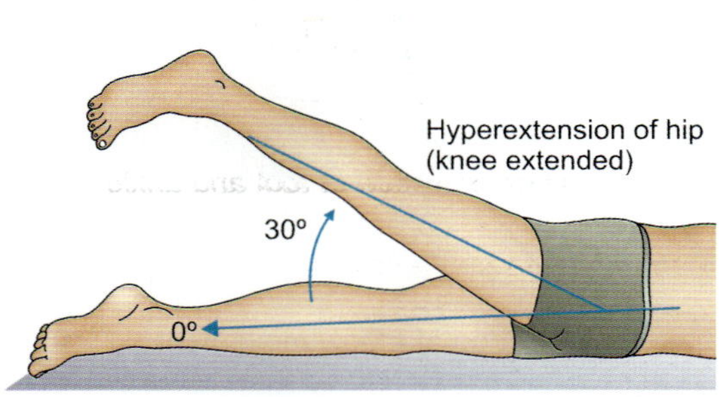

Movements of hip joints

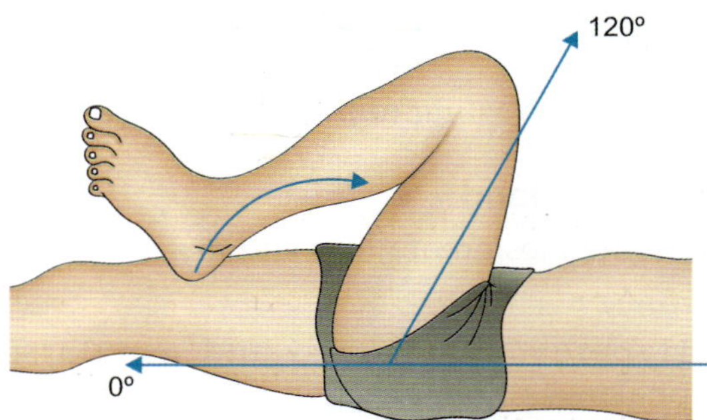

Hip flexion with knee flexed

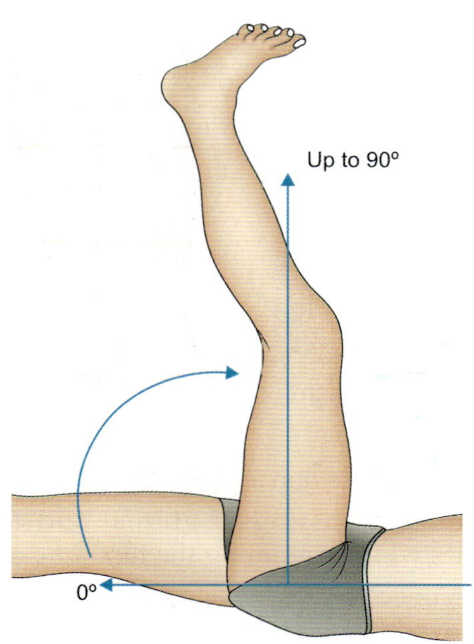

Flexion of hip—knee extended

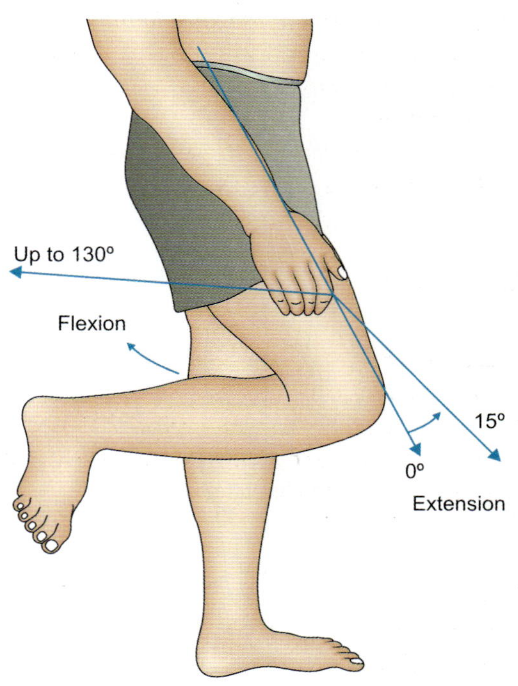

Range of movements of knee

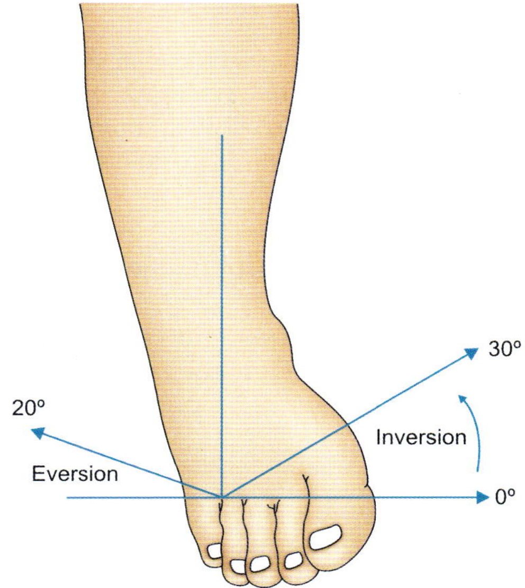

Range of motion of foot and ankle

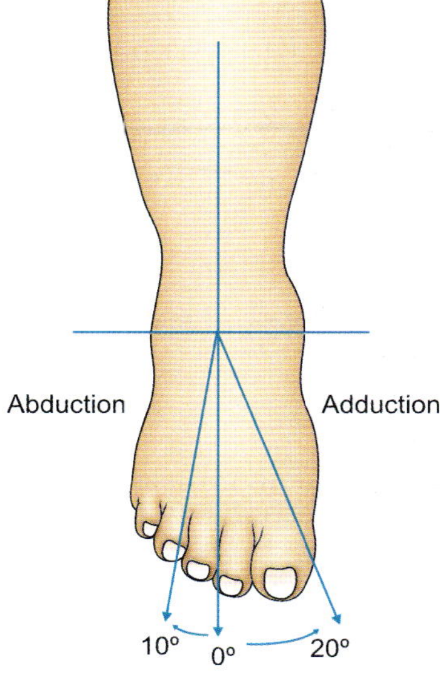

Range of motion of foot and ankle

- Apply downward pressure over the patella. Brisk downward pressure over the patella will result in sensation of fluctuation and also tapping sensation when patella knocks against the underlying femur.

Other abnormalities of the knee joint

- Medial and lateral angulation of the knee is called *varus* and *valgus* deformities respectively.
- Quadriceps wasting occurs in long-standing knee joint disease.
- Tenderness at joint margins.

Ankle Joint

Movements

- Dorsiflexion—20°
- Plantar flexion—50°
- Eversion (20°) and inversion (30°).
- Wasting of calf muscles occurs in long-standing ankle disease.

Foot

Movements

- *Metatarsophalangeal joint*
  - Flexion—40°
  - Extension—40°
- *Interphalangeal joint*
  - Eversion—15°
  - Inversion—5°
  - Flexion—90°
- *Check/or*
  - Hard skin over the pressure points like undersurface of metatarsal heads.

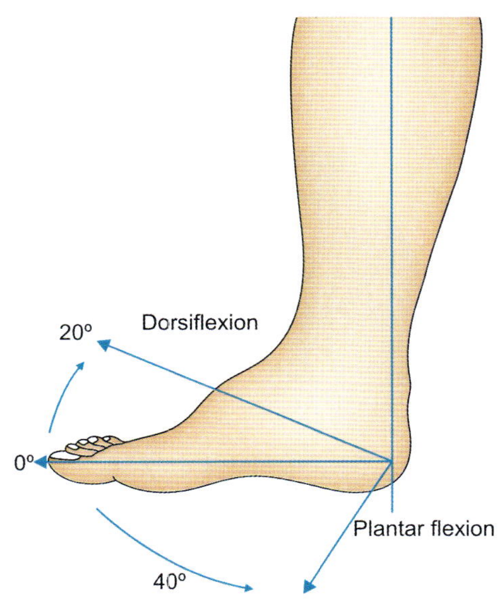

Range of motion of foot and ankle

- Lateral deviation of toes (hallux valgus).
- Claw toes—abnormal curvature and deformity of toes.
- Hammer toes—fixed flexion deformity of terminal joints.

EXAMINATION OF SPINE

Clinical Examination of Spine

Check for

- Curvature of spine
- Deformities of spine
- Localised projections over the spine.

Curvatures of spine

- *Lordosis*
  - Indicates anterior curvature of spine.
  - Cervical and lumbar spine are having normally minimal lordosis.
- *Kyphosis*
  - Indicates posterior curvature of spine.
  - Minimal kyphosis is common with thoracic spine.
- *Scoliosis*
  - Lateral bending of spine. Kyphosis and scoliosis may coexist.
  - Scoliosis may be due to spasm of muscles/bony abnormalities.

Key Points

- Inspect and palpate the spine with the patient standing with head erect.
- C_7 vertebra forms the vertebra prominence.
- Last rib articulates with T_{12} vertebra.

- *Gibbus*
  - Localised deformity of the spine with angulation.
  - Gibbus can be caused by TB spine (Pott's spine), secondary deposit in the spine or vertebral fracture.

Cervical Spine

Common disorders affecting the cervical spine

- Cervical spondylosis
- Ankylosing spondylitis
- Craniovertebral anomalies
- Occasionally rheumatoid arthritis

Movements

- Flexion (forward movement up to 45°): Person is asked to take the chin towards the Manubrium.
- Extension (up to 45°): Person is asked to look upwards.

Lateral movements

- Person is asked to touch the shoulder with the ear without raising the shoulder (around 40°).
- Rotation of spine: Person is asked to look towards the shoulder (around 70°).

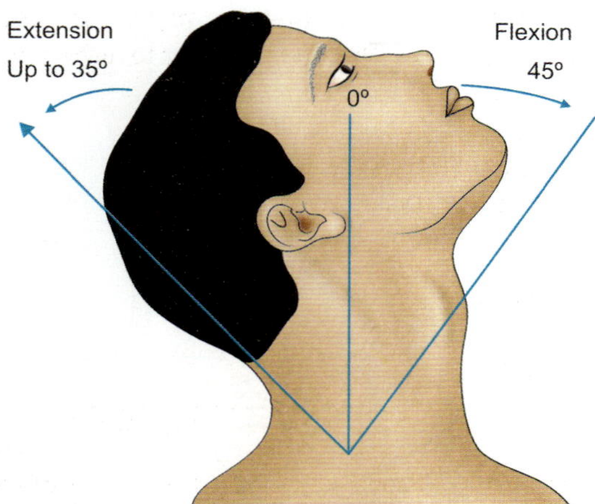

Cervical spine movement

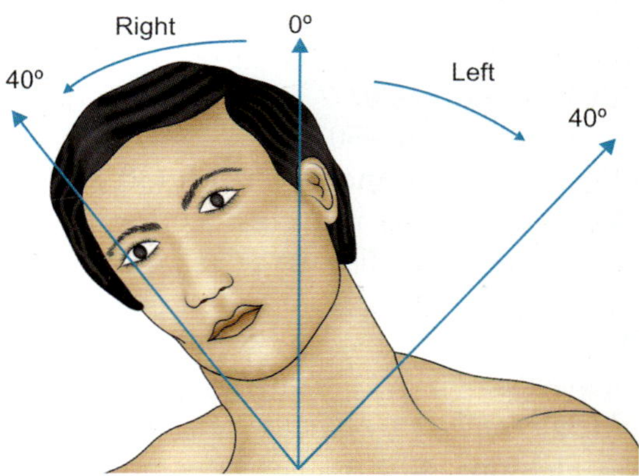

Cervical spine lateral movement

Note: In suspected cases of injury to the neck elicitation of neck movements is not advisable.

Thoracic Spine

Common disorders

- TB spine—produces gibbus
- Secondary deposits in the spine.

Movements

- *Flexion:* Forward bending to touch the toes without flexing the knee.
- *Extension:* Backward bending.
- *Lateral movement:* Touching the lower part of sides of the thigh.

Thoracic rotation: Turning to the right and left while the patient is sitting and the arms folded across the chest.

Causes of painful movements of the thoracic spine

- Intervertebral disc prolapse
- Trauma
- Infections
- Malignant deposits
- Ankylosing spondylitis

Lumbar Spine

Common disorders affecting the lumbar spine

- Osteoarthritis
- Secondary deposits
- Ankylosing spondylitis
- Acute disc prolapse

Movements

Check the movements as for thoracic spine.

Note: Rotational movements take place predominantly at lumbar spine than thoracic spine.

Straight Leg Raising (SLR) Test

Method of elicitation

- With the patient lying on his back, is asked to raise the fully extended lower limb from the bed.
- *Normal:* Full flexion of hip (around 90°) without discomfort.
- *Abnormal test:* Restriction of raising the lower limb due to pain.

Significance

Irritation/compression of sciatic nerve roots, e.g. intervertebral disc prolapse causing compression of sciatic nerve roots (L5, S1).

Lasegue's Sign

While performing the SLR, when the person feels initial pain, foot is dorsiflexed.

This causes: Aggravation of pain due to further traction on sciatic nerve roots.

Significance: SLR may be positive in sacroiliac joint disease but pain will not become aggravated due to dorsiflexion of foot in sacro iliac disease.

Schober's Test

Performed to make out lumbar spine flexion movement.

Mark a vertical line of 10 cm in the midline over the lumbar spines (level of sacral dimples becoming the lower limit of the spine).

Person is asked to bend forwards.

Observation: For the movement of the upper limit of the central line.

Normal: Upper limit of the line moves more than 5 cm (lumbar flexion of more than 5 cm).

Sacroiliac Joints

Tests for sacroiliac joint tenderness:

1. Compression of two iliac bones together.
2. Elicitation of tenderness by applying finger pressure over the sacral dimple when the person is bending forwards.

Differential Diagnosis of Common Joint Disorders

Rheumatic Fever

Severe pain

Key Points

- Early involvement of sacroiliac joints occurs in ankylosing spondylitis.
- Dimples on either side in the lower lumbar region represent the sacroiliac joints.

- Major joints arthritis
- Asymmetrical arthritis
- Flitting (migratory) arthritis
- Deformities rare
- Cardiac involvement common.

Rheumatoid Arthritis

- Symmetrical arthritis
- Polyarticular involvement
- Early involvement of proximal interphalangeal joints
- Deformities common.

Infective Arthritis

- Single joint involved
- Signs and symptoms of infection.

Osteoarthritis

- Weight bearing joints are involved
- Gradual increase of pain over months or years
- Minimal morning stiffness
- Loss of movements of joints.

Gout

- Small peripheral joints (1st metatarsophalangeal joint) are involved.
- Recurrent attacks
- Tophi may be present.
- *Severe attack:* Patient cannot bear even bedclothes.
- Skin over the joint is hot and dry.

Psoriatic Arthritis

- Proximal and distal interphalangeal joints are more commonly involved.
- Skin and nail changes are invariably associated.
- Occasionally, may present with symmetrical arthritis.

Arthritis associated with HLA-B27 Positivity

- Reactive arthritis
- Ankylosing spondylitis
- Reiter's syndrome
- Psoriatic arthritis
- Enteropathic arthritis
- Juvenile onset spondyloarthropathy.

Endocrine Disorders

10

CHECKLIST FOR GENERAL PHYSICAL EXAMINATION

- Symptoms and history of present illness
- Past history
- Family history
- Personal and socioeconomic history
- Menstrual history and history of previous pregnancies
- General physical examination
- Examination of height, body weight, face, eyes, neck, hands and feet in relation to endocrine system
- Systemic examination including genitalia

PHYSIOLOGICAL CONTROL OF ENDOCRINE SYSTEM

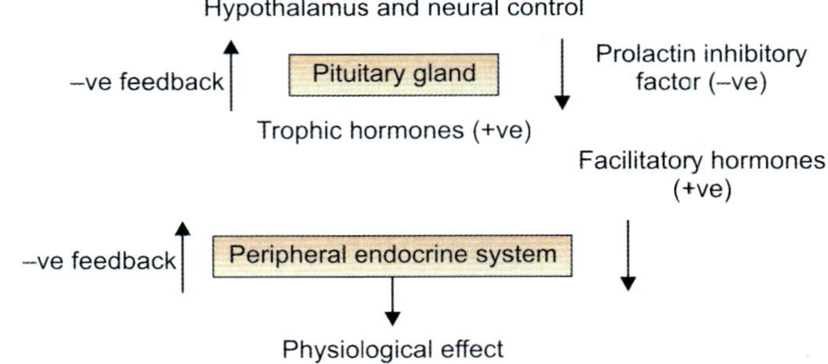

Hormones from hypothalamus

- GHRH–growth hormone releasing hormone
- CRF–corticotrophin releasing factor
- Prolactin inhibitory factor
- TRH–thyrotrophin releasing hormone
- GnRH–gonadotrophin releasing hormone
- Vasopressin
- Oxytocin stored in the posterior pituitary
- Stomatostatin

Trophic hormones from pituitary

- Adrenocortico trophic hormone (ACTH) along with
- Melanocyte stimulating hormone (MSH)
- Thyroid stimulating hormone (TSH)
- Follicle stimulating hormone (FSH)
- Luteinizing hormone (LH)
- Growth hormone (GH)
- Prolactin (PRL)

APPROACH TO A PATIENT OF ENDOCRINE AND METABOLIC DISTURBANCE

SCHEME OF HISTORY TAKING

Symptoms and History of Present Illness

Symptoms in general

- Easy fatigability

- Intolerance to heat/cold
- Alteration in body weight and appetite
- Neck pain, neck swelling and change of voice
- Alteration in body size and shape
- Flushing episodes
- Disturbance in sweating and body temperature.

Systemic Symptoms

- *Cardiovascular:* Chest pain, palpitation, dyspnea and edema.
- *Neuropsychiatric:* Headache, muscle weakness and cramps, tremors, faintness, paresthesia and higher mental function abnormalities.
- *Gastrointestinal:* Vomiting, constipation, diarrhea and abdominal pain.
- *Renal and urogenital:* Polyuria, polydipsia, gynaecomastia, galactorrhea and menstrual irregularities.
- *Disturbance in the sexual function and maturation:* Impotence. altered libido, infertility and pubertal abnormalities.
- *Musculoskeletal:* Bony pain and muscle cramps.

Past History

- Previous surgery
- Previous radiation and chemotherapy
- Previous drug history
- Previous pregnancies
- Developmental milestones in childhood.

Family History

- Family details of height, weight, body habitus, hair growth and sexual development.
- History of autoimmune disorders like diabetes mellitus, thyroid disorders, etc. in the family.

Socioeconomic

Alcoholism, drug abuse, occupational and dietary history.

REVIEW OF SYMPTOMS OF ENDOCRINE DISORDERS

Easy Fatigability

Following endocrine disorders may present with easy fatigability:

- Thyrotoxicosis
- Addison's disease
- Hypothyroidism

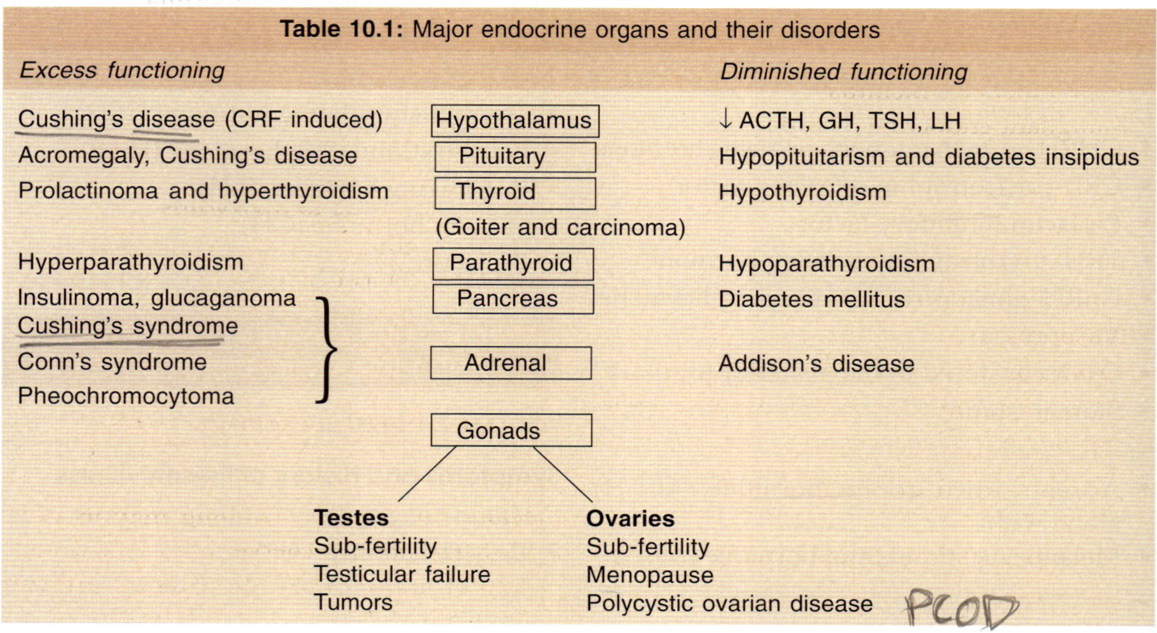

Table 10.1: Major endocrine organs and their disorders

Excess functioning		*Diminished functioning*
Cushing's disease (CRF induced)	Hypothalamus	↓ ACTH, GH, TSH, LH
Acromegaly, Cushing's disease	Pituitary	Hypopituitarism and diabetes insipidus
Prolactinoma and hyperthyroidism	Thyroid (Goiter and carcinoma)	Hypothyroidism
Hyperparathyroidism	Parathyroid	Hypoparathyroidism
Insulinoma, glucaganoma	Pancreas	Diabetes mellitus
Cushing's syndrome, Conn's syndrome, Pheochromocytoma	Adrenal	Addison's disease
	Gonads	
Testes: Sub-fertility, Testicular failure, Tumors		**Ovaries**: Sub-fertility, Menopause, Polycystic ovarian disease

- Hypogonadism
- Cushing's syndrome
- Conn's syndrome

Alteration in Body Weight and Appetite

Weight gain is a dominant manifestation of:

- Cushing's syndrome
- Hypothyroidism (associated with loss of appetite)
- Hypothalamic disorders
- Insulinoma

Note: Patients with primary obesity present with obesity since childhood with very strong positive family history (energy spent is less compared to the calorie consumed).

Cushing's disease will be having characteristic truncal obesity, moon face, fat deposition in the upper part of face and Buffalo hump (fat deposition in the interscapular area)—"Lemon on match stick appearance".

Type II diabetes mellitus has got strong association with obesity.

Weight Loss

Endocrine disorders presenting with weight loss:

- Thyrotoxicosis*
- Addison's disease
- Type I diabetes mellitus*
- Malignant endocrine disorders
- Hypopituitarism
- Anorexia nervosa

* Associated with excessive appetite

Disturbance in Sweating

Thyrotoxicosis and attacks of hypoglycemia cause excessive sweating.

Gustatory sweating: Circumoral sweating while eating and excessive sweating after food may be associated with diabetes mellitus (may be a manifestation of autonomic neuropathy).

Note: Autonomic neuropathy may also cause decreased sweating.

Hypoglycemia, thyrotoxicosis and pheochromocytomas may present with attacks of palpitation and sweating especially on fasting.

Alteration in Body Size and Shape

Hypopituitarism, hypothyroidism and Cushing's syndrome in childhood cause short stature.

Excessive growth hormone secretion in childhood and adolescence (prior to epiphyseal fusion) may result in increase in total height and gigantism.

Hypogonadism presents with tall stature (delayed epiphyseal fusion).

Note: Hormonal or systemic illness causes short stature with delayed bone age.

Genetic growth plate defect results in short stature with normal bone age.

Intolerance to Heat, Cold and Altered Body Temperature

- Thyrotoxicosis causes heat intolerance.
- Hypothyroidism causes cold intolerance.
- Hyperthyroidism and hypothalamic disorders may cause increased body temperature and hyperthermia.
- Hypothermia may be a consequence of myxedema coma.

Neck Pain and Swelling and Change of Voice

- Neck pain—due to thyroiditis
- Neck swelling due to enlarged thyroid (goiter) cervical lymphadenopathy (carcinoma of thyroid).

Voice Changes

- Hypothyroidism causes hoarseness of voice (due to accumulation of fluid in the vocal cords).
- Malignant thyroid swelling may involve recurrent laryngeal nerve and voice changes.
- Acromegalias may have deep hollow sounds to voice.

Flushing Episodes

Endocrine disorders presenting with episodes of flushing

- Carcinoid syndrome
- Menopausal syndrome
- Pheochromocytoma

SYSTEMIC SYMPTOMS

Cardiovascular Symptoms

Palpitation

Endocrine causes of palpation

- Thyrotoxicosis
- Pheochromocytoma (recurrent attacks)
- Endocrine hypertension with heart disease
- Hypoglycemic attack

Chest Pain

Thyrotoxicosis: Precipitates angina in patients with underlying coronary artery disease especially in the presence of hypertension.

Hypothyroidism: Deranged lipid metabolism causes hyperlipidemia in a hypothyroid with aggravation of coronary atherosclerosis and angina.

> *Note:* Precipitation of angina can occur in a hypothyroid with coronary artery disease after starting therapy with L-thyroxine.

Dyspnea

Endocrine hypertension can cause left ventricular dysfunction and dyspnea.

Uncontrolled thyrotoxicosis results in high output cardiac failure and dyspnea.

Dyspnea in a hypothyroid may be due

- Decreased respiratory drive
- Sleep apnea
- Impaired respiratory muscle function
- Accumulation of pleural fluid
- Cardiac dysfunction

Edema

Hypothyroidism: Person will have puffiness of face, periorbital edema and swelling of feet.

Cushing's syndrome may also produce facial puffiness.

Neuropsychiatric Symptoms

Headache

Headache may be a manifestation of pituitary tumors.

Features of headache due to pituitary tumors:

- Variable, more in the morning
- Frontal or occipital

Headache caused by the pituitary tumor is due to dural (diaphragm sellae stretch) or obstructive hydrocephalus caused by the pituitary tumors.

Endocrine hypertension and hypoglycemia can also cause headache.

Muscle Weakness

Endocrine disorders presenting with muscle weakness (non-neurological)

- Hypothyroidism
- Acromegaly
- Cushing's syndrome
- Steroid therapy

Tremors

Following endocrine disorders will be associated with tremors:

- Thyrotoxicosis (fine and rapid)
- Hypoglycemic attack
- Pheochromocytoma

Faintness

Postural unsteadiness and faintness on standing may be due to postural hypotension caused by:

- Diabetes mellitus with autonomic neuropathy
- Addison's disease

Paresthesia

Paresthesia may be a manifestation of:

- Diabetes mellitus with peripheral neuropathy.

- Carpal tunnel syndrome (due to hypothyroidism and acromegaly).

Higher mental function abnormalities

Agitation and anxiety may be caused by:

- Thyrotoxicosis
- Pheochromocytoma

Depression and psychosis may be the manifestation of

- Hypothyroidism
- Cushing's syndrome
- Recurrent hypoglycemia
- Hypercalcemia

Eye and Visual Disturbances

Endocrine Disorders Producing Eye and Visual Disturbances

Pituitary tumors

Visual field defect (bitemporal hemianopia):

- Due to direct compression on optic chiasma
- Direct compression on optic nerve (supra sellar extension of tumor).

Hyperthyroidism

- Proptosis (eyeball prominence)
- Visual loss (Graves' disease—due to ophthalmopathy/direct compression of the optic nerve).
- Diplopia—due to extraocular muscle involvement.

Diabetes mellitus

- Disturbances of vision due to cataract retinopathy
- Diplopia—due to external ophthalmoplegia.

Gastrointestinal Symptoms

Genitourinary Symptoms

- Polyuria and polydipsia is a predominant manifestation of:
  - Diabetes mellitus
  - Diabetes insipidus
  - Hypercalcemia
- Polyuria is also a manifestation of hypokalemic disorders.

DISTURBANCE IN SEXUAL FUNCTION AND MATURATION

Abnormalities of Sexual Function

Impotence and Loss of Libido

Impotence: Inability to perform the sexual act due to failure of sustained penile erection.

Loss of libido: Decrease in the drive towards opposite sex.

Causes of erectile impotence

1. *Endocrinal*
   - Testicular failure (especially in elderly)
   - Hyperprolactinemia
   - Diabetic—vascular and autonomic dysfunction.
2. *Vascular disorders*: Damage to the penile blood vessels—traumatic/atherosclerosis.
3. *Neurological*: Dysfunction of sacral spinal cord or autonomic fibre dysfunction of penis.
4. *Drug induced*
   - Cimetidine
   - Calcium channel blockers
   - β-blockers
   - Digoxin
   - Progesterone
5. *Psychogenic*

Table 10.2: Gastrointestinal manifestations of endocrine disorders

Symptoms	*Associated endocrine disorders*
Nausea and vomiting	Diabetic ketoacidosis and Addison's disease
Hyperdefecation	Thyrotoxicosis (due to hypermotility of intestine)
Diarrhea	Diabetic autonomic neuropathy, Zollinger-ellison syndrome, Addison's disease, carcinoid syndrome and medullary carcinoma of thyroid (severe)
Constipation	Hypothyroidism and hypercalcemic disorders
Abdominal pain	Diabetic autonomic neuropathy and hypercalcemic disorders

Note: Normal level of testosterone is important for normal erection of penis especially in older males.

Hyperprolactinemia and testosterone deficiency cause early loss of libido and erectile dysfunction.

Pituitary dysfunction and hypothyroidism can also cause loss of libido and infertility.

Infertility

If pregnancy does not result after one year of unprotected sexual intercourse by the couple it requires investigation for infertility.

- *Primary infertility:* Conception has never occurred.
- *Secondary infertility:* Pregnancy fails to result after producing a child or definite miscarriage.

Causes

- *Male factors*
  - Semen abnormalities (including volume, sperm concentration, sperm motility)
- *Female factors*
  - Ovulatory disorders
  - Tubal factors: Injury, block
  - Adhesions: Endometriosis mechanical
  - Cervical factors: Abnormalities in the cervical mucus
- *Miscellaneous causes*
  - Immunological abnormalities, rarer uterine abnormalities and infections.
  - Unexplained infertility.

Galactorrhea

Indicates milk or milk like substance inappropriately secreted from the breast.

Causes of galactorrhea

Due to excess prolactin:

- Prolactinomas
- Hypothyroidism (increased prolactin release)
-  Bronchogenic carcinoma—ectopic prolactin production
- Hydatidiform mole—ectopic prolactin production
- Drugs
  - Metoclopramide (inhibition of prolactin inhibitory factor)
  - Phenothiazines
  - Reserpine

Note: Exclude parturition while defining galactorrhea. Secretion of milk in a mother who is not nursing the child after 6 months of post-parturition is also called galactorrhea.

Gynaecomastia: Indicates enlargement of glandular breast tissue in a male.

Lipomastia: Enlargement of breast due to fat deposition (exclude lipomastia in all patients with gynaecomastia).

Gynaecomastia may indicate the presence of endocrinal disorder.

Causes of gynaecomastia

- *Physiological:* Newborn infants, adolescents and elderly ↑E states
- *Common pathological causes*
  - Viral infection of the testis
  - Trauma to testis
  - Bronchogenic carcinoma
  - Liver disease
- *Rare causes*
  - Klinefelter's syndrome
  - True hermaphroditism
- *Common drugs causing gynaecomastia*
  - Estrogen containing preparations
  - Spironolactone
  - Cimetidine
  - Antidepressants

Physiological Gynaecomastia

Adolescents: Appearance of gynaecomastia occurs around 14 years of age and regression occurs by 20 years.

Elderly: Excess conversion of androgens to estrogens in extraglandular tissues causes gynaecomastia in elderly.

Note: All breast masses in males which are > 4 cm in size and tender (indicates rapid growth) especially in the absence of relevant drug therapy ideally requires evaluation.

Malignant lesions of male breast may cause firm to hard breast mass.

Amenorrhea

Term indicates failure of onset of menstrual cycles.

- *Primary:* Failure to attain menarche (requires evaluation if not by age of 16 yrs).
- *Secondary:* Stoppage of menstruation in a woman who had previous regular menstrual cycles (absence of menstruation for 6 months/3 menstrual cycles).

Causes

- *Physiological*: Before puberty, pregnancy, lactation and menopause.
- *Pathological*

  Primary: Congenital or developmental defect of female genital tract.

  Secondary
  - Hypothalamopituitary dysfunction
  - Cushing's disease
  - Pituitary apoplexy
  - Ovarian failure
  - Tuberculosis
  - Chronic systemic diseases
  - Prolactinoma
  - Malnutrition
  - Hypothyroidism

Note: Delay in the onset of menstruation may be occasionally physiological and severe physical exertion can cause scanty menstrual flow. Defective development of female genital tract can also cause amenorrhea.

Disturbances in the Sexual Maturation

Puberty: Onset of secondary sexual characters marks the onset of puberty.

Puberty in Males

Age of onset of puberty: 9–14 yrs (mean 11.5 yrs)

Characteristics: Growth of testes [size over 2.5 cm (4 ml)], increase in the muscle growth, deepening of voice.

Puberty in Females

Age of onset of puberty: 8–12 years (mean 10 yrs).

Characteristics: Breast development occurs first, followed by axillary and pubic hair development and pelvic bone growth.

Delayed Puberty

Failure of onset of sexual maturation

- In boys: If not by 13.5 yrs.
- In girls: If not by 13 yrs.

Delayed puberty is also defined as sexual maturation manifestations have not occurred at a chronological age that is 2.5 SD above the mean age of onset of puberty.

Causes of delayed puberty

Endocrine causes

- Hypothalamopituitary dysfunction
- Gonadal failure:
  - Tumors
  - Chemotherapy
  - Radiation
- Males:
  - Orchitis
  - Undescended testes
- Genetical abnormalities
  - Turner's syndrome
  - Klinefelter's syndrome

Nonendocrine causes

- Chronic systemic illness
- Malnutrition
- Excessive exercise

Precocious Puberty

Development of sexual function occurring at an earlier age (boys: Less than 9 years, girls: Less than 8 years). Precocious puberty may be a manifestation of endocrine dysfunction.

Causes

- Females: Congenital adrenal hyperplasia, hyperthyroidism

- Males: Congenital adrenal hyperplasia, hyperthyroidism.

Hypothalamic and CNS disease can also cause precocious puberty.

Virilisation

Virilisation indicates development of masculine features in a female. Virilisation is invariably due to endocrine abnormality.

Characteristics

- Loss of female body contour
- Increase of muscle bulk
- Clitoromegaly
- Deepening of voice
- Temporal recession of hair

Causes

- Ovarian/adrenal tumors
- Congenital adrenal hyperplasia CAH

Disturbance in the Hair Growth and Distribution

Enquire recent development of excess hair in a female or loss of hair in both sexes.

Hair distribution in normal female

Predominantly pubic, axillary (apart form scalp/eyebrow).

Excess androgen production in a female results in hair growth (hirsutism).

Sites: Face, back, chest, lower abdomen, inner thighs—with male pattern of hair distribution.

Hirsutism

Development of excessive (male pattern) hair growth in women.

Key Points

- Look for distribution of hair in a female patient of suspected hirsutism.
- Check also for other evidences of virilisation.
- Sudden rapid development of hairs in a female and virilisation—rule out ovarian adrenal androgen producing tumors.
- Pelvic examination is essential in all patients with hirsutism with amenorrhea.
- Enquire always the history of drug intake in all patients with hirsutism.

Causes

- Endocrine disorders
- Polycystic ovarian disease
- Congenital adrenal hyperplasia
- Cushing's syndrome
- Idiopathic
- Drug induced—phenytoin, minoxidil, diazoxide, etc.

Loss of Hair

Endocrine causes of loss of hair

- Hypopituitarism
- Hypogonadism
- Hypothyroidism (diffuse alopecia and also loss of outer 1/3rd of eyebrow).

Dermatological Symptoms

- Enquire any recent change in the skin appearance.
- Excessive pigmentation of skin occurs due to Addison's disease and ACTH induced Cushing's syndrome.
- Pale appearance may be due to hypopituitarism and hypothyroidism.
- Primary hypothyroidism can also cause thick dry skin.

Bony Pain and Muscle Cramps

Symptoms of excessive bony pain may be due to hyperparathyroidism. Occurrence of muscle cramps and spasm of hands, feet (carpopedal spasm) may be due to hypocalcemia.

Past History

- *Previous surgery:* History of previous thyroid surgery is important in patients with:
  - Hypothyroidism.
  - History of orchidopexy may be suggestive of previous undescended testis.
- *Radiation:* Neck irradiation (for malignant lymph glands) may cause hypothyroidism at a later date. Radiation to gonads can cause ovarian and testicular failure.

- *Drug therapy:* Enquire previous cytotoxic drug therapy in all patients with evidence of gonadal failure.
- Therapy with sex hormones and oral contraceptive pills interferes with menstrual and sexual function. Long-term therapy with lithium, amiodarone and ^{131}I therapy can cause hypothyroidism.
- Details of previous pregnancies and time of conception is important in assessing hypothalamopituitary and gonadal dysfunction.
- Postpartum hemorrhage can cause hypopituitarism (Sheehan's syndrome) due to ischemic infarction of pituitary (pituitary apoplexy).
- Enquire details of developmental milestones while evaluating congenital/early age endocrine dysfunction.

Family History

Endocrine disorders having familial occurrence

- Diabetes mellitus type II
- Autoimmune disorders–thyroid abnormalities, etc.
- Hyperparathyroidism
- Multiple endocrine neoplasia syndromes.

It is beneficial to enquire the height, weight, body habitus, hair growth and distribution, sexual development and onset of menstruation in other siblings while evaluating respective endocrine disturbances.

Socioeconomic and Dietary History

Sub fertility may be a consequence of excessive intake of nicotine, alcohol or cannabis.

Iodine deficient diet intake can result in goiter and hypothyroidism.

EXAMINATION

General Physical Examination

Body habitus and nourishment (height, weight and body mass index)

- Pallor
- Clubbing
- Icterus
- Lymphadenopathy
- Cyanosis
- Edema

Vital signs, pulse, BP, temperature and respiratory rate.

Examination of face, eyes, neck, hands, feet, hairs, genitals, skin in relation to endocrine disorders.

Systemic Examination

Cardiovascular, gastrointestinal, respiratory, nervous system and other related systems.

General Physical Examination

Height and Body Weight

Measure the total height, weight and body mass index in all patients with suspected growth abnormalities. (*See* Chapter 1, general physical examination).

Causes of short stature (*see* Chapter 1, general physical examination).

Endocrine causes of tall stature (*see* Chapter 1, general physical examination).

Body weight: Check the body weight and look for evidence of obesity and distribution of body fat (*see* Chapter 1, general physical examination for further details).

Pallor

Endocrine disorders associated with pallor

Hypothyroidism and hypopituitarism

Pallor may be due to development of anemia or due to endocrine disease itself.

ACTH decrease (associated MSH decrease) causes pallor in patients with hypopituitarism and pituitary induced adrenal insufficiency.

Mechanism of Anemia in Hypothyroidism

- Decreased oxygen demand causes decreased erythropoietin production and decreased RBC mass resulting in normochromic normocytic anemia.

- Autoimmune hypothyroidism with pernicious anemia causes B_{12} deficiency (macrocytic anemia).
- Menorrhagia and decreased iron absorption causes iron deficiency (microcytic hypochromic).
- Decreased folate absorption can also cause macrocytic anemia.

Icterus

Jaundice may not be a primary manifestation of endocrine disorders.

Hypercarotenemia in hypothyroidism can cause yellowish discoloration of skin.

Clubbing

Thyroid Acropachy

Clubbing like appearance in the fingers and toes but the pathological changes in the bone are different from that of hypertrophic pulmonary osteoarthropathy.

Thyroid acropachy is strongly associated with dermopathy.

Plummer's nail: *See* next page.

Lymphadenopathy: Cervical lymphadenopathy occurs due to thyroid malignancy.

Generalised lymphadenopathy occurs due to Graves' disease.

Edema

Non-pitting edema

Cause

Myxedema (due to trapping of water by accumulated glycosaminoglycans).

Examination of Face

Facial appearance in different endocrine disorders:

- *Acromegaly:* Increased nasolabial and scalp folds.
  Soft tissues of lips and tongue thickened.
  Excess growth of mandible with jaw protuberance (prognathism).
  Overgrowth of zygoma and orbital margins.
- *Hypothyroidism:* Facial fullness and periorbital edema. Thinning of outer 1/3rd of eyebrows.
- *Cushing's disease:* Moon face with plethoric appearance.
- *Thyrotoxicosis:* Widened palpebral fissure with startled appearance.

Examination of Eyes

Eye Abnormalities in Endocrine Disorders

- *Cataract:* Causes—diabetes mellitus and hypo-parathyroidism
- *Corneal calcification:* Caused by hyperparathyroidism
- *Visual field defect:* Bitemporal hemianopia caused by pituitary tumors
- *Visual loss:* Causes—Graves' disease and diabetes mellitus
- *Diplopia:* Ophthalmoplegia due to diabetes mellitus and occasionally pituitary tumors.
  Extraocular muscle swelling due to Graves' disease can also cause diplopia.
- *Proptosis:* Caused by Graves' disease.

Eye Abnormalities in Thyroid Disease

Exophthalmos (proptosis) is a classical manifestation of Graves' disease.

Eye Abnormalities in Thyrotoxicosis

Wide opening of eye occurs due to retraction and spasm of upper eyelid (due to sympathetic overactivity).

While looking downwards upper eyelid lags behind exposing the sclera and on looking upwards eyeball lags behind the lid.

Specific Eye Signs of Thyrotoxicosis

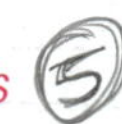

- *von Graefe's sign:* Lid lag
- *Stellwag's sign:* Infrequent blinking
- *Jeffroy's sign:* Absence of forehead wrinkling on upward gaze
- *Mobius sign:* Weakness of convergence
- *Darlymple's sign:* Retraction of upper eyelid.

Exophthalmos of Graves' Disease

Usually bilateral but may be asymmetrical.

Detection of exophthalmos: Keep the eye in primary position. Sclera becomes visible between the lower lid and lower part of iris.

Assessment of exophthalmos

- Patient is sitting comfortably.
- Examiner is standing behind and looks downwards from above.
- Assess the forward protrusion of the eye beyond the plane of forehead by looking downwards from above.

Measurement of exophthalmos

Instrument used: exophthalmometer (Hertel/ Leudde).

Draw an imaginary tangent to the most anterior curvature of the cornea and measure the distance between the imaginary tangent and lateral angle of the bony orbit.

Normal: 18 to 22 mm.

Pathogenesis of Ophthalmopathy of Graves' Disease

- T cells which are antigen specific are supposed to be responsible for initiating the disorder.
- The site of antigen is supposed to be retro-orbital and skin fibroblasts (for dermopathy).
- Infiltrating T cells and macrophages secrete cytokines activating fibroblasts in the extra-ocular muscles. There will be accumulation of glycosaminoglycans with trapping of water leading onto edema. As the disease advances fibrosis becomes prominent.

Eye Involvement

- Excess retro-orbital connective tissue and increased mass of ocular muscles cause increase in the volume of orbital contents.
- Accumulation of hydrophilic glycosaminoglycans cause edema of muscle. There will be lymphocyte infiltration of extraocular muscles with inflammation and muscle dysfunction. Lid retraction may be due to exaggerated sympathetic activity.

Eye involvement in thyrotoxicosis may result in

- Proptosis may cause exposure and corneal damage
- Periorbital edema
- Scleral redness
- Conjunctival chemosis

Extraocular Muscle Involvement in Graves' Disease

Inferior rectus is the first muscle to be involved followed by medial rectus, etc.

Ophthalmic Fundus in Endocrine Disorders

Check for the evidence of:

- Diabetic retinopathy
- Hypertensive retinopathy
- Papilledema (Graves' disease and pituitary tumors).

Examination of Hands and Feet

Endocrine Disorders with Hand and Feet Abnormalities

Thyrotoxicosis

- Palmar erythema
- Clubbing like appearance (thyroid acro-pachy)
- Warm and sweaty palm

Plummer's Nails

Recession of the junction of the nail with distal margin of the nail getting separated from the nail bed (onycholysis).

Acromegaly

- Increased hand and feet size with thickening.
- Increased heel pad thickness
- *Diabetes mellitus:* Dupuytren's contracture
- *Addison's disease:* Pigmentation of palmar creases and knuckles
- *Pseudohypoparathyroidism:* Short 4th and 5th metacarpals and metatarsals.

Examination of Breast

Check for evidence of gynaecomastia, galacto-rrhea.

Sheehan's syndrome can result in depigmented areola and breast atrophy.

Examination of Skin

Check for: Hyperpigmentation, bruises, striae, skin texture in suspected endocrine disorders.

Dermatological Manifestations of Endocrine Disorders

Addison's Disease

Brownish discoloration of palmar crease, elbow, oral cavity and other mucous membranes. Pigmentation can also occur over the areas of trauma, friction and pressure.

Cushing's Syndrome

Striae: Numerous broad (> 1 cm) voilaceous striae over the lower flanks and abdomen.

Stretching of the skin and weakening and rupture of collagen exposes the dermal capillaries and venous blood columns causing violaceous striae.

Bruises: Easy bruisability and ecchymoses can occur due to rupture of collagen.

Hyperpigmentation: Occurs in patients with ACTH induced Cushing's syndrome.

Nelson's Syndrome

Hyperpigmentation occurs due to excess ACTH after bilateral adrenalectomy (in patients with Cushing's disease).

Diabetes Mellitus

Acanthosis nigricans: May be present in patients with insulin resistance.

Vitiligo: Diabetes mellitus type I and autoimmune adrenalitis may be associated with vitiligo.

Necrobiosis lipoidica diabeticorum: Ulcerating skin lesions over the anterior tibial region in patients with diabetes mellitus.

Dermatological Manifestations of Specific Endocrine Disorders

Hypothyroidism: Skin is dry, coarse and thickened.

Vitiligo may be present in patients with autoimmune thyroiditis.

Graves' Disease

- *Pretibial myxedema*
  - Purplish or pink colored indurated lesions over the anterior aspect of the leg (may have orange skin appearance).
  - Pretibial myxedema usually coexists with dermopathy.
- *Pathogenesis oj pretibial myxedema*
  - Pretibial myxedema may be a consequence of deposition of hyaluronic acid and chondroitin sulphate. Lymphatic drainage becomes inadequate due to compression of dermal lymphatics.
  - Dermopathy of Graves' has got same immunological mechanism as ophthalmopathy.

Examination of Neck and Thyroid

Method of examination of thyroid (see Chapter 1, general physical examination*)*

- Patient is seated comfortably and minimal neck flexion is beneficial.
- Examiner stands behind the patient/front and encircles the patients neck with the fingertips of both hands at the level of cricoid cartilage to identify the isthmus of the thyroid (lower borders of isthmus is just above the cricoid).
- Examiner moves the right thumb laterally to identify the right lobe as he compresses it against the trachea. Same procedure is repeated with the left thumb to identify the left lobe.
- Check for the movement of mass on swallowing while examining the thyroid.

Note: Isthmus is a band of tissue running across in front of trachea connecting two lobes.
Right lobe of the thyroid is usually larger than the left lobe.
Thyroid swelling moves with deglutition.
Check always for lymph node enlargement in the neck while examining the thyroid.

Retrosternal Goiter

Characteristics

- Inability to make out the lower border of the swelling.

- Evidence of upper mediastinal widening may be present.

Pemberton's Sign

Ask the patient to raise both his hands above the shoulders so as to touch the ears. Facial congestion and venous distension of neck occurs in patients with retrosternal goiter.

Note: Raising both arms causes further narrowing of the thoracic inlet which has already been narrowed by the retrosternal goiter.

Thrills and Bruit over the Thyroid

Increased blood flow to the thyroid results in thrills and bruit over the thyroid in patients with hyperthyroidism.

Thyroid bruit/thrill: Usually present over the upper pole of the thyroid. Bruit is heard as a systolic continuous sound.

Characteristic Features of Different Thyroid Swellings

- Diffuse enlargement of thyroid, Graves disease (usually soft), colloidal goiter, puberty goiter, dyshormonogenesis
- Single nodule: Thyroid adenoma, thyroid cyst (transillumination positive)
- Firm enlargement: Hashimoto's thyroiditis
- Hard goiter: Carcinoma and Reidel's thyroiditis.

Bone Age in Endocrine Disease

- Appearance of ossification centers and skeletal growth depends on normal endocrine function.
  Hypothyroidism and deficiency of growth hormone in early age causes severe delay in the bone age advancement.
- Excess levels of circulating sex steroids cause premature fusion of epiphyses with a short adult.
  Exogenous or endogenous steroid excess retards or stops advancement of bone growth.
- Hypoparathyroidism in early age retards bone growth.

Note: Bone age estimation requires radiological examination of hand and wrist (for ossification centers and epiphyseal fusion) and comparison with the X-rays of normal individual.

Vital Signs

Pulse

Record the rate, rhythm, volume and character of pulse. Pulse abnormalities in endocrine disorders:

- *Thyrotoxicosis*
  - Tachycardia
  - Irregularly irregular pulse (multiple ectopics/atrial fibrillation)
  - High volume pulse
- *Hypothyroidism*
  - Bradycardia

Blood Pressure

Record both supine and standing blood pressure and check for postural hypotension.

Endocrine causes of Hypertension

- Adrenocortical hyperfunction
- Acromegaly
- Oral contraceptive therapy
- Paroxysmal hypertension with crises pheochromocytoma
- Primary hyperaldosteronism

Postural Hypotension

Causes

- Diabetes mellitus with autonomic neuropathy
- Pheochromocytoma
- Addison's disease (may be an early sign)

Postural hypotension in pheochromocytoma possible mechanisms

- Excess catecholamines—decreased plasma volume.
- Prolonged increase of catecholamines—blunted response to maintain the blood pressure in the up-right position.
- Release of neuropeptide (adrenomedullin)—vasodilatation.

All the above mechanisms together may be responsible for postural hypotension in a patient of pheochromocytoma.

Temperature

- Thyrotoxic crisis—causes hyperthermia
- Myxedema coma—can cause hypothermia.

Respiration

Severe respiratory depression can occur due to myxedema coma.

SYSTEMIC EXAMINATION

Cardiovascular System

Thyrotoxicosis: Check for:

- Cardiomegaly
- Ejection systolic flow murmur
- Atrial fibrillation
- Congestive cardiac failure

Means-Lerman scratch

- Scratching or clicking systolic sound heard in patients with thyrotoxicosis
- Heard in the left 2nd intercostal space
- Occurs due to rubbing together of normal pleural or pericardial surfaces because of hyperdynamic heart.

Note: Cardiac manifestations of thyrotoxicosis may be due to the direct effect of thyroxine on the myocardium and may also due to the effect on sympathetic nervous system. Hypermetabolism in patients with thyrotoxicosis results in overproduction of body heat causing vasodilatation to facilitate heat loss.

Hypothyroidism: Check for cardiomegaly and pericardial effusion.

Pericardial effusion: Myxedema can result in altered permeability of capillaries with protein leaking into the interstitial space causing pericardial and pleural effusion.

Cardiac muscle dysfunction can occur in patients with hypothyroidism.

Endocrine Disorders Associated with Hypertension can Produce Signs of Hypertensive Heart Disease

Respiratory System

Check for—retrosternal goiter, pleural effusion (hypothyroidism).

Gastrointestinal Tract and Abdomen

Check for—oral cavity hyperpigmentation (Addison's disease). Abdominal striae (Cushing's syndrome).

Note: Vigorous palpation of the abdomen may initiate an attack of hypertension paroxysm in a patient of pheochromocytoma.

Nervous System Abnormalities and Associated Endocrine Disorders

Higher Mental Function Alteration

- *Agitation and anxiety*
  - Thyrotoxicosis
  - Hypoglycemia
  - Pheochromocytoma
- *Depression and psychosis*
  - Myxedema
  - Cushing's syndrome
  - Hypercalcemia
- *Coma*
  - Myxedema coma
  - Addisonian crisis
  - Hypoglycemia/hyperglycemia

Cranial Nerves

- Ophthalmoplegia (3rd, 4th and 6th nerve palsy):
  - Diabetes mellitus
  - Pituitary tumors

Graves' disease—can cause ophthalmoplegia due to extraocular muscle involvement.

Motor System

- *Proximal muscle weakness*
  - Thyrotoxicosis
  - Diabetes mellitus
  - Steroid therapy

- *Pseudo myotonia*
  - Hypothyroidism

Sensory System

- Peripheral neuropathy: Diabetes mellitus
- Entrapment neuropathy: Hypothyrodism, acromegaly.

Reflexes Abnormalities

- Hyperreflexia—thyrotoxicosis
- Delayed relaxation of ankle jerk—hypothyroidism (hung up reflex).

Note: Hypothyroidism can be associated with cerebellar ataxia.

Examination of Genitalia (*See* urogenital system)

Male External Genitalia

Normal adult testicular size:

- Length: Average 4.5 cm (3.6–5.5 cm)
- Width: Average 2.6 cm (2.1–3.2 cm)
- Volume: Average 15 ml (18 ± 4 ml)

Testicular volume is measured with the help of Prader orchidometer.

Testicular Consistency

- *Prepubertal male:* Small and rubbery.
- *Klinefelter' s syndrome:* Firm and very small.
- *Post pubertal testicular atrophy:* Soft and small

Testicular torsion may result in small fibrous testes with loss of testicular sensation.

Loss of testicular sensation can occur in the following conditions

- Testicular tumor
- Gumma of the testis
- Leprosy

Check for—evidence of varicocoele and hydrocoele.

Examination of Penis (See urogenital system)

Normal adult length of penis: Average 12–16 cm

- *Measurement*
  - Measure the penile length when its fully stretched and flaccid.
  - Measure the distance from the junction of penis with the pubis to the glans.
- Check for evidence of:
  - Epispadiasis
  - Hypospadiasis
  - Phimosis
  - Chordee (abnormal curvature of penis due to fibrous plaque).

Above penile abnormalities may result in erectile impotence in males.

Examine vas deferens and seminal vesicles for abnormalities.

11 Unconscious Patient

CHECKLIST FOR GENERAL PHYSICAL EXAMINATION

- Different terminologies and their descriptions
- Approach to a patient of altered sensorium
- History review in a patient of altered sensorium
- General physical examination
- Vital signs
- Examination of head, neck, spine and eyes in a patient of altered sensorium
- Systemic examination
- Diagnosis of brain death

TERMINOLOGIES AND THEIR DESCRIPTIONS

Coma

Person cannot be aroused by any form of stimuli and appears to be in a state of sleep.

Drowsiness

Person is easily arousable and alertness is maintained for a short period of time.

Akinetic Mutism

Person is lying in an inert and mute state. Patient may follow movement of examiner with his eyes. (Patient's eyes may be open.)

Site of lesion: Bilateral infarction in the region supplied by anterior cerebral artery.

Coma Vigil: (Vigilant coma)

French terminology, it was first used to describe the altered mental state seen in patients with typhus and typhoid fevers.

Significance

- Coma vigil and akinetic mutism have almost same significance.
- Coma vigil is a rare form of apparent vigilance, but patient is unresponsive.

Abulia

Milder form of akinetic mutism with same anatomical significance. Person will have change in behavior with decreased rate and complexity of language and speech.

Locked in State

Person is awake but does not move any part of his body. Person is unable to speak.

Site of lesion: ventral pons (corticospinal and corticobulbar tracts are disconnected).

Decortication

Features

Attitude of limbs

- Arms are flexed and adducted, supinated
- Legs are extended

Site of lesion: Internal capsule/thalamus/cerebral white matter.

Decerebration (Decerebrate state)

Features

Attitude of limbs:

- All four limbs or arm and leg on one side are extended.

- Limbs are stiff, arms extended and pronated and feet are plantar flexed.

Above attitude of limbs may occur either spontaneously/on manipulation of limbs/or by application of painful stimuli.

Site of lesion: Midbrain at intercollicular level.

Due to the derangement of functions of the structures in the brainstem (midbrain).

Causes

- Hemispheric mass compressing the midbrain
- Posterior fossa/cerebellar lesions
- Can also occur due to anoxic/hypoxic/hepatic encephalopathies or severe intoxications.

Persistent Vegetative State

- Appearance of state of wakeful unresponsiveness.
- No meaningful response to painful or environmental stimuli.
- Preservation of respiratory and autonomic functions.
- Person appears awake with eyes open, may have blinking and slow movement of eyes.
- Person is immobile and may have decerebrate/decorticate posturing but with swallowing and gag reflex intact.
- Persistence of vegetative state for more than six months carries bad prognosis.

Different Mechanisms Leading onto Development of Coma

a. Due to diffuse cerebral dysfunction, e.g. drugs/metabolic/toxins.
b. Direct structural damage to the brainstem.
c. Pressure effect on the brainstem and ascending reticular activating system.

Causes of Unconsciousness

Common in Younger Age Group

- Head injury*
- Post epileptic*
- Intracranial infection
- Drugs/Intoxication*
- Hypo/hyperglycemia*
- Cerebral embolism*
- Subarachnoid hemorrhage*

Elderly Age Group

- Cerebrovascular accident*
- Intracranial infection
- Head injury*
- Hypo/hyperglycemia*
- Cardiac arrhythmias*

* Causes of sudden onset of coma

Note: Renal/hepatic/metabolic disorders can cause coma in all age groups.

Approach to a Patient of Altered Sensorium

Key Points

- Ensure adequate ventilation and circulation and the care of bleeding if any before examination proper.
- Cardiopulmonary resuscitation may be required if the person is pulseless with dilated fixed pupils.
- Suspected injury to the neck and spine—splint and immobilize the neck.
- Enquire the onset, duration and the events leading onto coma either with the relatives, bystanders or paramedical personnel.
- Search for the empty containers of the drugs/poisons in a suspected case of poisoning or drug overdosage (more likely in a patient of psychiatric illness).
- It is useful to identify bracelets, necklaces or cards in patient's pockets as necessary clues may be obtained in-patients of diabetes mellitus, Addison's disease, hypo/hyperthyroidism or epileptic disorder.
- Take care of raised intracranial pressure if required and arrange for metabolic parameters.
- Do CT scan/MRI brain whenever necessary.

EXAMINATION OF A PATIENT OF ALTERED SENSORIUM

SCHEME OF EXAMINATION

General Physical Examination

- Build and nourishment
- Vital signs

Examination of

- Breath odor
- Nose
- Ear
- Tongue
- Skin

Systemic Examination

Central Nervous System

a. Degree of altered sensorium
b. Examination of head, neck and spine
c. Examination of eye:
   - Conjunctiva
   - Pupils
   - Ocular movements
   - Ophthalmic fundus
d. Lateralising signs:
   - Examination of cranial nerves
   - Motor, sensory systems and cerebellum
e. Abnormalities in patients postures
f. Brainstem reflexes:
   - Corneal reflex
   - Doll's head movement
   - Caloric test
g. Examination of other systems.

History Review in a Patient of Altered Sensorium

- Conditions like sub-arachnoid and intracerebral hemorrhage will be sudden in onset with severe headache.
- History of head injury is significant as it may cause subdural and extradural hematoma with lucid interval.
- Lucid interval is a classical feature of extradural hematoma. There will be an initial period of concussion causing altered sensorium, followed by a period of recovery and again deterioration in the level of consciousness (due to enlarging intracranial hematoma).
- Occurrence of seizure prior to the onset of altered sensorium is common in patients with encephalitis and intracranial space occupying lesions (ICSOLs) like tumors, abscess (usually associated with severe headache and vomiting).
- Febrile illness prior to the altered sensorium may be suggestive of intracranial infections or systemic infections secondarily involving the nervous system (e.g. malaria) or post infectious demyelination.
- Consider and rule out renal, hepatic, respiratory, cardiovascular, endocrinal and electrolyte abnormalities in all patients with altered sensorium.
- Suspect drug overdosage and poisoning in all patients of unexplained altered sensorium especially in younger age groups.

General Physical Examination

Build and Nourishment

Severe emaciation with altered sensorium may be associated with following disorders:

- Tuberculosis
- HIV infection
- Internal malignancy
- Diabetes mellitus and Addison's disease
- Chronic systemic illness with nutritional deficiency.

Vital Signs

Pulse and Blood Pressure

- Increased intracranial tension with tentorial herniation can result in—bradycardia and transient systolic hypertension (Cushing's response occurs as a result of raised intracranial tension induced lower brainstem distortion).
- Altered rate and rhythm of pulse signifies primary cardiac cause causing altered sensorium, e.g. atrial fibrillation with embolism, complete AV block.
- Extreme degree of hypertension is associated with:
  - Hypertensive encephalopathy
  - Intracranial/subarachnoid hemorrhage
- Presence of hypotension with altered sensorium may be due to:
  - Alcohol/barbiturate intoxication
  - Internal bleed/myocardial infarction/sepsis

Temperature

Causes of altered sensorium with temperature raise

- Systemic infections with nervous system involvement
- Intracranial infection
- High body temperature with heat stroke.

Hyperpyrexia with Altered Sensorium

Causes

- Cerebral malaria
- Pontine hemorrhage
- Anti-cholinergic overdosage
- Neuroleptic administration

Hypothermia with Altered Sensorium

Causes

- Myxedema coma
- Extensive structural brain damage
- Alcohol/barbiturate intoxication
- Peripheral circulatory failure.

Respiration

Observe the rhythm and depth of respiration in all patients with altered sensorium.

Pathogenesis and Characteristic Features of Abnormal Respiratory Rhythms

- *Kussmaul breathing:* Due to stimulation of respiratory center by metabolic acidosis.
- *Cheyne-Stokes breathing:* There will be loss of normal inhibition on the control of breathing with over responsiveness of the control system to pCO_2 level, e.g.: Bilateral pyramidal disease.

  Hypoxia (low pO_2) induced excess respiratory drive on the depressed respiratory center may be also responsible for Cheyne-Stokes breathing.
- *Biot's breathing:* Respiratory rhythm is irregular and becomes interrupted. There will be variation of rate and depth of respiration. Biot's breathing usually progresses to apnea.

  It may be due to release of reflex mechanisms of respiratory centre in the lower part of brainstem.
- *Apneustic breathing:* There will be few rapid breaths alternating with apnea (2–3 secs).
- *Central neurogenic hyperventilation*
  - Deep regular breathing with increased rate and depth of respiration.
  - Suggests lower part of the brain stem respiratory centers are released from the higher control.

SYSTEMIC EXAMINATION

Examination of Nervous System

Degree of Altered Sensorium

Assess the depth of altered sensorium as per the Glasgow coma scale.

Table 11.1: Abnormal respiratory rhythms with altered sensorium

Pattern of breathing	*Associated disorders*
• Slow depressed breathing	• Opiates, barbiturate intoxication and hypothyroid coma
• Rapid shallow breathing alternating with apnea.	• Lower pontine lesion
• Kussmaul breathing (regular breathing which is deep sighing with a rapid rate)	Metabolic acidosis (diabetic ketoacidosis, uremia, hepatic failure)
• *Cheyne-Stokes breathing* Temporary stoppage of respiration (apnea), followed by respirations which slowly increase in magnitude to maximum and then decrease till the appearance of apnea again	• Coma of any cause Massive supratentorial lesion Metabolic brain disturbance
• Central neurogenic hyperventilation	• Lower midbrain/upper pontine lesion
• Biot's breathing	• Lesion in dorsomedial part of medulla
• Apneustic breathing	• Lesion in the lower pons

Examination of facial structures, breath odour and skin in a patient of altered sensorium

Abnormalities	*Associated disorders*
Breath odour	
Smell of alcohol	• Alcohol intoxication
Ketones (fruity odour)	• Ketoacidosis
Hepatic/uremic fetor	• Hepatic/uremic encephalopathy
Smell of particular poison	• Intoxication and poisoning
Smell of bitter almond	• Cyanide poisoning
Examination of tongue	
Central cyanosis	• Inadequate oxygenation due to respiratory/ cardiac disease/poisoning
Dry tongue	• Severe dehydration
Tongue bite	• Seizure disorder
Examination of nose	
Fracture of nasal bones and CSF rhinorrhea	• Anterior cranial fossa injury
Examination of ear	
Battle' s sign: Discoloration over the mastoid due to bruising) Discoloration of tympanic membrane due to collection of blood behind:	• Middle cranial fossa fracture and fracture petrous bone
Ear discharge/pus	• Possible cerebral abscess
Bleeding from the ear	• Cranial trauma Fracture base of skull
CSF otorrhea	Basal fracture, disruption of dura matter over the petrous bone with rupture of tympanic membrane

Glasgow Coma Scale

Eye opening

- Spontaneous–4
- To speech–3
- To pain–2
- None–1

Best motor response

- Obeying–5
- Localising–4
- Flexion–3
- Extending–2
- None–1

Best verbal response

- Oriented–5
- Confused–4
- Inappropriate words–3
- Incomprehensible sounds–2
- None–1

Significance of Glasgow coma scale

- Usually useful in assessment of patients with head injuries.
- Lower the score on the Glasgow coma scale and longer the time taken for the memories to comeback more likely is the patient to suffer from higher mental function abnormalities.

Examination of Head, Neck and Spine

Examination of Head

Check for

- Scalp edema and hematoma.
- Palpate the orbital margin for zygomatic or malar bone fracture.

Examination of Neck

Examine the neck for

- Evidence of trauma

Abnormalities	Associated disorder
Examination of skin in a patient of altered sensorium	
Loss of skin turgor	• Severe dehydration/shock conditions
Coarse dry skin	• Hypothyroid coma
Cherry red color	• CO poisoning
Jaundice and stigmata of liver disease	• Hepatobiliary disease
Blisters	• Barbiturate overdosage
Pigmentation	• Addison's disease
Purpuric spots	• DIC Bleeding/clotting disorder with intracranial bleed
Skin rash	• Meningococcal meningitis Staph/typhus infections, etc.
Injection and needle marks	• Drug addiction with drug overdosage
Multiple bruises	• Check for indirect evidence of head injury or internal bleed
Pallor	• Internal bleed/Addison's disease
Increased sweating	• Hypoglycemia/shock

- Neck stiffness may suggest meningitis, subarachnoid hemorrhage or neck trauma.

Note: Rule out neck injury before checking for neck stiffness.

Passive flexion of the neck may be limited by temporal lobe or cerebellar pressure cone or decerebrate rigidity.

Examination of Spine

Spine should be examined for evidence of injury especially in-patients with lower limb weakness.

Examination of Eyes

Conjunctiva

- Presence of sub-conjunctival hemorrhage may suggest bleeding disorder, trauma or possible leptospirosis.
- Periorbital hematoma (raccoon eyes) can occur in sub-galeal hemorrhage or base of the skull fracture.

Pupil

Pupillary abnormalities in a patient with altered sensorium

Fixed Dilated Pupil

Unilateral

- 3rd nerve paralysis (due to stretching/compression) due to ipsilateral intracranial mass lesion/spontaneous intracranial bleed or ipsilateral traumatic hematoma.
- Initially there may be only loss of light reflex. Continued compression of the 3rd nerve causes pupillary dilatation.

Bilateral

- Bilateral 3rd nerve palsy
- Midbrain displacement/damage
- Tentorial herniation
- Anti-depressant/atropine overdosage.

Pinpoint Pupil

Less than 1 mm size with very sluggish reaction to strong light.

Causes

- Pontine bleed (sluggish reaction or no reaction to light)
- Narcotic over dosage
- Organophosphorus poisoning

Note: Pinpoint pupil with eyes deviated downwards and towards patient's own nose occurs in patients with thalamic hemorrhage.

Over dosage of barbiturate causes constricted pupils (1 mm or more) but may react to light.

Horner's Syndrome with Miosis

- Unilateral Horner's syndrome occurs with ipsilateral pons/medullary or hypothalamic lesion.

- Ciliospinal reflex induced pupillary dilatation is lost in brainstem lesions.

Key Points

- Normal pupillary reaction and hippus with altered sensorium is a common manifestation of metabolic causes of coma (till late) and usually not due to mass lesion.
- Usage of mydriatics can interfere with pupillary size and reaction.
- Extensive brain damage results in mid position of pupil with failure of reaction (complete sympathetic and parasympathetic paralysis).
- Massive midbrain lesion causes dilated pupils (5 mm) with no reaction to light.

Fundoscopic Examination

In all patients with altered sensorium ophthalmic fundus should be checked for the presence of:

- Papilledema (suggests raised intracranial tension of any cause)
- Hemorrhage (subhyaloid suggests sub-arachnoid hemorrhage)
- Diabetic/hypertensive/uremic retinopathy.

Important Brainstem Reflexes in a Patient with Altered Sensorium

Check for

- Corneal reflex
- Oculocephalic reflex (doll's head movement)
- Vestibulocular reflex (caloric test).

Corneal Reflex

Corneal reflex is usually lost in late stages of coma and loss of corneal reflex is a bad prognostic sign (except in the absence of drug overdosage).

Corneal reflex may also be lost due to focal abnormalities of 5th nerve.

Note: Corneal and pharyngeal reflex may be transiently lost on the side of acute hemiplegia.

Oculocephalic Reflex (Doll's head movement)

Reflex elicitation

- Patient is lying in the supine position.
- Hold the patient's head with both hands while using the thumbs to hold the eyelids open.
- Move the patient's head from side-to-side and also passively flex and extend the neck.

Observation: Observe the patients eye position during the movement of the head.

Normal response: Eye moves in the direction opposite to the passive movement of the head.

Eyeball movements: Significance of different types of eyeball movements in an unconscious patient

Type of abnormal eyeball movement	*Significance*
Sustained conjugate deviation to the opposite side	• Irritative lesion in the opposite frontal lobe
Conjugate deviation of eyes to the same side	• Destructive lesion in the opposite frontal lobe
Brainstem and cerebellar lesion	
Sustained conjugate deviation away from the lesion	Lesion in the pons
Skew deviation (one eye upward with the other eye downward)	Brainstem/cerebellar lesion Cerebellar bleed/tumor
Conjugate downward bobbing	• Pontine lesion
Abducted eye: 3rd nerve palsy due to medial rectus involvement	
Adducted eye: 6th nerve palsy (may be a false localising sign)	
Ocular dipping—diffuse anoxic cortical damage (slow downward movement of eyes with faster upward movement)	

Key Points

- Nystagmus as such cannot occur in an unconscious patient (requires ocular fixation to develop fast phase).
- Metabolic coma and drug overdosage may not abolish eyeball movements till late stage.
- Most of the conjugate eye movements are lost in cases of coma with brainstem lesions.

Normal response suggests: Intact vestibular reflex, its central connection with brainstem and MLF, vestibular nuclei, and 3rd, 4th and 6th cranial nerve nuclei.

Abnormal response

- Ipsilateral pontine lesion—reflex is absent on that side.
- Total absence of doll's eye movement—severe structural lesion in the brainstem or deep metabolic coma.

Note: Severe sedative and anti-convulsant overdosage with coma call abolish oculocephalic and even oculovestibular reflex.

Following clinical signs may indicate deepening of coma

- Lack of spontaneous blinking
- Loss of corneal reflex
- Loss of blink in response to touching the eyelashes.

Vestibulocular Reflex (Caloric test)

Key Points

- Avoid doing the caloric test if there is otitis media or perforation of tympanic membrane.
- Keep a gap of few minutes between testing each ear.

Reflex elicitation

Head position: Head is tilted for about 30° to make the horizontal semicircular canal—vertical (for maximal thermal stimulation).

Irrigation of each ear: 10 to 30 ml of ice-cold water and observe for eye movements.

Observations

- *In a conscious patient:* Tonic deviation of eyes towards the stimulated side with corrective nystagmus towards the opposite side.
- *In unconscious patient:* Only slow conjugate deviation of eyes towards the irrigated side after few seconds of delay (if the brainstem is intact).
- *Brainstem lesion:* Caloric reflexes are lost or disrupted (there will be absence of eye deviation).

Localising Neurological Signs in a Patient with Altered Sensorium

Occurrence of focal seizures and myoclonic jerks

- Focal become generalised–structural cortical lesion
- May suggest metabolic encephalopathy (hepatic/hypoxic/uremic)

Note: Convulsions indicate intact pyramidal tract.

Response to menace/visual threat

- Observe for the rapid eye closure while giving the visual threat
- Defective eye closure on one side may suggest the presence of hemianopia on that side.

Movements of limbs: Absence of spontaneous movements on one side suggests paralysis of that side.

Induced movements

- Pinch the skin of thigh or forearm or apply pressure over the supraorbital ridge or stemum.
- Observe for any difference of response on one side (paralysed side may not have any movement).

Reflex movements

In deep structural lesions of brain there may be decorticate/decerebrate postures.

Facial weakness

Unilateral facial weakness is suggested by:

- Facial asymmetry on one side.
- Drooling of saliva on one side.
- Puffing out of cheeks and lips on expiration on the affected side.

Hemiplegia

Presence of hemiplegia is evidenced by:

- Paralysed lower limbs—externally rotated, thigh flat and wider than the normal.
- Paralysed limb is slack with lack of restless movement.
- Exaggerated deep reflexes on one side.
- Extensor plantar response on one side.

Note: Plantars can be bilaterally extensor in a comatose patient.

Hemianaesthesia

- Moaning or grimacing provoked by painful stimuli is lost on one side.
- Temporal lobe herniation causes compression of the opposite cerebral peduncle against the tentorium and results in arm and leg weakness (horizontal mass effect) extensor plantar on the side ipsilateral to the lesion (Kernohon's Wattman's sign).

Examination of other systems

- Examine cardiovascular, respiratory, gastrointestinal and other related systems in all patients with altered sensorium to find the cause of altered sensorium.

Clinical Characteristics of Different Types of Coma apart from Coma due to Primary CNS Disease

Metabolic

- Altered sensorium
- No focal neurological deficit
- No signs of meningeal irritation
- Doll's head movement normal till late

Drug induced

Altered sensorium

Pupillary changes depending on the drug consumed

1. Opium overdosage: Pinpoint pupil—very minimal reaction light
2. High dose barbiturate: 1 mm pupil
3. Atropine group of drugs: Dilated and fixed pupil
4. Tricyclic antidepressants: Dilated pupils

Evidence of repeated IV injections/venous thrombosis of antecubital veins—suggests IV drug abuse.

Psychological

- Closed eyes
- Normal pupillary reflex and eyeball movement
- Resists eye opening
- Facial grimacing for pain present.

Brain Death

Before declaring brain death ensure the following circumstances are ruled out. Unconsciousness is not because of:

- Depressant drugs/muscle relaxants
- Primary hypothermia
- Metabolic/Endocrine disorder

Brain death is usually considered in the presence of structural brain damage (patient is on ventilator with adequate ventilation).

Diagnostic Tests for Brain Death

- Pupillary light reflexes and corneal reflexes are absent
- No response to caloric stimulation
- Coughing and gag reflexes are absent
- Motor response within the cranial nerve territory is absent
- Respiratory movements are absent (after disconnecting the ventilator and $PaCO_2$ > 60 mm Hg).

Evidences for Brain Death

1. *Loss of cerebral function:* Deep coma (no response to any form of stimuli).
2. *Total loss of brainstem function*
   - Fixed dilated pupil.
   - No response to doll's head movement.
   - No response to caloric testing.
3. Presence of complete apnea (lower brainstem damage).

Demonstration of Apnea before Declaring Brain Death

- Administer 100% oxygen before disconnecting the patient from ventilator.

- Disconnect the patient from ventilator (continuously administer oxygen through tracheal cannula).
- Make sure arterial $pCO_2 > 50$ to 60 mm of Hg for adequate medullary respiratory stimulation.
- Observe for respiratory movement, no respiratory movement suggests brain death.

Other Requirements for Declaring Brain Death

- Examination should be performed by two experienced clinicians.
- Tests are performed either together or separately.
- Tests are usually repeated after an interval (interval depends on the clinical situation).

Note: Body temperature should not be less than 35°C while performing the tests.

EEG shows flat isoelectric lines and not necessary to be carried out.

Intact spinal cord reflexes are not against brain death.

12 Examination of the Eye

CHECKLIST FOR GENERAL PHYSICAL EXAMINATION

- Different types of eye disturbances
- Lacrimal glands
- Abnormalities of different parts of the eye
- Ophthalmoscopy
- Ophthalmoscopic appearances in different disorders
- Retinopathies

APPROACH TO COMMON EYE DISTURBANCES

Red Eye

Causes

- Conjunctivitis
- Scleritis
- Acute glaucoma
- Iridocyclitis
- Sub-conjunctival hemorrhage
- Trauma

Painful Red Eye with Impairment of Vision

Causes

- Corneal inflammation
- Uveitis
- Acute glaucoma
- Trauma
- Burns

Painless Eye with Impairment of Vision (Painless white eye)

Causes

- Disease of intracranial optic pathways
- Diseases of optic nerve
- Errors of refraction
- Opacities in the media
- Chronic simple glaucoma

Eye Discharge

Causes

Excessive lacrimation: All local eye diseases.

Epiphora: Lacrimal drainage system defect results in painless outflow of tears called **epiphora**.

Infective and inflammatory disorders of eye can also produce eye discharge.

Disorders associated with insufficient production of tears will result in dry eyes.

Pain in the Eye

Causes

- Iridocyclitis
- Endophthalmitis
- Scleritis
- Acute congestive glaucoma
- Herpes zoster of the trigeminal nerve with eye involvement.

Note: Foreign body sensation in the eye can occur due to dry eyes, corneal inflammation and exposure to ultraviolet light.
Refractive defects, visual field defects and tension headache can cause feeling of tiredness in the eyes with frontal headache (eye strain).

Abnormal Appearance of Eyes

Prominent Eyes (Proptosis-outward displacement eyes)

Pulsating proptosis, e.g. caroticocavernous fistula and saccular aneurysm of ophthalmic artery.

Causes of proptosis

Unilateral

- Orbital cellulitis
- Hemorrhage into the orbit
- Cyst/Tumor of orbit
- Graves' disease.

Bilateral

- Graves' disease.
- Cavernous sinus thrombosis
- Lymphoma/Malignant tumor of the naso-pharynx.

Enophthalmos (Inward displacement of eyeball)

Causes

- Severe emaciation
- Phthisis bulbi
- Horner's syndrome

Squint: See Chapter 5, nervous system.

Loss of Vision

Sudden Loss of Vision

Unilateral

- Amaurosis fugax (transient)
- Central retinal artery occlusion
- Ischemia of optic nerve
- Retinal detachment

Bilateral loss of vision

- Pituitary apoplexy
- Bilateral occipital lobe infarction
- Psychogenic (pupillary light reflex normal).

Night Blindness (Nyctalopia)

- Congenital and hereditary night blindness
- Retinitis pigmentosa
- Peripheral chorioretinitis
- Vitamin A deficiency

Day Blindness (Hemeralopia)

Vision is poor in bright light than dim light, e.g. congenital central opacity of lens/cornea and pathological changes in the macula.

Lacrimal Gland

Examination of the Lacrimal Gland

Ask the patient to look downwards and medially, while simultaneously pulling up the outer aspect of the upper eyelid—look for the visibility of the gland.

Enlargement of the Lacrimal Gland

Causes

- Viral infection (mumps)
- Lymphoma
- Sarcoidosis

Dacryoadenitis: Lacrimal gland inflammation resulting in swelling of the gland with tenderness.

Dacryocystitis: Inflammation of the lacrimal sac usually secondary to the obstruction in the nasolacrimal duct.

Visual Acuity

Distant vision: Tested by using Snellen's charts.

Chart contains series of letters arranged in a line.

Each line of letters are formed in such a way that, an individual with normal acuity of vision can read those lines at a distance of 60, 24, 18, 12, 9 and 6 meters from top to the bottom line respectively.

Testing the visual acuity

- Visual acuity in each eye is tested separately.
- Close the eye, which is not being tested.
- Ask the patient to read the letters in the Snellen's chart at six meters distance as far as possible.
- Normal person can read up to the last line and visual acuity (VA) is expressed as 6/6.

$$\text{VA } 6/6 = \frac{\text{At 6 meters distance (distance between patient and test chart)}}{\text{Smallest line of the letters read}}$$

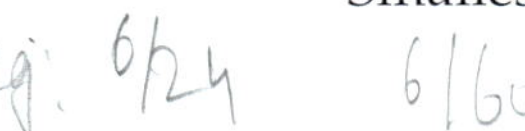

If the patient cannot read at six meters, he can be brought near and acuity can be estimated.

If the vision is very poor–vision is tested for finger counting/hand movements perception of light sensation.

The last line of the chart can be read at 60 meters. If only top line is read the vision is read as 6/60.

Near Vision

Use standard near vision chart.

For near vision testing special reading test types are available, e.g. Jaeger types, Snellen's chart.

Test types have a notation of different sizes, e.g. J1, J2/N5, N6.

Smallest print of newspaper can also be used to test near vision if near vision charts are not available.

Scotomas

Scotomas are defects in the visual field, surrounding an area of normal vision.

Causes

- Glaucoma (arcuate scotoma)
- Diseases of the macula (central scotoma)
- Toxic damage to the optic nerve (centro-caecal scotoma)
- Retinitis pigmentosa (ring scotoma)

Hemianopias

See Chapter 5, nervous system.

Different Types of Refractory Defects

Myopia

- Short-sighted eye.
- With the accommodation at rest parallel rays from a distant object are brought to a focus in front of the retina.

Hypermetropia

- Long-sighted eye.
- With the accommodation at rest parallel rays from a distant object are brought to a focus behind the retina.

Astigmatism

Refractive condition of the eye in which the refraction differs in the different meridians of the eye.

Colour Vision

- Usually red, green and blue colour vision is tested.
- Ishihara's pseudoisochromatic charts are used to test the color vision.

Defects of the colour vision

- Congenital: Red green defect
- Acquired: Optic nerve disease
- Age related macular diseases.

Glaucoma

Features

- Severe pain in the eye and headache
- Vomiting
- Marked disturbance in the vision
- Ciliary congestion

Abnormalities of Different Parts of the Eye

Eyelids

Periorbital edema

Causes

- *Renal:* Acute glomerulonephritis and nephrotic syndrome
- *Hypoprotienemia:* Hypoalbuminemic states
- *Hepatic:* Cirrhosis
- *Cardiovascular:* CCF and SVC obstruction
- *Endocrinal:* Myxedema, Cushing's syndrome
- *Allergic:* Angioneurotic edema

Blepharitis (Inflammation of eyelids)

Features

- Redness of lid margins
- Formation of scales around the bases of eyelashes at the lid margins.

Entropion

Lid margins become inverted, eyelashes may rub over the cornea due to their malposition.

Ectropion

Lid margins become everted usually associated with epiphora.

Pupil

Normal pupil: Both pupil are equal in size, round with regular margin.

Anisocoria

Pupil size varies from one eye to other.

Causes

- Physiological
- Third nerve palsy (pupils dilated)
- Homer's syndrome (pupil constricted).

> *Note:* Sleep, aging and exposure to bright light causes pupillary constriction.
> Exposure to darkness, sympathetic stimulation and mydriatics cause pupillary dilatation.

Conjunctiva (Conjunctivitis)

Features

- Redness of conjunctiva
- Painful/painless
- Normal vision
- Normal pupil

Causes

- Viral (associated with serous discharge)
- Allergic (white discharge)
- Bacterial (purulent discharge)
- Trachoma (presence of follicles in the upper part of conjunctiva).

Sub-conjunctival Hemorrhage

Causes

- Trauma
- Bleeding diathesis
- Leptospirosis
- Vigorous coughing

Conjunctival Chemosis (Edema)

Causes

- SVC obstruction
- Respiratory failure type II
- Graves' disease

Bitot's Spots

Occurs in patients with vitamin A deficiency.

Features

Triangular patches which are dirty grey in colour, appear in the bulbar conjunctiva especially in the temporal side of the cornea.

Cornea

Keratitis (Inflammation of the cornea)

Causes

- Trauma–causes corneal opacity
- Bacterial–pus formation in the anterior chamber leads to hypopyon
- Interstitial–viral/syphilis

Features

- Pain in the eye
- Circumcorneal congestion
- Photophobia
- Visual loss
- Pupils are normal

Severe Damage to the Cornea

Causes

- Chemical injury to cornea
- Vitamin A deficiency
- Severe exophthalmos
- Conditions associated with dry eyes.

Arcus Senilis

Present in the elderly: Characteristic circular opacity seen surrounding the cornea.

Sclera

Scleritis

- Inflammation of deeper scleral lamellas
- Causes painful eye with redness.

Causes

- Connective tissue disorder
- TB, syphilis, etc.
- In rheumatoid arthritis perforation of sclera can occur (scleromalacia perforans).
- Blue sclera/yellow sclera (*see* Chapter 1, general physical examination).

Episcleritis

Inflammation of deeper sub-conjunctival layer and superficial lamellae of sclera.

Causes: See scleritis.

Iris

Iritis/Iridocyclitis

Characteristics

- Severe pain in the eye
- Circumcorneal congestion
- Irregular constricted pupil
- Dimness of vision
- Synechiae (adhesion) between pupil and lens

Causes

- Trauma
- Corneal ulcer
- TB
- Syphilis
- Allergy
- Gout/Diabetes, etc.

Lens

Cataract: Recognised as opacity in the lens.

Common causes: Aging

Secondary causes

- Diabetes mellitus
- Post-traumatic
- Steroid therapy

Intraocular Pressure

Digital estimation of intraocular pressure

- Elicit fluctuation over the eyes with two forefingers.
- Note the degree of fluctuation.

Correct estimation of intraocular pressure can be done by Tonometer (Schiotz).

Dehydration can decrease intraocular pressure and glaucoma causes rise in the intraocular pressure.

OPHTHALMOSCOPY

Key Points for ideal ophthalmoscopy

- Correct position of the patient and the examiner
- Adequate ophthalmoscopic light
- Dark examination room
- Expert examiner

Note: Usually dilatation of the pupil is not required before ophthalmoscopy. Note the size of the pupil and pupillary reaction before dilating the pupil (if required).

Pupillary dilators used

- Tropicamide–0.5% to 1.0%
- Cyclopentolate 1%

Sequence of Ophthalmoscopic Examination

- Patient is sitting/lying down and is asked to look at a distant object.
- Examiner holds the ophthalmoscope in the hand and the scope is brought as near the eye as possible.
- It is ideal to use the examiners right eye to the patient's right eye and vice versa.

Check for the following points while performing ophthalmoscopy

- Optic disc
- Retinal blood vessels
- Macular region
- Periphery of the retina

Normal Ophthalmic Fundus Appearance (Fig. 12.1)

Normal retinal color: Pale pink to reddish black.

Normal optic disc: Pink in color (except for temporal pallor). Normally temporal side of the optic disc is pallor than the nasal side.

Margin: Round and well-defined.

Physiological cup: An area of depression in the center of the disc. Blood vessels appear to enter/exit from the eye through the cup.

Retinal Blood Vessels

Arteries	*Veins*
Thinner than veins	Larger than arteries
Bright red colour	Pulsations normal
No pulsations	

Macula

- Darker in color compared to the remaining part of the retina.
- Lies temporal to the optic disc.
- Fovea lies to the center of the macula.
- Macula contains two or more layers of ganglion cells.

Note: Macular involvement results in a greater visual damage compared to other parts of the retina.

Abnormal Ophthalmic Fundal Appearances

Papilledema (Fig. 12.2)

Suggests edema of the optic nerve head.

Characteristics: Disc is swollen and pink, vessels are congested, hemorrhages may be present.

Disc margins are blurred with obliteration of the physiological cup. Vision is normal till late.

Causes

- All cases of intracranial space occupying lesions
- Optic nerve inflammation–papillitis
- Chronic meningitis
- Malignant hypertension

Papillitis

Suggests inflammation of the optic nerve head.

Features

- Optic disc is swollen
- Blurring of disc margins
- Veins are engorged
- Marked visual loss

Causes

- Multiple sclerosis
- Focal infection (tonsillitis, sinusitis)
- Febrile illness
- Syphilis

Retrobulbar Neuritis

Features

- Inflammation of the optic nerve behind the eyeball
- Optic disc mayor may not be involved
- Marked impairment of central vision
- Pain in and around the orbit
- Backward pressure on the eyeball results in tenderness
- Ill sustained and sluggish pupillary light reflex.

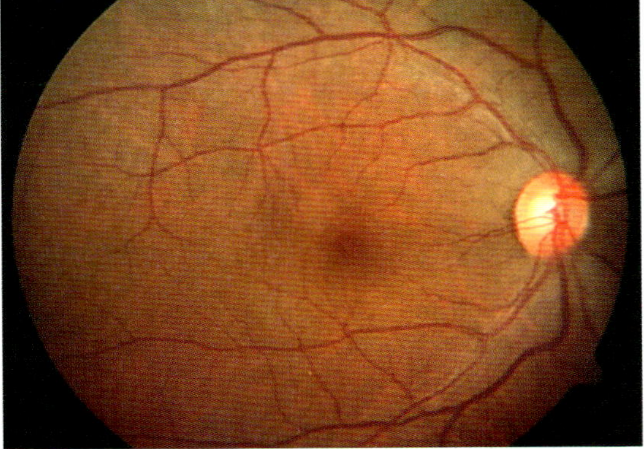

Fig. 12.1: Normal ophthalmic fundus

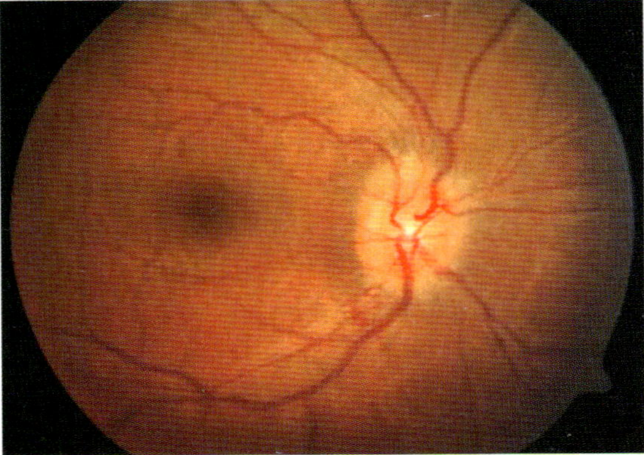

Fig. 12.2: Papilledema

Table 12.1: Differences between papillitis and papilledema

	Papillitis	*Papilledema*
Vision	Lost	Usually not lost
Pain on eyeball movement	Present	Absent
Swelling of optic disc	Minimal	Marked
Retinal vessels	Minimally distended	Markedly distended
Hemorrhages and exudates	Absent	Present
Unilateral/Bilateral	Usually unilateral	Usually bilateral

Causes

- Multiple sclerosis MS
- Orbital periostitis
- Inflammation of the sinus–frontal/maxillary spreading on to optic nerve
- Syphilis

Optic Atrophy (Fig. 12.3)

Characteristics: Disc is pale (white) with decreased number of capillaries.

Primary optic atrophy: Distinct disc margins (primary optic nerve disease/papillitis).

Secondary optic atrophy: Blurred disc margins (*see* papilloedema).

Causes of optic atrophy

- Chorioretinitis, retinitis pigmentosa
- Secondary to papillitis/papilloedema
- Multiple sclerosis
- Syphilis
- Ischemia to the optic nerve
- Optic nerve disease
- Hereditary neurological diseases

Retinal Artery Occlusion

Characteristics

- Pale and swollen retina
- **Cherry red spot** in the macular region
- Sudden total loss of vision

Retinal Vein Occlusion

Retinal hemorrhages appear to be splashing over the fundus (stormy fundus)—blood and thunder appearance of the fundus

Optic disc margin is significantly swollen.

Hypertensive Retinopathy

Grade I: Arterial thickening and tortuosity, localised or focal spasm AV ratio 1:2

Grade II: Grade I changes

- Generalised arterial spasm
- AV nipping
- AV ratio 1:3

Grade III: Grade II

- Exudates and hemorrhages
- AV ratio 1:4

Grade IV: Grade III + papilloedema

Note: AV ratio is the ratio between the diameter of the arterioles and the vein.

AV Nipping

Arteries press over the veins (due to high pressure) making them to constrict and may also disappear from the view.

Retinal hemorrhages

Type of bleed	*Structures involved*
Large dark red margins of hemorrhages	• Choroidal hemorrhages
Flame shaped hemorrhages	• Superficial retinal hemorrhages
Round dark red blots	• Deep retinal hemorrhages

Flat topped with fluid level situated in front of the retina suggests: Subhyaloid hemorrhage (due to subarachnoid bleed or bleeding from the retinal nerve vessels)

Hazy fundus/absent fundal glare: Vitreous hemorrhage (abnormal red reflex)

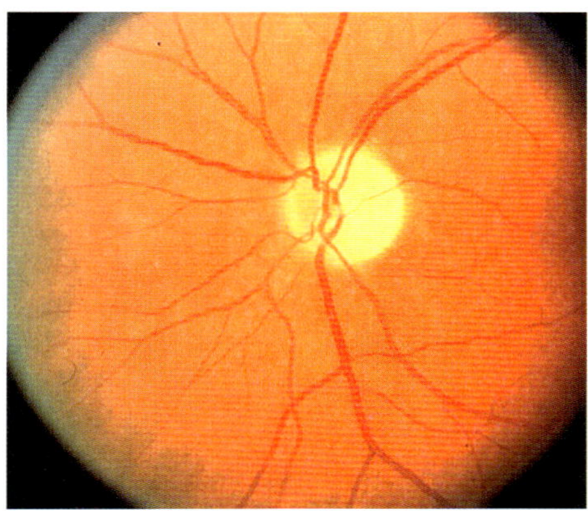

Fig. 12.3: Optic atrophy

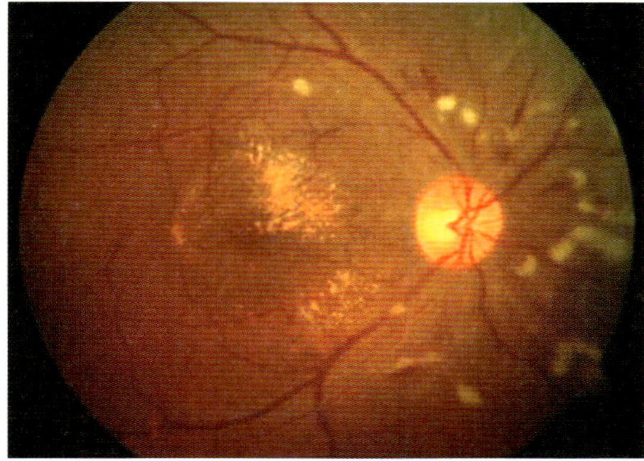

Fig. 12.4: Grade III retinopathy with hemorrhages and cotton wool spots and macular edema

Diabetic Retinopathy

Early background NPDR (non-proliferative diabetic retinopathy)

- Micro-aneurysms (appear as small dark red dots around the macula).
- Dot and blot hemorrhages.
- Cotton wool spots.

Proliferative diabetic retinopathy (PDR): New vessel formation (neovascularisation) at macula and optic nerve. Extension of these vessels can occur into the vitreous and their bleeding causes vitreous hemorrhage and visual loss.

Exudates in the Retina

Hard Exudates

Yellowish white deposits which are well defined. May be arranged in rings.

Hard exudates are due to

- Altered permeability of blood vessels with lipoprotein leaking out into the retinal layers.
- At macula they form a star like appearance.
- Seen in hypertension, diabetes mellitus and retinal vascular occlusion.

CRVO/CRAO

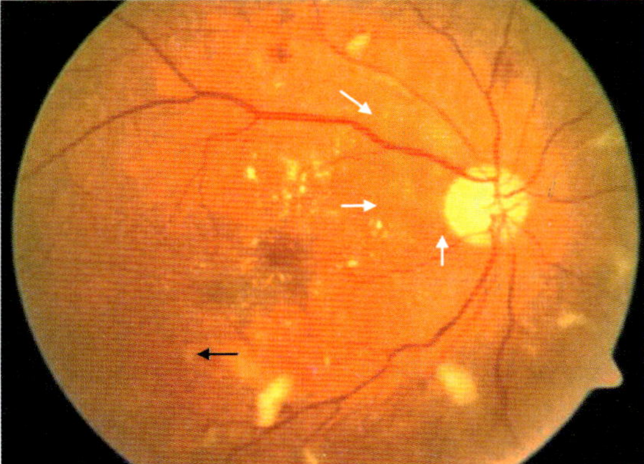

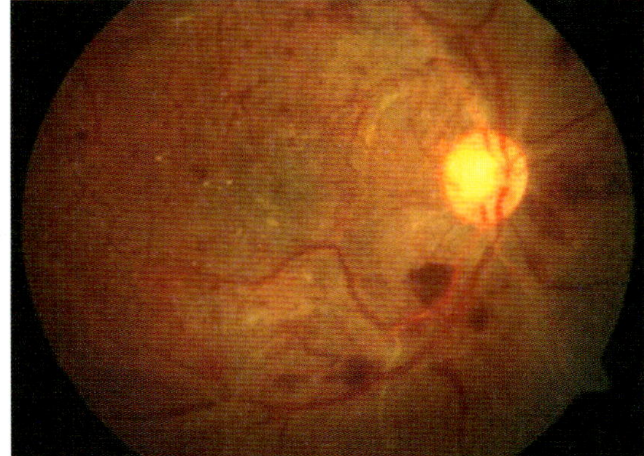

Fig. 12.5: Moderate-to-severe NPDR with cotton wool spots, and macular edema. PDR with neovascularization of the disc (arrows) and neovascularization elsewhere (black arrow)

Soft Exudates

- Due to retinal ischemia and swelling of the nerve fiber layer with focal infarcts.
- Appear as cotton wool deposits in the superficial retina called "cotton wool spots".
- Seen in hypertension/diabetes mellitus.

Choroid Tubercle

Characteristics

- Small yellowish white spots surrounded by edematous hazy retina and dilated retinal vessels.
- Seen in disseminated tuberculosis.

Arteriosclerotic Retinopathy

Normal arterioles appear as fine yellow lines with red blood column.

- *Grade I:* Minimal AV compression. Red blood column visible with broad yellow lines.
- *Grade II:* AV crossing changes are more prominent. Copper wire appearance (reddish brown), no blood column visible. Broad yellow line.
- *Grade III:* Blood column not visible. Broad white line–silver wire appearance.
- *Grade IV:* No visible blood column. Only fibrous cords are seen.

Cytoid Body in Ophthalmic Fundus

- Commonest retinal lesion in SLE
- It represents–while swollen nerve fibres
- It occurs due to vasculitis of the retinal capillaries causing localised microinfarction of the superficial nerve fibre layer of the retina.

Common Radiological Abnormalities

13

CHECKLIST FOR GENERAL PHYSICAL EXAMINATION

- General informations
- Interpretation of chest X-ray
- Different abnormalities in the chest X-ray
- X-ray skull and abdomen

Interpretation of Chest X-ray

Demographic details of the patient:

Name: Sex:

Age: Date of the X-ray:

General Informations while Interpreting the Chest X-ray

- View of the chest X-ray
- Positioning of the patient including rotation
- Exposure of the X-ray film
- Inspiratory/Expiratory film

Structural Details of Clinical Significance while Interpreting the Chest X-ray

- Neck shoulder
- Breast tissue
- Part of the abdomen
- Bony cage
- Costophrenic and cardiophrenic angles
- Diaphragm
- *Mediastinum:* Trachea, airways, cardiac shadow, major blood vessels and lung fields.

Different Chest X-ray Views

PA View (Posteroanterior view)

In PA view X-ray beam passes from posterior aspect of the chest and exists through the anterior aspect of the chest. Identification of PA view:

- Most common view taken while taking chest X-ray
- Cardiac shadow is not magnified
- There will be no overlapping of scapulae over the lung fields.

AP View (Anteroposterior view)

In AP view X-ray beam enters through the anterior aspect of the chest and exists through the posterior aspect of chest.

AP view is usually reserved for bedridden patients.

Identification of AP View

- There will be cranial projections of the clavicles over the lung apices
- Cardiac shadow is magnified with shortening of lung fields.

In PA view and AP view of the chest X-ray positioning of the structure are made out whether they are placed medially or laterally.

Other Chest X-ray Views

Lateral view: Left lateral and right lateral views.

In lateral views positions of the structure are made out whether they are placed anteriorly or posteriorly.

Lateral view is helpful in following circumstances:

- For posterior costophrenic recess
- For anterior and posterior mediastinum
- To localise the lesion suspected in the frontal view.

Decubitus Views

Patient is positioned in the right or left decubitus position. Decubitus view can differentiate pleural effusion/consolidation and loculated effusion/free fluid in the pleural cavity.

Lordotic View (Apicogram)

Lordotic view is useful for better visualization of the apex of the lung E—for Pancoast's tumor. LAO (left anterior oblique) and RAO (right anterior oblique) view are taken for delineation of cardiac chamber enlargement.

Inspiratory/Expiratory Film

Most of the chest X-rays are taken on full inspiration. On full inspiration posterior ribs 9 and 10 are clearly seen bilaterally.

Chest X–ray characteristics of well centralized patient without rotation:

- Clavicles are seen in the same horizontal plane on either side
- Medial end of the clavicles are equidistant from the vertebral spine

Exposure of the Chest X-ray Film

Following features suggest adequate chest X-ray film exposure:

- Vertebral column shadow is fully visible
- Translucent tracheal shadow will be visible up to the medial end of the clavicles
- Inter vertebral disc spaces are not clearly visible
- Vascular markings of the lungs are well made out.

Radiological Signs of Overpenetrated (Overexposed) Chest X-ray

- Cardiac shadow becomes decreased and heart becomes central and narrowed
- Hyperlucency of lung fields
- Spines of vertebrae and vertebral column will be clearly visible
- Tracheal translucency will be visible up to the bifurcation of trachea.

Airways: In a normality positioned and adequately exposed chest X-ray film tracheal lucency can be traced downwards in the midline and branches of bronchi can be made out.

Bony Structures

Observe for the following bony structures in the chest film:

- Chest wall including bony thorax and spines.
- Contour of ribs, placement of ribs and any abnormality like fracture/discontinuation of ribs.
- Check also for abnormality of shoulder joint.
- Look also for abnormality of soft tissue lesion, lytic lesion in the bone and free air in the thoracic cavity.

Cardiac shadow: Check for the cardiac borders and dimension of the cardiac shadow.

Measurement of Cardiac Dimension (Fig. 13.1)

Drop a perpendicular line at the centre of the chest from above downwards till the diaphragm in between the two medial ends of clavicles.

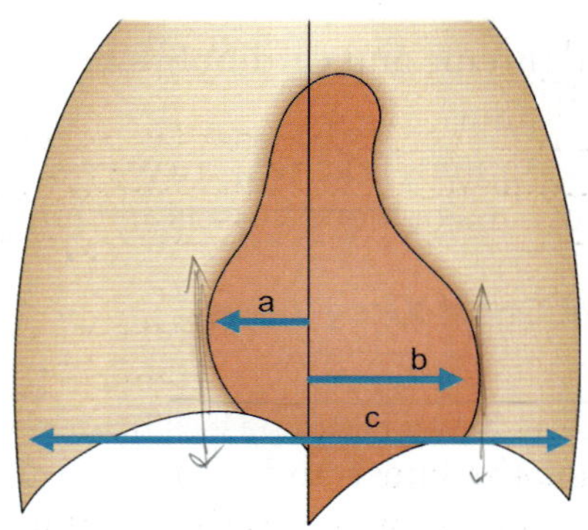

Fig. 13.1: Measurement of cardiac dimension

Drop another perpendicular line to the central line touching the left cardiac border (b) and right cardiac border (a) at their maximum distance from the central line.

Draw an intrathoracic horizontal line just above the diaphragm touching the rib cage on either side (c). Normally the sum of (a) and (b) is less than 50% of line (c).

It the sum of (a) and (b) is more than 50% of (c), it is suggestive of cardiomegaly.

Important causes of massive cardiomegaly

- Severe AR
- Severe MR
- Pericardial effusion
- Dilated cardio myopathy

While examining the cardiac shadow observe for the following

- Size and shape of the heart and cardiac borders
- Evidence for cardiac chamber enlargement
- Look for contour of aorta, positioning of arch of aorta and pulmonary arteries.

Cardiac Borders

Left cardiac border

Following structure represent left cardiac border from above downwards.

- Aortic knuckle
- Pulmonary artery
- Left atrial appendage
- Left ventricle

Right cardiac border: Normally, right cardiac border is mainly represented by the right atrium. A small portion of inferior vena cava and superior vena cava, can contribute to the right cardiac border.

If the right cardiac borders is > 5 cm from the midline it is indicative of right atrial enlargement. Cardiophrenic and costophrenic angles:

- Normally, cardiophrenic and costophrenic angles should be sharply delineated
- Blunting of costophrenic angle occurs in pleural effusion
- Pericardial effusion results in blunting of cardiophrenic angle

Diaphragm

Observe for the right and left (doom) of the diaphragm. Right doom of the diaphragm is about 2.5 cm above the level of left doom of the diaphragm.

3 cm or greater than 3 cm difference in the height between 2 sides of the diaphrgm is clinically significant.

Elevated doom of the diaphragm occurs in following conditions:

- *Supradiaphragmatic disorders:* Due to loss of lung volume—fibrosis or collapse of lower lobe.
- *Infradiaphragmatic pathology*
  - Massive ascites
  - Subdiaphragmatic abscess
  - Hepatic and splenic disorders

Flattening of diaphragm occurs in patients with hyperinflation of lung fields as in emphysema.

Lung Fields

Radiologically lung fields are divided to 3 zones

- Upper zone: Up to the 2nd costal cartilage
- Mid zone: From 2nd to 4th costal cartilage
- Lower zone: Below the 4th costal cartilage

Observe for the following structures while examining the lung fields in the chest X-ray

- Airways (right upper lobe bronchus is higher than left upper lobe bronchus)
- Interstitium of lungs
- Blood vessels
- Fissure location and thickening
- Pleural margins

Look for following abnormalities while inspecting the lung fields

- Abnormal densities/opacities
- Lucencies (trapping of air/bulla)
- Mass lesion
- Infiltrations
- Calcifications

Hilum of the Lung

This is the part or root of the lung where great arteries/veins and airways enter and exit from the lung.

Blood Vessels

- Trace the blood vessels (pulmonary arteries) from hilum of the lung.
- Look for the size and location and distribution of pulmonary arteries.
- The left pulmonary airways artery is always at a higher level than the right.

Pulmonary Artery

- Right pulmonary artery is anterior to the right main bronchus
- Left pulmonary artery lies above the left main bronchus
- Maximum size of descending pulmonary artery measured (1 cm medial and 1 cm lateral) to the hilar point—in males 16 mm. In females—15 mm.

Aortopulmonary Window (Pulmonary bay)

Aortopulmonary window is made out in PA view. It is formed by the overlap of the aortic arch and left pulmonary artery. Space should be clear and concave. If there is convexity in the region of aortopulmonary window, it may be indicative of enlarged lymph nodes, mass lesions or enlarged pulmonary artery.

Extrathoracic Structures

Observe for any abnormality of breast tissue and soft tissues of the upper part of the abdomen.

Gastric bubble: Fundal gas shadow: presence of lucency in the upper quadrant of the abdomen on the left side.

Hardwears: Chest X-ray may reveal presence of Ryle's tube, endotracheal tube, monitor leads and central venous lines, etc.

DIFFERENTIAL DIAGNOSIS OF IMPORTANT RADIOLOGICAL ABNORMALITIES IN THE CHEST X-RAY

Nodular Lesions (Pulmonary nodules)

Causes

- Granuloma—tuberculosis, fungal infection
- Benign and malignant neoplasm
- Pulmonary infection and pneumonia
- Wegener's granulomatosis
- Sarcoidosis
- Metastasis
- Multiple cannonball shadows: Due to tumor embolisation into the lungs (from breast, thyroid, prostate, renal cell carcinoma).

Ground glass appearance in the chest X-ray

Causes

- Diffuse interstitial pneumonia
- Extrinsic allergic alveolitis
- Alveolar proteinosis

Miliary Mottling in the Lung (Fig. 13.2)

Presence of mottling opacities (like millet seed sized 2–4 mm) in the lung fields.

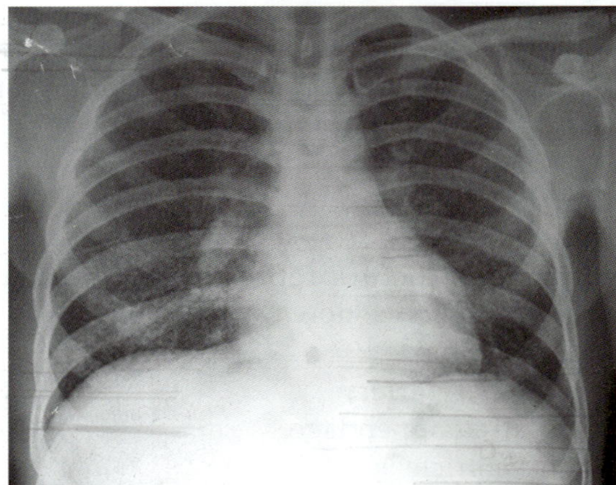

Fig. 13.2: Miliary mottling in the lung

Causes

- Miliary tuberculosis
- Pulmonary Eosinophilia
- Lymphangitis carcinomatosis
- Sarcoidosis

Pulmonary Nodules (Figs 13.3 and 13.4)

- *Nodule*: Opacity in the lung parenchyma which is less than 3 cm in diameter.
- *Mass lesion*: Opacity in the lung parenchyma which is 3 cm or more than 3 cm in diameter.

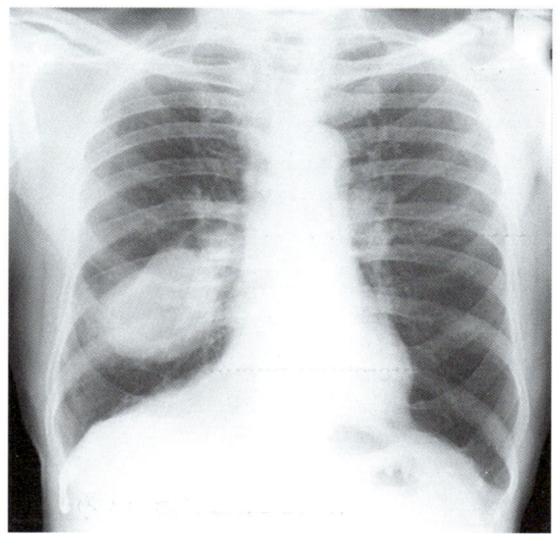

Fig. 13.3: Pulmonary mass lesion

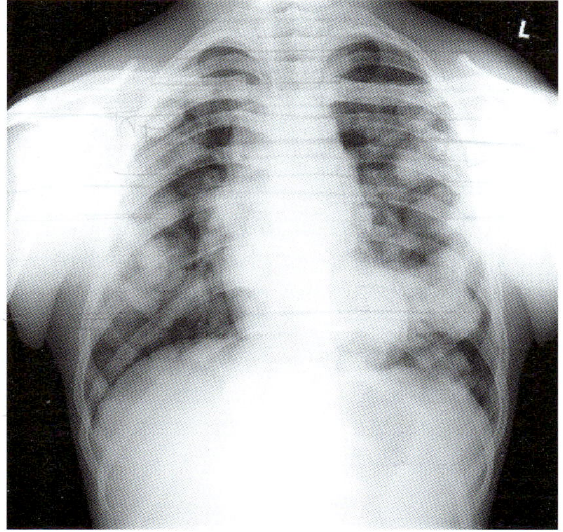

Fig. 13.4: Multiple cannonball shadows

- *Tumor doubling time*: time taken by the mass to become double of its previous volume.
- *Malignant lesions*: Usual doubling times 1–6 months
- If nodule size has not changed for 18 months it is usually benign. Important clinical aspects of a pulmonary nodular lesion
- Masses greater than 4 cm are usually malignant
- Calcification of the nodule favours a benign lesion
- Malignant nodules have notched or spiculated margins and are irregular in shape
- Hamartomas have classically popcorn calcification
- Granulomatous nodules can calcify and they are multiple and are usually similar in size.

Solitary pulmonary nodule: Well circumscribed nodular opacity in the lung of 1 to 6 cm size with normal surrounding lung parenchyma.

Pulmonary Collapse (Fig. 13.5)

Radiological signs

- Homogeneous opacity corresponding to a lobe/segment of the lung.
- Mediastinum shifted to the same side.
- No visible airbronchogram or bronchovascular markings.

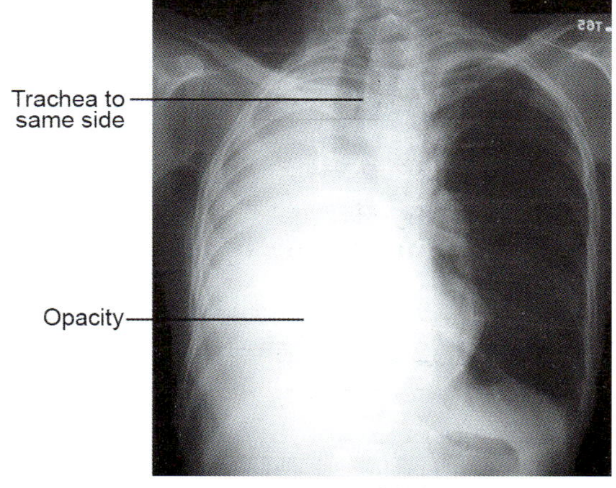

Fig. 13.5: Pulmonary collapse (atelectasis) of right lung

Pulmonary Cavity (Fig. 13.6)

Pulmonary cavity is a gas filled space, in the pulmonary parenchyma which is surrounded by complete wall which is 3 mm or more in its thickness.

Observe for the following findings while inspecting for a cavity in the chest X-ray.

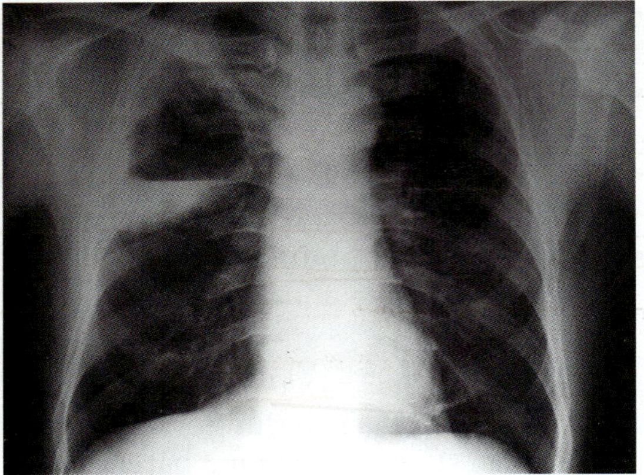

Fig. 13.6: Pulmonary cavity

- Structure of the cavity wall
- Contents of the cavity: Empty cavity/ presence of collection/aspergilloma
- Changes in the lung parenchyma around the cavity.

Causes of Cavity in the Lung

- Pulmonary tuberculosis
- Lung abscess
- Cavitating malignancy
- Cystic disease of the lung
- Cavitating granuloma (Wegener's granulomatosis)
- Cystic bronchiectasis

Thick walled cavities in the lung, e.g.

- Acute lung abscess
- Cavitating squamous cell carcinoma
- Wegener's granulomatosis

Thin walled cavities in the lung, e.g.

- Pneumatocoeles and hydatid cysts
- Pneumatocoeles are thin walled cavities which are produced secondary to Staphylococcal pneumonia.

Fluid levels: Common in cavities secondary to lung abscess, tumor cavities with necrotic mass or blood clot.

Air Crescent (Meniscus) Sign

- This is typical of aspergilloma inside a cavity
- Fungal ball inside a cavity is surrounded by a crescent of air.

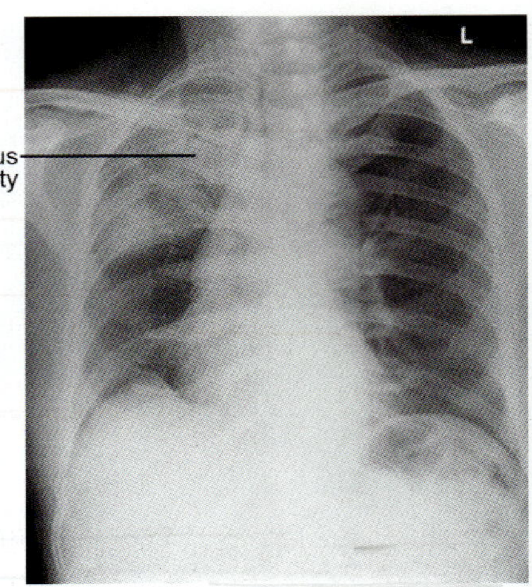

Fig. 13.7: Pulmonary consolidation right upper lobe

Consolidation of Lung

Radiological signs

- Homogeneous opacity corresponding to a lobe or bronchopulmonary segment
- Mediastinum is central
- Presence of air bronchogram
- Costophrenic angle is not blunted.

Air bronchogram: Presence of branching translucency corresponding to the bronchi and division of bronchi seen within the opacity. Air bronchogram is suggestive of consolidation.

Silhoutte sign: This is a radiological sign of right middle lobe consolidation. Right cardiac border is not able to be differentiated from the opacity (consolidation).

Pleural Effusion

Radiological signs

- Dense homogeneous opacity not corresponding to a lobe or segment of the lung
- Mediastinal shift to the opposite side
- Blunting of costophrenic angle on the side of the opacity.

Minimal of 75 ml of fluid is required to blunt the costophrenic angle on lateral X-ray

Minimum of 200 ml of fluid is required to produce blunting of costophrenic angle in the PA view.

Table 13.1: Characteristic chest X-ray appearances of certain congenital heart diseases

Congenital heart disease	*Chest X-ray appearance*
Tetralogy of Fallot	Boot shaped heart
Ebstein's anomaly	Box-like heart
Transposition of great arteries	Ovoid or egg shaped heart
Total anomalous pulmonary Venous connection	Figure of 8 or cottage leaf or snowman appearance
Coarctation of aorta	Figure of 3 sign (dilated left subclavian artery above, narrowing due to coarctation and dilated descending aorta)

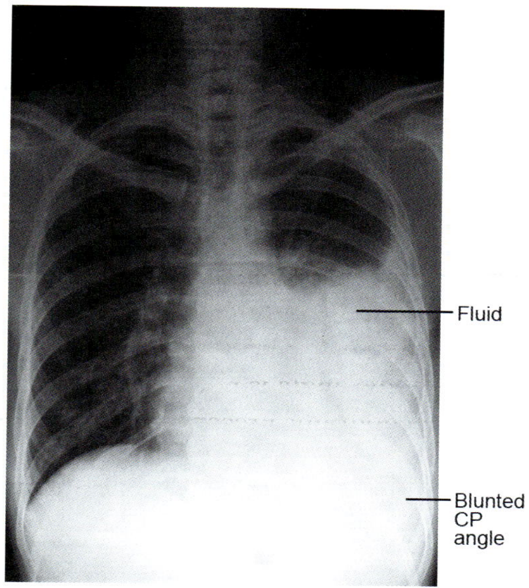

Fig. 13.8: Pleural effusion left side

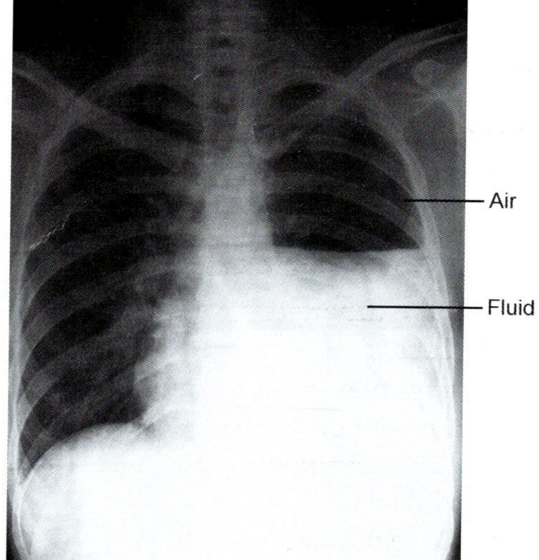

Fig. 13.9: Hydropneumothorax left side

Pleural effusion will present as a meniscus at its upper border on the upright chest X-ray.

Hydropneumothorax

- Hydropneumothorax presence of air (above) and fluid (below) in the pleural cavity
- There will be straight level of fluid other features will be pleural effusion.

Causes

- Tuberculosis
- Trauma to the chest
- Iatrogenic (after tapping of pleural effusion)

Pleural Thickening

Chest X-ray appearance: Costophrenic angle is blunted. Shadows/opacities appear to be vertically ascending linear shadows clinging onto the ribs.

Recticulonodular Shadows in the Chest X-ray

Causes

- Crytptogenic/idiopathic pulmonary fibrosis
- Connective tissue disorders
- Sarcoidosis
- Asbestosis
- Pneumocystis pneumonia

Chronic Bronchitis and Emphysema

Chronic bronchitis: Radiological signs: Prominent bronchovascular markings may give dirty lung appearance.

Emphysema (Fig. 13.10)

Radiological signs

- Hyperlucent lung fields
- Tubular heart shadow
- Low flat diaphragm
- Widening of intercostal spaces
- Presence of emphysematous bulla (usually in the apices of lung)

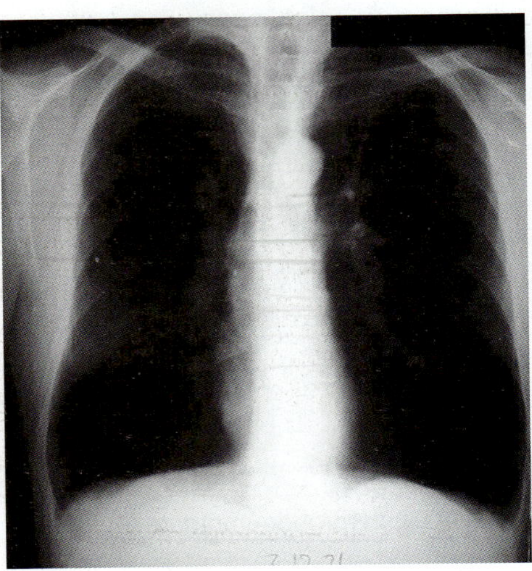

Fig. 13.10: Pulmonary emphysema

Emphysematous bulla: This is an airspace of more than 1 cm in diameter with complete destruction of lung parenchyma producing an emphysematous area.

Pneumothorax (Fig. 13.11)

- Presence of air in the pleural cavity–visible as hyperlucency with visible collapsed lung margin.
- Bronchovascular markings are absent inside the translucency
- Mediastinum is shifted to the opposite side

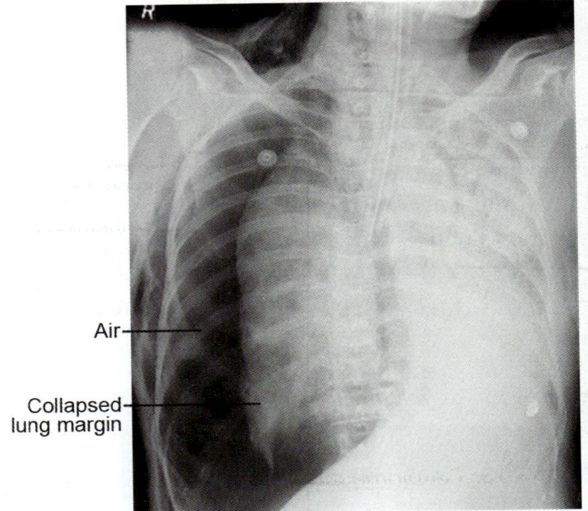

Fig. 13.11: Pneumothorax right side

Pulmonary Fibrosis (Fig. 13.12)

Radiological signs

- Homogeneous/nonhomogeneous opacities in the lung fields
- Evidence of volume loss on the side of fibrosis
- Mediastinum shifted to the side of fibrosis.

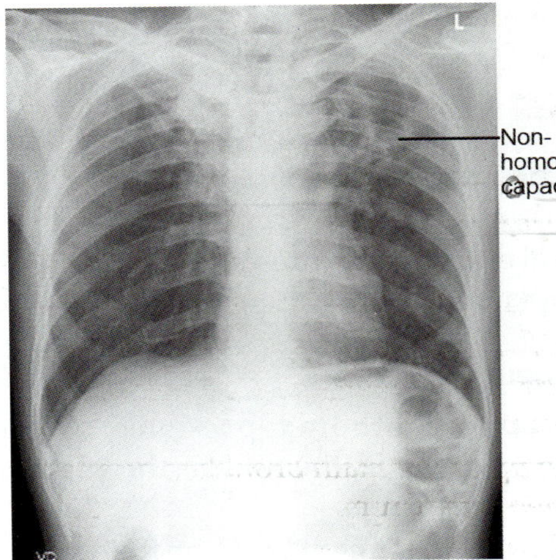

Fig. 13.12: Pulmonary fibrosis left upper lobe

Chest X-ray Findings in Patients with Rheumatic Mitral Stenosis (Fig. 13.13)

a. *Mitralisation of left cardiac border:* Straightening of the left heart border occurs due to

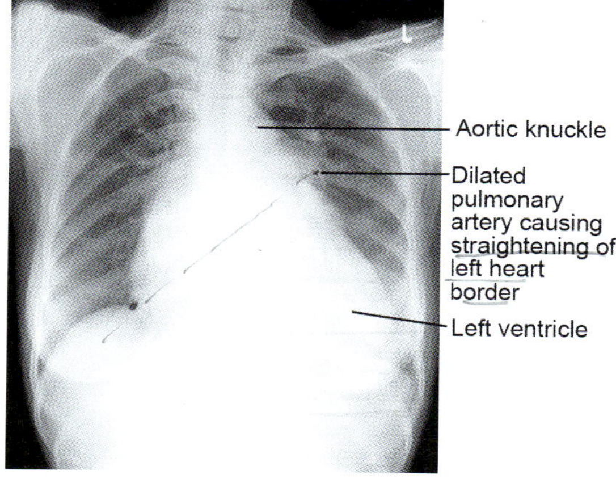

Fig. 13.13: Cardiomegaly with mitral valve disease

dilatation of pulmonary artery and dilated left atrium. Concavity of the pulmonary bay becomes obliterated.

b. *Hilar congestion:* Congestion of the pulmonary hilum (haziness on either side of the hilum) indicates early left heart failure.

c. *Batwing appearance*
   - Haziness of the lung fields starting from hilum to the periphery in a winged manner. This is indicative of severe pulmonary edema.
   - Prominent upper lobe veins: Veins of the upper lobe of the lung become prominent and dilated indicating chronic pulmonary venous hypertension.
   - Kerley B lines: Thickened horizontal lines delineated near the costophrenic angle indicates chromic pulmonary venous hypertension.

Other chest X-ray findings in a patient of mitral valve disease

- Lifting up of left main bronchus due to the enlarged left atrium.
- Double right atrial border: Due to massively enlarged left atrium, border of the left atrium can be made out as a separate shadow inside the right cardiac border.

Calcification of valve

- Calcified mitral valve: Made out below the level of imaginary oblique line which joins right cardiophrenic angle to the left pulmonary hilum.
- Calcified aortic valve: Made out above the level of abovesaid imaginary oblique line.

Bronchiectasis: Chest X-ray may be normal in early stages.

Later stages:

- Appear as thickening of bronchi
- Cystic shadows or may appear as cavities
- Lateral view may show tram track appearance due to parallel thickened wall of bronchi.

Pericardial Effusion (Fig. 13.14)

Radiological signs

- Cardiomegaly with narrow hilum (water bottle/money bag appearance)
- Obliteration of cardiophrenic angle.

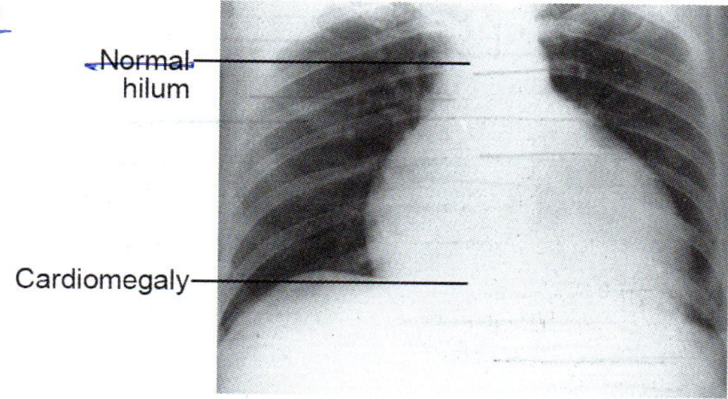

Fig. 13.14: Pericardial effusion

Multiple Punched out Lesion in the Skull (Fig. 13.15)

Causes

- Multiple myeloma
- Metastases into the skull
- Eosinophilic granuloma

X-ray Skull Appearance in Hyperparathyroidism

- Skull will have tiny granular appearance (salt and pepper skull/pepper pot skull)
- Skull can have small punched out lesions and there will be loss of differentiation between outer and inner table of the skull.

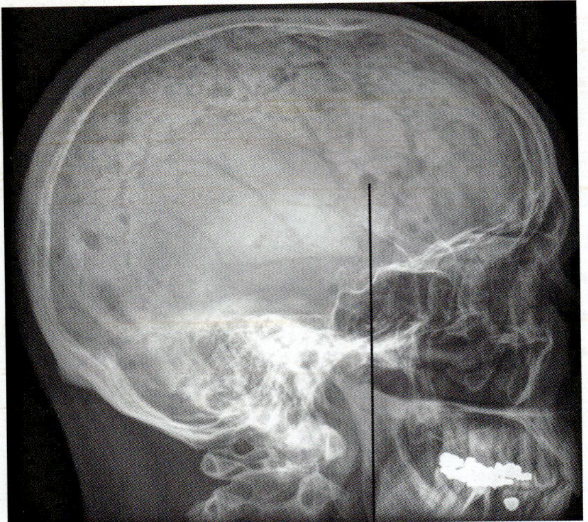

Fig. 13.15: Skull X-ray lateral view showing multiple punched out lesions—multiple myeloma

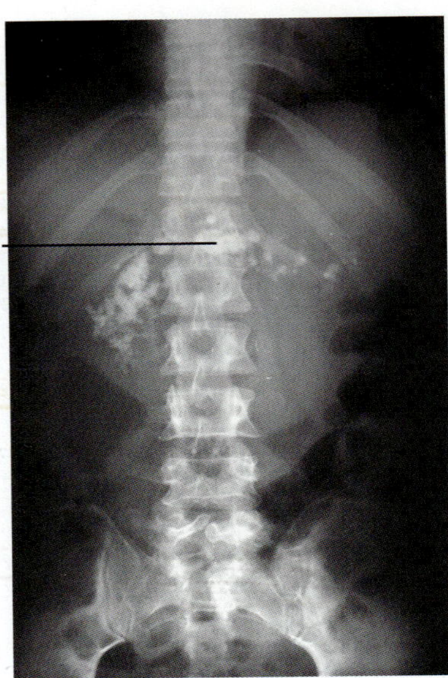

Fig. 13.16: Abdominal X-ray showing opacities across L1 vertebra suggestive of pancreatic calcification

Pancreatic Calcification

Opacities across L1 vertebra suggestive of pancreatic calcification.

Other cause of intra-abdominal opacities

- Renal calculi (on either side of vertebra)
- Calcified lymph nodes
- Faecoliths

Common Bedside Procedures in Medicine

14

CHECKLIST FOR GENERAL PHYSICAL EXAMINATION

- Ascitic tap (paracentesis of the abdomen)
- Bone marrow examination
- Liver biopsy
- Lumbar puncture
- Pleural tap (thoracentesis)

Ascitic Tap (Paracentesis of the abdomen)

Indications

Diagnostic: For diagnosis of causes of ascites, to differentiate between transudative and exudative causes of ascites.

Therapeutic

- In patients with refractory ascites in cirrhosis
- Massive abdominal distention with respiratory difficulty due to ascites.

Massive paracentesis of the abdomen to be avoided if

- Serum bilirubin >10 mg/dl
- Platelet count < 40,000/cmm
- Serumcreatinine > 3 mg/dl
- Impending hepatic encephalopathy

Prerequisites for ascetic tap

- Empty the urinary bladder
- Position of the patient supine

Site of Tapping (Fig. 14.1)

Left lower quadrant of the abdomen: Point selected at the junction of lateral 1/3rd to the medial 2/3rds of the line joining the anterior superior iliac spine and umbilicus.

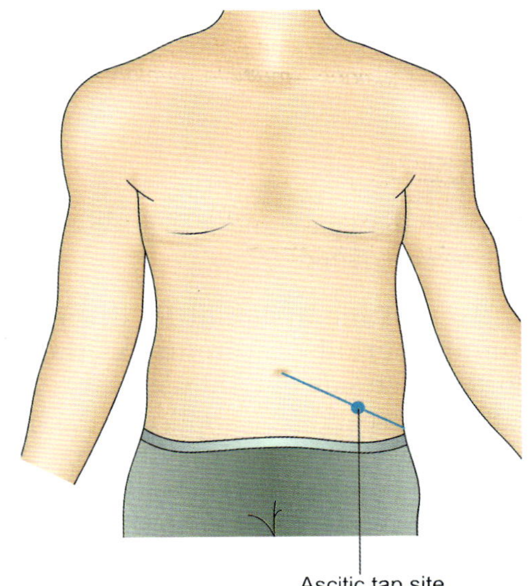

Fig. 14.1: Site for ascitic tap

Local anesthesia: Infiltrate the skin and subcutaneous tissue with 2% lignocaine.

Needle used: A large bore needle of sufficient length.

Procedure: Introduce the needle through the skin and subcutaneous tissue into the peritoneal cavity (ascitic fluid starts draining through the needle).

Connect needle to the syringe and fluid is aspirated.

If the fluid is not draining out properly needle position can be adjusted within the peritoneal cavity with gentle mobilization and patient's position can be shifted to the left lateral side.

Complications of Ascitic Fluid Aspiration

- Relatively a safe procedure
- Syncope can occur due to removal of large amount of fluid
- Bleeding into the peritoneal cavity
- perforation of viscus
- precipitation of hepatic encephalopathy

Note: Ascitic fluid is sent for analysis for the following parameters:
- Biochemistry
- Cytology
- AFB
- Gram stain
- Culture sensitivity
- Amylase and lipase and malignant cytology whenever required

Aftercare: Patient should lie down for a minimum period of 2 hours on the side opposite to the side of fluid removal.

- A Benzoin seal can be applied at the site of aspiration.
- A tight abdominal binder can be applied if there is leakage of ascitic fluid.

Large amount of ascitic fluid can be removed (5–10 liters at a time) in therapeutic paracentesis in patients with cirrhosis (replace 8 gm of albumin/liter of fluid removed) and in patient with massive ascites to relieve the discomfort and to increase renal blood flow.

Causes of Ascites

Transudative ascites

Features

- Clear fluid
- Fluid protein < 3 gr/dl
- Fluid LDH is less than 60% of serum LDH
- Fluid cell count < 250 cells/cmm

Causes

- CCF
- Cirrhosis of liver
- Nephrotic syndrome

Exudative Ascites

Features

- Straw colored/hemorrhagic/purulent
- Fluid protein > 3 gr/dl
- Fluid LDH > 60% of serum LDH
- Fluid cell count > 250 cells/cmm

Causes

- Peritonitis (pyogenic/tubercular)
- Primary/secondary abdominal malignancy
- Lymphomas
- Connective tissue diseases.

BONE MARROW EXAMINATION

Bone marrow examination is carried out by aspiration and biopsy of the bone marrow.

Aspiration of the marrow is helpful in following circumstances

- For forming smear of marrow cells and examination of morphology of marrow cells.
- For examination of marrow cellular elements.
- Biopsy of the bone and associated marrow by the biopsy needle is performed for following examinations: For cellularity, infection, infiltration and fibrosis of the bone marrow.

Indication of Bone Marrow Aspiration and Biopsy

- Bone marrow culture and sensitivity: For infections like Salmonella, Brucella, Mycobacterium, etc.
- Evaluation of fever of undetermined origin, e.g. tuberculosis, fungal infections, granulomas, malaria, kala-azar.
- In the diagnosis of primary hematological malignacies, e.g. leukemias, lymphomas.
- For metastasis of the marrow by primary malignancies

- In the diagnosis of systemic disorders like iron overload, storage disorders, systemic mastocytosis
- For follow-up and treatment of hematological disorders:
  - Post radiation and chemotherapy
  - Bone marrow transplantation

Sites of Bone Marrow Aspiration

- *In children:* Anterior medial tibial area, spines of L1 and L2 vertebrae
- *In adults—most preferred site:* Posterior iliac crest.

Anterior iliac crest: Its posterior iliac crest is not approachable due to pain, surgery or radiation.

Sternal Aspiration

- Aspiration is performed at 2nd intercostal space. Bone biopsy is not possible at sternum, only bone marrow aspiration is possible.
- While performing sternal puncture penetration of the inner table of the sternum is possible with damage to the great arteries.

Bone Marrow Aspiration and Biopsy Needle (Fig. 14.2)

Parts of the needle: 14–18 guaze needle, has got removable obturator which prevents plugging of the needle.

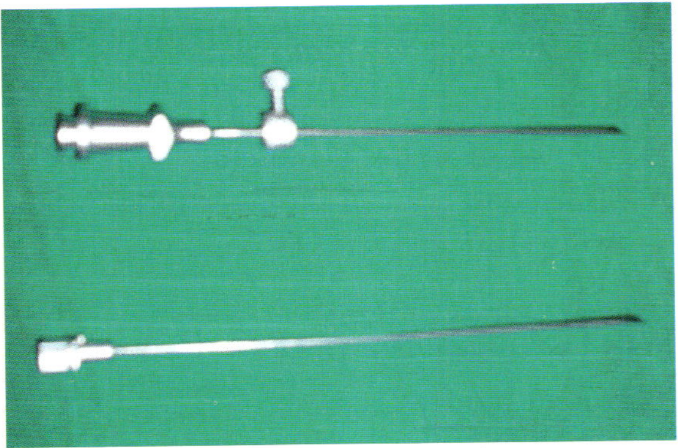

Fig. 14.2: Bone marrow aspirations needle

Stylet: To express the bone marrow biopsy sample from the needle. Marrow material can be aspirated from a syringe connected to the needle.

Bone Marrow Biopsy Needle (Fig. 14.3)

- *Name*: **Jemshedi** needle
- *Parts*: Hollow needle with beveled tip obturator and stylet.

Sternal puncture needle has a guard to limit the penetration of the needle.

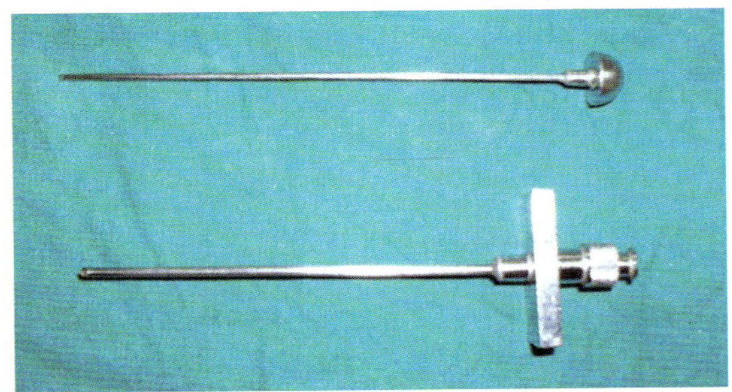

Fig. 14.3: Bone marrow biopsy needle

Procedure of Bone Marrow Aspiration (Fig. 14.4)

- Select the site (usually) posterior iliac crest
- Disinfect the area with antiseptic lotion.

Local Anesthesia

Anesthetise the skin, subcutaneous tissue and periosteum (most pain sensitive) with 1% lignocaine and achieve anesthesia effect.

Technique of Bone Marrow Aspiration

- Patient is in prone position. Introduce the bone marrow aspiration or biopsy needle

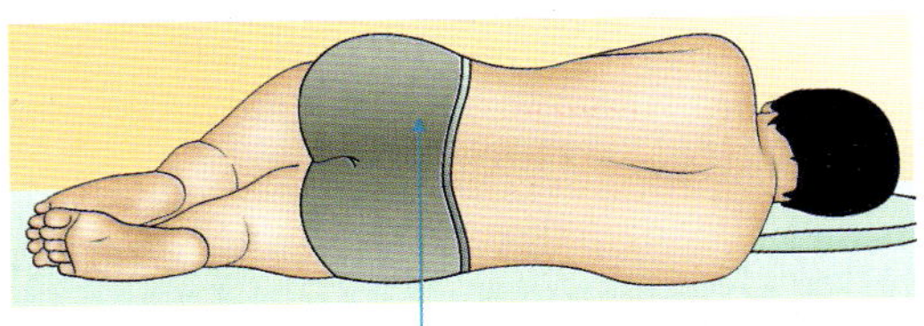

Fig. 14.4: Bone marrow aspiration site–iliac crest

through the skin, subcutaneous tissue and bone cortex with a rotatory motion (a small cut can be made through the skin)

- A give away sensation is felt once the needle enters into the marrow cavity.
- Remove the obturator and connect a 10–20 ml syringe to the needle and rapid suctioning of the marrow is made through the syringe—obtain 1 to 2 ml of bloody fluid.

If no marrow is obtained— rotate the needle again and do the suction through the syringe or relocate the area and repeat the procedure. Marrow material is used for:

- Making the smear
- Culture of the material
- Cytology and cytogenetic study

Bone Marrow Biopsy

- After obtaining the bone marrow aspiration as described above, needle is further rotated and advanced with more pressure and rotating movements (repositioning of the needle is preferred to prevent artifacts). Once the needle is in the bone, needle becomes stable. Needle is removed and biopsy is expressed from the stylet.
- Biopsy specimen is fixed, decalcified and processed.

Aftercare, After Bone Marrow Aspiration and Biopsy

- Apply manual pressure for several minutes to prevent bleed, patient is to lie down in recumbent position for 60 minutes and the site is bandaged.
- Pressure bandage is applied in the presence of thrombocytopenia and coagulation disorders.

Complication of Bone Marrow Aspiration and Biopsy

- Pain at the site of biopsy
- Hematoma formation
- Introduction of infection

Dry Bone Marrow Tap (Unable to obtain aspiration and biopsy)

- Defective technique
- Infiltration and too much cellular marrow, e.g. leukemias)
- Marrow fibrosis.

LIVER BIOPSY

Indication for Liver Biopsy

- Pyrexia of undetermined origin
- Unexplained jaundice
- Aetiological diagnosis of cirrhosis of liver
- Hepatic malignancies
- Storage disease/Wilson disease

Contraindications for Liver Biopsy

Absolute contraindications

- Bleeding Tendencies
- Hemangioma/hydatid cyst of the liver
- Chronic passive congestion of the liver
- Hepatic encephalopathy

Relative contraindications

- Massive ascites
- Infection at the biopsy site
- Severe jaundice
- May precipitate hepatic encephalopathy

Prerequisite for liver biopsy

- Informed consent
- Tests for bleeding parameters like bleeding time, clotting time, prothrombin time, activated partial prothrombin time and platelet count
- Stand by blood transfusion
- Tapping of ascites if present
- Ultrasound scan of the liver to know the architecture and liver size.

Different Types of Liver Biopsy Needles (Fig. 14.5)

- Tru-cut biopsy
- Menghini aspiration biopsy
- Vim Silverman needle biopsy

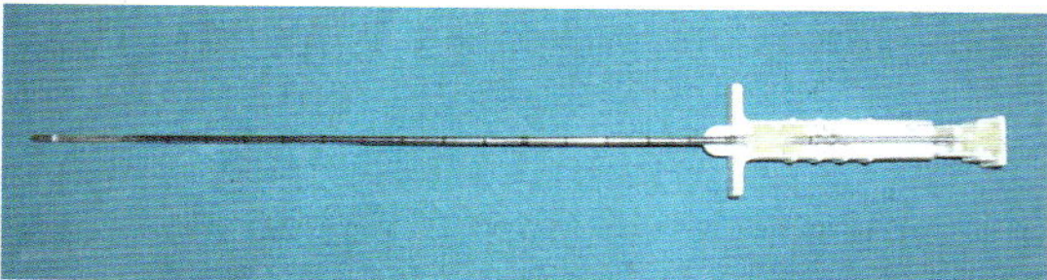

Fig. 14.5: Liver biopsy needle tru-cut

Technique of Liver Biopsy

Vim Silverman Needle Biopsy Procedure (*Fig. 14.6*)

Premedication

- If the patient is very anxious –IM diazepam 10 mg along with 1 amp. inj—atropine
- Local application of antiseptics
- Local anaesthesia with 1% lignocaine (5 to 10 ml). Infiltrate the skin, subcutaneous tissues and up to the liver capsule.

Site of needle introduction: 8th or 9th intercostal space in the midaxillary line—right side.

Technique

- Needle is introduced through the skin, subcutaneous tissues into the liver.
- Direction of the needle is held posterior and cranially to avoid injury to the gall bladder
- Needle moves with respiration if the needle is inside the liver.
- Patient is asked to hold the breath on expiration.
- Once the needle is inside the liver trocar is removed and bifurcated needle is introduced into the cannula. Once the bifurcated needle enters the liver tissue outer cannula is rotated over the bifurcated needle so that the cut liver tissue remains inside the needle.

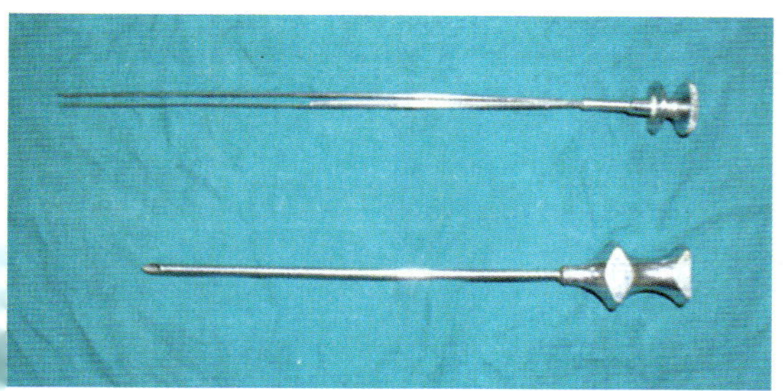

Fig. 14.6: Vim Silverman needle

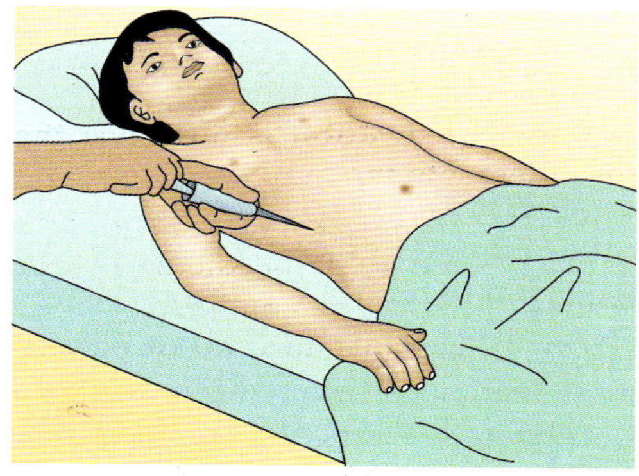

Fig. 14.7: Site for liver biopsy

- Now both the outer cannula and bifurcated needle are rotated together and both are withdrawn. Tissue which is present in the bifurcated needle is collected into the collecting fluid.
- Menghini's aspiration biopsy
- Saline is injected into liver substance through the needle and liver material is aspirated. This causes less destruction of the liver substance and minimal distress for the patient.

Aftercare

- Apply benzoin seal at the puncture site
- Bed rest for 24 hours
- Regular monitoring of pulse and blood pressure every 15 minutes for first 2 hours
- Observe the patient for 24 hours.

Complications

- Vasovagal attack (give atropine for bradycardia and sweating)
- Pain—at the biopsy site for the 24 hours in the right hypochondrium.
- Referred pain from diaphragm to the shoulder, occasionally pain also may be due to subcapsular hematoma/biliary peritonitis.

Bleeding

- Bleeding can occur inside the liver/or to the biliary tract. If severe bleeding—blood transfusion should be administered.

- If severe hypotension, abdominal distension and ultrasound showing intraperitoneal collection of blood—surgical intervention is required.

Other forms of biopsy of the liver
- Ultrasound/CT guided biopsy
- Using biopsy gun
- FNAC liver

Transjugular biopsy *(preferred) in patients with*
- Uncooperative patients
- Massive ascites
- Coagulation disorders
- Smaller sized liver

LUMBAR PUNCTURE

Lumbar puncture is a procedure where in there is aspiration of cerebrospinal fluid from spinal subarachnoid space by puncturing the lumbar subarachnoid space.

Indications of Lumbar Puncture (Fig. 14.8)

Diagnostic
- For measuring the CSF pressure
- Obtaining CSF sample for cytology, chemical and bacteriological examination.
- To inject radiopaque substance in myelography, radioactive agent as in radionuclide cysternography.

Therapeutic
- For reduction of CSF pressure, e.g. in normal pressure hydrocephalus.
- For administration of spinal anesthesia, antibiotics, anti-tumor agents.

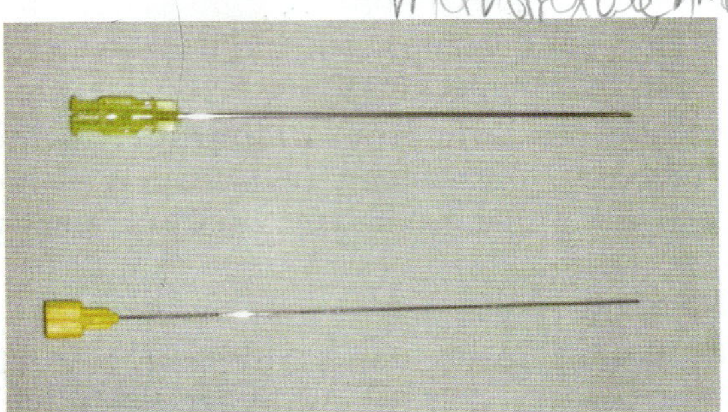

Fig. 14.8: Lumbar puncture needle

Contraindications for lumbar puncture (CI)

Absolute: Raised intracranial tension.

Relative: Local infection at the site of lumbar puncture site, significant deformity of spine.

Technique of Lumbar Puncture (Fig. 14.9)

Patient position
- Positioned on his side.
- Axis of hips vertical, hip and knee flexed.
- Knee is flexed as close to the head as possible.
- Patient is positioned near to the edge of the bed.
- Pillow can be kept beneath the ear.

Site of puncture
- Easiest at L3–L4 vertebral interspace (at the level of highest level of iliac crest. Spinal cord ends at the level of lower part of L1 vertebra).
- One space above or below can also be chosen (above L3–L4 vertebra).

Local anesthesia and sterilization
- Skin over the back is sterilized with spirit (from lower dorsal vertebra up to coccyx).
- Infiltrate the skin, subcutaneous tissue and deeper structures (up to ligamentum flavum) with 2% lignocaine.

Lumbar Puncture Needle and the Procedure

Smallest possible/atraumatic needle to be used. Needle with stylet is introduced into the space.

Needle is introduced in the direction upwards and forwards through the supraspinous and interspinous ligament.

After piercing the ligaments (about 4 to 7 cm) give in sensation is felt when the needle

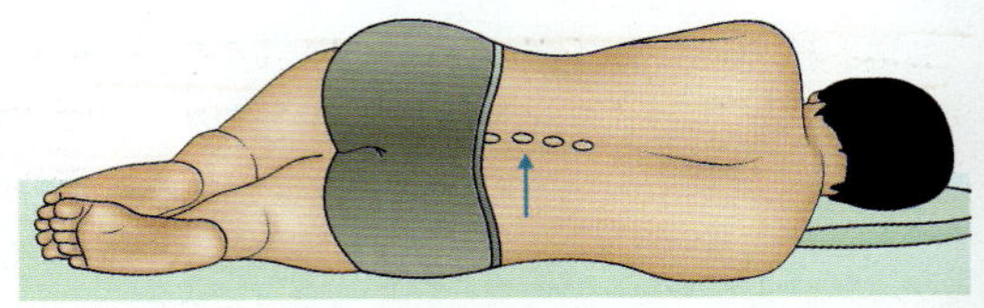

Fig. 14.9: Position of patient and site for lumbar puncture

pierces the dura and enters into the subarachnoid space. Remove the stylet slowly and collect the CSF in different containers.

Note: Rapid removal of stylet can injure nerve roots.

Occurrence of sciatica pain indicates needle is too lateral. If CSF flow is slow elevate the head of the patient.

Complications and Risks of Lumbar Puncture

- In case of raised intracranial tension (evidenced by headache and papilledema) fatal cerebellar and transtentorial herniation can occur.
- Transtentorial herniation risk is high in patients with intracranial mass lesion with displacement of brain tissue.
- Except in patients with pyogenic meningitis (CSF examination is mandatory) it is preferable to perform CT/MRI of brain before lumbar puncture if intracranial pressure elevation is suspected.
- In patients with suspected elevation of raised intracranial tension following precautions are preferable before performing lumbar puncture.
  - Perform LP with thin bore— no 22 or 24 gauge needle.
  - Administer IV mannitol before performing lumbar puncture.
  - Inj. dexamethasone IV 10 mg and then 4 mg to 6 mg QID to reduce the intracranial pressure.

In patients with spinal block—cysternal puncture/lateral cervical subarachnoid puncture can be performed.

Note: If there is failure to obtain CSF in lying down position try, in sitting position and then patient can be asked to lie down while removing CSF.

Dry tap of CSF: Failure to obtain CSF may be due to:

Faulty technique

- Chronic adhesive arachnoiditis
- Obliteration of subarachnoid space by compressive lesion of cauda equina.

Complications of Lumbar Puncture

- Post lumbar puncture headache (due to lower CSF pressure)
- Bleeding into the meningeal space if bleeding/clotting disorder is present.
- Rarely bacterial meningitis/disc space infection with nonsterile technique.

Examination of CSF

CSF obtained is examined for

- CSF pressure
- Color of CSF
- Cell type, cell count and tumor cells
- Gram stain, AFB, culture sensitivity, bacteria and fungus.

Special circumstances: Viral PCR, TB PCR, cryptococcus antigen and virus isolation.

CSF Pressure

- CSF pressure is measured by manometer attached to the LP needle.
- Normal CSF open pressure in adult: 100–180 mm of H_2O (8–14 mm of Hg).
- Raised CSF pressure: Above 200 mm H_2O
- Low CSF pressure: Less than 50 mm of H_2O, e.g. leak of CSF and systemic hypotension.

Normal CSF Analysis

Color: Clear

Pressure: 100–180 mm of H_2O

Protein: 45 mg/dl or less

Glucose: 60% of corresponding blood glucose

Chloride: Around 720 mEq/l

Cells: 5 lymphocytes/mononuclear cells/cmm

Quickenstedt's Test

- *Significance*: To detect the block between the intracranial and spinal subarachnoid space.
- *Procedure*: Connect the manometer to the LP

needle and note the CSF pressure during the lumbar puncture.

Apply pressure over the jugular veins and note the change in the CSF pressure in the manometer.

Normally, CSF pressure raises while applying pressure over the jugular veins because of transmission of intracranial pressure to the spinal subarachnoid space. If there is no significant raise in the CSF pressure while compressing the jugular vein indicates block in the CSF pathway.

Appearance of CSF

Normal CSF: Clear

Several hundred WBCs in the CSF (pleocytosis)–CSF color can become opaque.

Traumatic Tap (Bloody tap)

Blood gets into CSF from blood from epidural venous plexus. Collection of samples of CSF to be done in 3 separate containers. In a traumatic tap 2nd and 3rd sample of the CSF color decreases.

Presence of large amount of blood in the CSF—clot or fibrin web may be formed.

Usually there will be 2 WBCs/1000 RBCs in a traumatic tap of CSF.

Subarachnoid Hemorrhage

- All samples of CSF are equal in color
- Color of CSF becomes pinkish to red due to hemolysis of RBCs (erythrochromasia).

In subarachnoid hemorrhage: If CSF is allowed to stay for day CSF color becomes yellow-brown. This is called xanthochromia of the CSF. There may be presence of crenated RBCs in the CSF.

Causes of Xanthochromia of CSF

- Bleeding into the CSF with hemolysis of RBCs
- Hyperbilirubinemia
- Significant elevation of CSF protein (> 150 mg/dl), xanthochromia occurs due to albumin bound fraction of bilirubin.
- Hypercarotenemia.

Cellularity of CSF: Normal CSF may contain 5 lymphocytes/Mononuclear cells/cmm.

Abnormal cellularity of CSF

- Neutrophilia in CSF (normally neutrophils are absent in CSF): Pyogenic/bacterial infection of meninges.
- Lymphocytosis in CSF: TB, fungal/viral infection of meninges.
- Eosinophils in CSF (Hodgkin's disease/parasitic infection)
- India ink stain positive in CSF can occur in cryptococcal meningitis.
- Occasionally tumor cells can be identified.
- Gram stain, acid fast bacilli and culture sensitivity of CSF may demonstrate the pathogenic organism.

CSF Protein

- Normal CSF protein : 45 mg/dl or less
- Excess of CSF protein indicates: Meningeal/ependymal pathology.
- Traumatic tap–CSF protein raise by 1 mg/1000 RBCs
- Subarachnoid hemorrhage

In subarachnoid hemorrhage protein raises in the CSF due to chemical irritation of the meninges by hemolysed RBCs.

In pyogenic meningitis: CSF protein may be around 500 mg/dl.

In viral meningitis CSF protein may reach around 200 mg/dl.

Albuminocytological dissociation: Significant raise in CSF protein (500 mg/dl) without cellular response, e.g. Guillain-Barré syndrome.

CSF protein > 1000 mg/dl: Can occur in patients with CSF block/CSF loculation.

Froin syndrome: Deep yellow CSF with very high protein content and CSF can clot (due to high content of fibrinogen), e.g. CSF block/spinal block.

> *Note:* Meningismus is the term used for occurrence of febrile illness with signs of meningeal irritation with normal CSF analysis.

CSF chloride: Normal CSF chloride is around 119 mEq/L. CSF chloride can be low in bacterial meningitis.

CSF Glucose

- Normal CSF glucose—45 to 80 mg/dl
- CSF glucose less than 35 mg/dl abnormal
- Low CSF glucose—pyogenic/tubercular, fungal and neoplastic meningitis
- In viral meningitis invariably CSF glucose is normal.

Significance of CSF glucose in pyogenic meningitis

- CSF glucose decreases less than 60% of corresponding blood glucose in pyogenic meningitis
- If CSF glucose becomes less than 40% of blood glucose it is more definitive of pyogenic meningitis.
- CSF sugar may be zero in pyogenic meningitis.

Very low sugar in CSF in pyogenic meningitis is considered to be due to impaired membrane transfer system causing inhibition of glucose transport into the CSF.

Characteristics of CSF in Different CNS Disorders

Bacterial Meningitis

- Colour may be opaque
- Pressure is increased
- Glucose is greatly reduced
- Protein around 100–250 mg/dl
- Cells neutrophils present

Gram stain and culture sensitive may demonstrate the organism in the CSF.

TB Meningitis

- CSF may clot on standing for 24 hrs (cob-web formation due to high protein content of the CSF)
- Pressure is increased
- Glucose minimally decreased
- CSF lymphocytosis
- AFB may be positive in the CSF/TB PCR may be positive in CSF.

Viral and Fungal Meningitis

- CSF pressure may be increased
- CSF glucose minimally reduced or normal
- CSF protein increased (around 50–200 mg/dl)
- Cells WBCs (lymphocytes) 10–100 cell/ cmm

Ischemic Stroke (CVA)

- CSF pressure may be normal or increased if cerebral edema occurs
- CSF glucose: Normal
- CSF protein: Normal
- Cellular content: Normal

Intracerebral Hemorrhage (Hypertensive)

- CSF pressure: Usually increased
- CSF glucose: Normal
- CSF protein may be elevated
- CSF cells: Excess of RBCs especially if blood is leaking into the ventricles.

Subarachnoid Hemorrhage

- CSF pressure is increased
- CSF color—xanthochromia present
- CSF glucose is normal
- CSF protein is increased (50–150 mg/dl)
- RBCs significantly increased (> 500 cells/ cmm)
- Presence of crenated RBCs.

PLEURAL FLUID ASPIRATION (THORACENTESIS)

Indicates for Thoracentesis

- *Diagnostic:* For pleural fluid analysis to determine the aetiology of pleural effusion.

Key Points

- In TB pleural effusion mesothelial cells are almost absent in the pleural fluid.
- Absence of mesothelial cells in the pleural fluid in tuberculosis is due to the formation of layer of fibrin over the pleural surface.
- In pyogenic pleural effusion lymphocytosis of pleural fluid can occur due to treatment.

- *Therapeutic:* To relieve dyspnea in a patient of massive pleural effusion.

Patient's Position (Fig. 14.10)

Patient is sitting upright. Arm and head supported by the adjustment table.

Site of aspiration

- Identify the upper border of the effusion by percussion.
- Mark the site of aspiration— usually 7th or 8th intercostal space in the midaxillary or scapular line. Select the upper border of the lower rib for aspiration (intercostal vessels and nerves run in the groove of the lower border of the rib).
- Site of aspiration should be free from disease.
- Loculated fluid—ultrasound guided aspiration is recommended.

Local anesthesia: Infiltrate the skin, subcutaneous tissue and parietal pleura with local anesthetic 2% lignocaine.

Procedure

- Aspiration needle is introduced at the site already marked. Advance the needle continuously with gentle pressure until the give way sensation is felt (parietal pleura is penetrated—fluid is obtained). Aspiration of air suggests penetration deep into the lung and needle to be withdrawn.
- If the tapping of fluid is attempted very low (below the 10th intercostals space) needle can injure the diaphragm, liver (right side) and spleen (left side). Patient will complain of pain at the shoulder if the diaphragm is irritated.
- Once the needle is in the pleural space (fluid is coming out) connect to the syringe and aspirate the fluid (50 to 100 ml of fluid is required for analysis).
- More than one liter of fluid should not be aspirated as it can cause unilateral pulmonary edema due to reperfusion injury.
- Reperfusion injury occurs due to release of free radicals causing increased permeability of the capillaries and also due to restoration of intrathoracic pressure.
- To avoid the reperfusion injury do the procedure slowly and stop the procedure when the patient complains of cough.

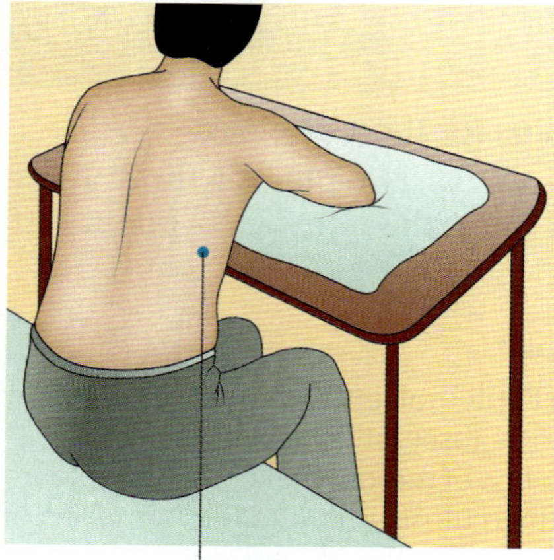

Fig. 14.10: Position of patient and site for pleural fluid aspiration

Complications of Thoracentesis

- Hemothorarx, pneumothorax, reexpansion pulmonary edema.

Pleural Fluid Analysis

Transudative Pleural Effusion

Characteristics

- Specific gravity less than 1.016
- LDH level < 60% of serum LDH.
- Pleural fluid protein < 3 gr/dl
- Cells < 250 cells/cmm.

Causes

- Cirrhosis of liver—nephrotic syndrome
- Congestive cardiac failure
- Hypoalbuminemic states.

Exudative Pleural Effusion

Characteristics

- Specific gravity > 1.016
- LDH level >60% of serum LDH
- Pleural fluid protein > 3 gr/dl
- Cells > 250 cells/cmm

Causes

- Tuberculosis
- Connective tissue disorders
- Primary/secondary malignancy of pleura
- Lymphomas
- Empyema thoracis.

Eosinophilia in the Pleural Fluid

Causes

- Presence of air/blood in the pleural fluid
- Resolving pleural effusion
- Asbestos pleural effusion

Increased levels of amylase in the pleural fluid.

Causes

- Malignant pleural effusion
- Pancreatic pleural effusion
- Oesophageal rupture

Chylous effusion

- Milky creamy appearance of pleural fluid
- Triglycerides > 100 mg/dl/ of pleural fluid
- Presence of chylomicrons in the fluid.

Pseudochylous effusion

- Milky appearance
- Presence of lecithin globulin complex
- Pleural fluid triglyceride level >50 mg/dl

Cholesterol effusion

- Pleural fluid cholesterol level >1000 mg/dl.
- Produced by the inflammatory cells in the pleural effusion, e.g. tuberculous pleural effusion and rheumatoid arthritis.

15 Common Therapeutic Agents

CHECKLIST FOR GENERAL PHYSICAL EXAMINATION

- Chemotherapeutic agents and antibiotics
- Antihypertensive drugs
- Cardiac glycosides
- Drugs used in the treatment of peptic ulcer
- Inotropic agents
- Drugs used in endocrine disorders
- Drugs used in parasite infections
- Sedatives, hypnotics and anticonvulsants
- Drugs used in viral infections
- Drugs used in treatment of anemias
- Drugs used in treatment of fungal infections

CHEMOTHERAPEUTIC AGENTS AND ANTIBIOTICS

Cotrimoxazole

- A chemotherapeutic agent
- Bactericidal
- Contains trimethoprim 80 mg + sultamethoxazole 400 mg (1:5) or double of that ratio.

Uses

- Gram-negative GIT infection
- Urinary tract infection
- Prostatitis
- Respiratory infection
- Typhoid fever
- Sexually transmitted diseases
- Pneumocystis infection

Adverse effects

- Allergic reactions
- Cytopenias
- Megaloblastic anemia

Nitrofurantoin

- Completely absorbed from the GIT
- Achieves bactericidal concentration in the urine
- Used predominantly in UTI
- Activity is less at alkaline pH
- Dose: 50 to 100 mg QID

Ciprofloxacin

- A fluoroquinolone
- Effective orally or parenterally
- Acts predominantly against gram-negative organisms, e.g. *E. coli. Klebsiella, Shigella, Pseudomonas.*

Uses

- Acute gastroenteritis
- Resistant typhoid
- Gram-negative respiratory infection
- Urinary tract infection
- Multidrug resistant tuberculosis

Adverse reactions

- Allergic reactions
- Gastrointestinal intolerance
- Can precipitate convulsions
- Can interfere with cartilage growth in pediatric age group
- Simultaneous intake of theophylline or INH along with ciprofloxacin increases the chances of seizures.

Common Fluoroquinolones used in Clinical Practice

- *Ciprofloxacin tab*: 500 mg 1-0-1, Inj 200 mg IV.BD
- *Ofloxacin tab*: 400 mg OD or BID, Inj. IV 400 mg BD
- *Levofloxacin tab*: 500 mg OD or IV 500 mg OD

  Other quinalones: Norfloxacin, gatifloxacin and sparfloxacin.

Penicillins

Penicillins belong to a group of antibiotics called β-lactam antibiotics.

Other β-lactam antibiotics: Cephalosporins, cephamycins, monobactams and carbapenems.

Basic structure of penicillins: Thiazolidine ring fused with β-lactam ring.

Mechanism of action of penicillins

- Bactericidal
- Prevent the synthesis and cross-linkage of bacterial cell wall peptidoglycans.

Classification of Penicillins

- Penicillin G and esters:
  - Benzyl penicillin
  - Procaine penicillin
  - Benzathine penicillin
- Penicillinase resistant penicillins:
  - Acid labile: Methicillin/cloxacillin
  - Acid resistant: Flucloxacillin

Acid Resistant Penicillins

- Phenoxymethylpenicillin
- Phenoxyethylpenicillin
- Penicillin effective against gram-positive and gram-negative organisms, e.g. ampicillin/ amoxycillin.

Extended spectrum penicillins (antipseudomonal)

- Carboxypenicillin: Carbenicillin, tricarcillin
- Ureidopenicillin: Piperacillin

Beta-lactamase inhibitors

- Clavulanic acid
- Sulbactam
- Tazobactam

Indications for Penicillin Use

- Streptococcal infection
- Pneumococcal infection
- Staphylococcal infection
- Meningococcal infection
- Syphilis and gonorrhea
- Actinomycosis
- Anthrax
- Diphtheria and tetanus

Oral Penicillins

- Phenoxymethylpenicillin
- Phenoxyethylpenicillin
- *Acid resistant*: Can be used as prophylaxis against rheumatic fever and meningococcal infection.

Carboxypenicillin and Ureidopenicillin (Piperacillin, Carbenicillin and Ticarcillin)

- Highly active against *Pseudomonas* and gram-negative infections.
- Act synergistically with aminoglycosides
- Active against anaerobes
- Not very effective against gram-positive organisms and staphylococci.

β–lactamase Inhibitors

Clavulanic acid: Weak antibacterial activity, potent and irreversible inhibitor of many beta-lactamases.

Other beta-lactamase inhibitors: Sulbactam and tazobactam.

Carbapenems: Carbapenems are β–lactam antibiotics, e.g. imipenem and meropenem

- They are bactericidal
- Active against gram-negative, gram-positive, aerobic, Pseudomonas and anaerobic infection.
- They are not active against methicillin resistant staphylococci (MRSA)
- Imipenem is hydrolysed in the kidney by the enzyme dehydropeptidase. Imipenem is combined with cilastin an inhibitor of the renal dehydropeptidase.

Meropenem

- Does not require combination with cilastin
- Active against imipenem resistant *Pseudomonas aeruginosa*
- Does not cause convulsions

Side effects of penicillins

- Allergy and anaphylaxis
- Arthritis
- Serum sickness like syndrome
- Renal dysfunction
- Hematopoetic disturbance
- Angioedema

Monobactams

Beta-lactam antibiotics, bactericidal non nephrotoxic, e.g. aztreonam.

Uses: In gram-negative infections, alternative to aminoglycosides, patients allergic to penicillins.

Cephalosporins

- Cephalosporins have 7-aminocephalosporanic acid nucleus. They contain beta-lactam and dihydrothaizine ring
- Bactericidal
- Active against gram-positive and gram-negative bacteria
- Inhibit bacterial cell wall synthesis.

First Generation Cephalosporins

Active against gram-positive organisms and less active against gram-negative organisms, e.g. cefalexin and cefadroxil.

Second Generation Cephalosporins

Act predominantly against gram-negative infections including *H. influenzae*, e.g. cefoxitin and cefuroxime.

Third Generation Cephalosporins

Act predominantly against gram-negative organisms and *Pseudomonas*, e.g. ceftriaxone, cefotaxime and cepaferazone.

Fourth Generation Cephalosporins

- Action similar to third generation cephalosporins.

  More active against streptococci, methicillin sensitive staphylococci.
- Resistant to some beta-lactamases, e.g. cefepime.

AMINOGLYCOSIDES

Aminoglycosides are active against aerobic gram-negative organisms.

- They are nephrotoxic, ototoxic and toxic to neuromuscular junction
- Have synergistic activity with beta-lactams
- Aminoglycosides inhibit protein synthesis function, e.g. streptomycin, gentamycin, amikacin, tobramycin, netilmycin, kanamycin and neomycin.

Uses

- Gram-negative infections
- Treatment of tuberculosis
- Treatment of brucellosis
- Treatment of plague

Side effects

- Damage to the 8th nerve
- Neuromuscular blockade
- Allergic reactions
- Renal failure

Dosage

- Inj. streptomycin 0.5 to 1 gm/day
- Gentamycin 2–5 mg/kg/day IM/IV
- Tobramycin 3–5 mg/kg/day
- Amikacin 15 mg/kg/day

MACROLIDES

Features of Macrolides

- Large lactone ring is present in their structure
- They inhibit protein synthesis by bacteria

Example of macrolides: Erythromycin, azithromycin and clarithromycin

Uses

- Mycoplasma and chlamydial infection
- Whooping cough
- Campylobacterial infection
- Legionella infection
- Gram-positive infection

Side effects

- Allergic reaction
- Gastrointestinal disturbances

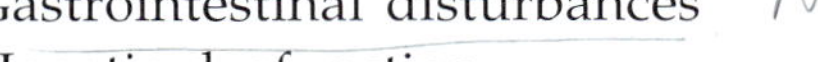

- Hepatic dysfunction

Dosage

- Erythromycin 500 mg QID
- Azithromycin 500 mg OD

TETRACYCLINES

Tetracyclines consist of fusion of four partially unsaturated cyclohexane radicals:

- Bacteriostatic
- Active against gram-positive and gram-negative organisms.

Tetracyclines are specifically active against following organisms

- Mycoplasma infections
- Leptospirosis
- Actinomycosis
- Nocardiosis
- Treponema infections

Adverse reactions

- Gastrointestinal intolerance
- Allergic reaction
- Hepatotoxicity
- Inhibit protein synthesis
- Nephrotoxicity
- Yellow staining of teeth in infants.

Doxycycline

Characteristics

- Has longer half-life
- Higher lipid solubility
- Better gastrointestinal absorption
- Can be used in patients with renal dysfunction
- Less tendency to cause diarrhea.

Uses of Tetracyclines Treatment

- Primary atypical pneumonia
- Chlamydial infection
- STDs
- Plague
- Acne vulgaris
- Drug resistant malaria
- Hepatic amoebiasis
- Rickettsial infection
- Cholera

Chloramphenicol

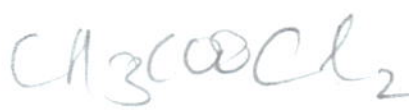

Chloramphenicol is derivative of dichloroacetic acid containing nitrobenzene moiety.

Acts by interfering with synthesis of bacterial proteins.

Chloramphenicol acts against: Rickettsiae, chlamydiae, mycoplasma, gram-positive and gram-negative organisms.

Adverse reactions

- Aplastic anemia
- Headache
- Drug allergy
- Gray baby syndrome

Therapeutic uses

- Treatment of typhoid fever
- Gram-negative infection
- Rickettsial infection
- Plague

Dosage: Cap 250 mg: 1 to 3 gm/day

Anti Fungal Drugs

Topically used anti fungal drugs, e.g. nystatin

- Nystatin is used for oral/vaginal candidiasis
- Nystatin is available as suspension, tablets and ointments.

Griseofulvin

- Anti fungal antibiotic
- Fungistatic
- Active against superficial mycoses
- Not active against deeper fungi and candidiasis

Uses

In the treatment of tinea capitis, cruris, tinea barbae and onychomycosis.

Dosage: 500 mg/day.

Amphotericin B

- Anti fungal antibiotic
- Fungicidal
- Active against
  - Candidiasis
  - Histoplasmosis
  - Cryptococcal infection
  - Coccidiodomycoses

Uses

- For topical anti fungal infection in candidiasis
- Treatment of deeper and systemic fungal infection

Adverse reactions

- Chills and rigors
- Anaphylaxis
- Nephrotoxicity
- Cytopenias

Dosage: 0.7 to 1 mg/kg body weight for 7–14 days.

Flucytosine

- Useful in systemic infection with yeasts
- Useful in the treatment of systemic fungal infection, e.g. cryptococcal infection.

Azole Derivatives

Azoles contain 5 member. Azole ring

Imidazoles

- *Clotrimazole*: For local application, e.g. vaginal candidiasis
- *Miconazole*: For local application of fungal infection. High dose can be used for trichomonal infection
- *Ketoconazole*: Topical antifungal agents can block the steroid synthesis.
- *Triazoles*, e.g. itraconazole
  - For both local and intravenous uses
  - In systemic candidiasis
  - Can be used in renal diseases.

Fluconazole

- Available as oral and intravenous preparations.
- Administered once daily
- Used for oral, local and systemic candidiasis

Miscellaneous fungal agents

Terbinafine: For superficial fungal infection can be given orally/topically.

Caspofung

- Active against *Candida* and *Aspergillosis*
- Given as intravenous preparation
- Causes severe phlebitis
- Expensive

Drug Therapy of Acquired Immune Deficiency Syndrome

Different types of antiretroviral drugs.

Nucleoside Reverse Transcriptase Inhibitors (NRTIs)

For example:

- Azidothymidine
- Didanosine
- Zalcitabine
- Stavudine
- Lamivudine
- Abacavir
- Emtricitabine

Non-nucleoside reverse transcriptase inhibitors (NNRTIs), e.g. nevirapine and efavirenz.

Protease inhibitors, e.g. saquinavir, retonavir and indinavir.

Fusion inhibitors: Enfuvirtide

Dosage

Azidothymidine: 200 mg/day oral, can cause myositis and cytopenia.

Lamivudine

- 150 1-0-1/day
- Best tolerated drug

- Rarely can cause lactic acidosis and liver failure

NRTIs can cause fatal lactic acidosis and hepatoxicity.

Nevirapine: Dosage 200 to 400 mg/day can cause allergic rashes and increase in liver enzymes.

Efavirenz

- Dosage 600 mg 0-0-1
- Crosses blood brain barrier
- Administered once daily
- Can cause dizziness and insomnia.

Indinavir

Dosage: 800 mg 1-1-1

Adverse effects: Nausea, vomiting, diarrhoea, hepatotoxicity, insulin resistance, hyperglycemia and hyperlipedemia.

Tenofovir: Given once daily, inhibitor of HIV replication.

Fusion inhibitors: For example, enfuvirtide, inhibits membrane fusion of HIV with cells.

Injection: Subcutaneous BID

Used in resistant HIV cases.

HAART (Highly active antiretroviral therapy)

Example of HAART

Two NRTIs + one NNRTIs or protease inhibitor = azidothymidine + lamivudine + nevirapine or efavirenz or indinavir.

Above drugs can be changed if there is treatment failure, drug interactions, adverse effects or patient incompliance.

Treatment of HIV infection is usually lifelong.

Antitubercular Drugs

INH (isonicotinic acid hydrazide)

- Bactericidal
- Inhibits the synthesis of mycolic acid component of cell wall of *Mycobacterium tuberculosis*
- Safe in renal failure

Dose: 5 mg/kg/day

Adverse reactions

- Allergic reaction
- Peripheral neuropathy
- Hepatitis
- Psychosis

Note: 20–40 mg of pyridoxine (vit B_6) should be administered along with INH to prevent peripheral neuropathy.

Rifampicin

- Bactericidal
- Inhibits bacterial DNA dependant RNA polymerase
- Food interferes with its absorption, to be given ½ an hour before break fast.

Dose: 10 mg/kg body weight

Adverse reactions

- Allergic reactions including flu-like syndrome
- Hepatitis
- Thrombocytopenia
- Orange discoloration of body fluids.

Uses: treatment of:

- *Mycobacterium tuberculosis*
- Leprosy
- Severe staphylococcal infection
- Legionella infection
- Brucellosis
- Prophylaxis against meningococcal infection.

Streptomycin

- Aminoglycoside antibiotics
- Only parenteral—intramuscular administration
- Bactericidal against TB bacillus
- Does not penetrate caseous material
- Less potent than INH and its CSF concentration is poor
- To be avoided in patients with renal failure.

Dosage: Inj streptomycin 0.75 gr to 1 gr/day

Pyrazinamide

- Bactericidal
- Only effective against human *Mycobacterium tuberculosis*

- Good meningeal penetration and also into the macrophages.

Dosage: 25 mg/kg/day

Adverse reactions

- Allergic reactions
- Hepatitis
- Hyperuricaemia

Ethambutol

- Bacteriostatic
- Inhibits synthesis of bacterial cell wall
- Does not penetrate the body fluids adequately.

Adverse reactions

- Retrobulbar neuritis—inability to see green color
- Optic neuritis disappears when the drug is discontinued

  Dosage: 15 to 25 mg/kg

Ethambutol to be avoided in children as they cannot complain of visual disturbance.

2nd Line Anti TB Drugs

Thiacetazone

- Bacteriostatic
- Should not be used in HIV patients as it can cause severe skin reaction
- Can cause cytopenia, Stevens-Johnson syndrome.

  Dosage: 150 mg/day.

Ethionamide

- Inhibits mycolic acid synthesis
- Effective against *Mycobacterium tuberculosis* and atypical mycobacteria
- Can cause allergic reactions, cytopenias, GIT disturbances and CNS disturbances.

  Dosage: 250 mg 1-0-1 up to 1 gr/day

Capreomycin

- Acts against mycobacteria resistant to other drugs
- It is an antibiotic
- Bactericidal
- Acts similar to streptomycin
- Dosage 15–20 mg/day

Kanamycin and amikacin can also be used in the treatment of tuberculosis.

Cycloserine

- Antibiotic
- Bacteriostatic
- Acts against resistant mycobacterial infection
- Causes severe psychosis. Peripheral neuropathy, ataxia and slurred speech.

  Dose: 0.5 to 1 gr/day

Fluoroquinolones, e.g: ciprofloxacin, ofloxacin, levofloxacin, etc. can be used in the treatment of *Mycobacterium tuberculosis*.

Macrolides: Azithromycin and clarithromycin can be used in resistant TB and atypical mycobacterial infection.

Different Drug Regimes Used in the Treatment of Tuberculosis

- *6 months regime:* Daily INH + rifampicin + ethambutol and pyrazinamide for 1st 2 months and daily INH + rifampicin for the next 4 months.
- *9 months regime:* Daily INH + rifampicin + either daily ethambutol or injection—streptomycin for 2 months and to continue INH and rifampicin daily for 7 months.

DOTS (Directly observed treatment short course)

DOTS regime of RNTCP (revised national tuberculosis control programme)

- *Category I:* Regime used: 2 months of HRZEs + 4 months of HR
  - Serious sputum +ve
  - Serious sputum –ve
  - Serious extrapulmonary
- *Category II:* Regime used: 2 months HRZEs + 1 month HRZE + 5 months HRE
  - Sputum (+ve) relapse
  - Sputum (+ve) failure
  - Sputum (+ve) defaulter

- *Category III:* Regime used: 2 months HRZ + 4 months HR
  - Not serious sputum (–ve)
  - Not serious extrapulmonary
- All drugs are used thrice weekly in patient in category I and II.
- Patient whose sputum is +ve after initial intensive treatment receive additional 1 month of intensive phase treatment.

H = INH, R = rifampicin, Z = pyrazinamide, E = ethambutol, S = streptomycin.

Serious forms of tuberculosis

- Meningitis
- Disseminated TB
- Pericarditis
- Intestinal TB
- Genitourinary TB
- Spinal TB
- Extensive parenchymal involvement of lung
- Extensive pleural, smear +ve or –ve tuberculosis.

DRUGS USED IN LEPROSY

Dapsone (Diamino diphenyl sulphone)

- Antileprosy drug
- Bacteriostatic—inhibits the synthesis of folic acid

Adverse reactions

- Skin reaction
- Hemolytic anemia
- Agranulocytosis
- Methemoglobinemia

Preparation and dosage: Dapsone 50–100 mg/day

Clofazamine

- Bactericidal
- Concentrates in reticuloendothelial system
- Inhibits mycobacterial DNA synthesis.
- Antileprosy drug
- Causes reddish black discoloration of skin which can persist for several months.

Dose: 100 to 300/day.

DRUGS USED IN THE TREATMENT OF MALARIA

Classification

Antifolate Drugs

- Diaminopyrimidines: Pyrimethamine.
- Biguanides: Proguanil
- Sulfonamides: Sulfadoxime.

Quinoline Derivatives

- *4-aminoquinolines*: Chloroquine and amodiaquine.
- 8-aminoquinolines: Primaquine
- Quinoline methanol: Mefloquine halofantrine

Cinchona alkaloids: Quinine and quinidine

Artemisinin compounds: Artesunate, arteether and artemether.

Antimicrobial drug: Doxycycline, clindamycin and atovaquone.

Chloroquine

Action: Chloroquine induces oxidative damage to digestive proteases and membranes of the parasite.

Kills schizonts of *Plasmodium vivax* and *falciparum*, effective against the gametes of *Plasmodium vivax*, *Plasmodium ovale* and *Plasmodium malariae.*

No action on sporozoites, preerythrocytic stage and persistent tissue forms.

- Safe during pregnancy
- Can depress the myocardium

Adverse reactions

- Allergic skin rashes
- Cytopenia
- Long-term use—retinopathy
- Insomnia and depression
- ST-T changes in the ECG.

Uses

- Acute attack of malaria
- Amoebic liver abscess
- Rheumatoid arthritis
- Skin manifestation of SLE
- Lepra reactions

Preparation and Dosage

- Chloroquine phosphate 250 mg (150 mg base of chloroquine)
- Hydroxychloroquine–less toxic
- Inj chloroquine 40 mg/ml

Primaquine

- Acts against persistent tissue forms of *Plasmodium vivax*
- Acts against pre erythrocytic (hepatic) and sexual forms (gametocytes) of all species of human malarial parasite
- Produces radical cure in *Plasmodium vivax* infection.

Adverse reactions

- Gastrointestinal discomfort
- Cytopenias
- In G6PD deficient patients–it can cause hemolysis

Dose: 0.3 to 0.5 mg/kg body weight × 15 days.

Prevents the relapse of *Plasmodium vivax* infection.

Antigametocidal action against *Plasmodium falciparum*–45 mg single dose.

Mefloquine

Acts on the erythrocytic stage of *Plasmodium falciparum*.

Highly effective against *Plasmodium falciparum* including chloroquine resistant strain and multidrug resistant strains.

Adverse effects

- Gastrointestinal disturbance
- Bradycardia and arrhythmias
- Neuropsychiatric disturbance

Dosage

- 25 mg/kg body weight
- 750 mg stat and after 12 hrs 500 mg

Note: Quinine should not be administered after administering mefloquine for at least 15 days, due to cardiac toxicity.

Halofantrine

- Schizonticidal drug
- Acts against resistant *falciparum* species
- Causes gastrointestinal disturbance, QT prolongation and ventricular arrhythmias. Should not be used in patients taking quinine.

Biguanides: Proguanil

- Acts against schizonts of *vivax* and *falciparum*
- Effective against primary pre erythrocytic form of *Plasmodium falciparum*.
- Prevents gametocyte development in the gut wall of the mosquito
- No action against persistent tissue forms of *Plasmodium vivax*.
- No hypoglycemic action

Use

For causal prophylaxis 100–200 mg daily.

Side effects

- Gastrointestinal side effects
- Stomatitis
- Oral ulcers

Pyrimethamine

- Active against erythrocytic forms of all types of malarial parasites.
- Active against pre erythrocytic form of *Plasmodium falciparum*.
- Prevents maturation of fertilized encysted gametes within the mosquito.
- Can cause megaloblastic anemia and cytopenia.

Dose

Pyrimethamine 25 mg + sulfadoxime (3 tabs single dose).

Uses

In the treatment of malaria and toxoplasmosis.

Artemisinin

From Chinese plant–Artemisia anneta.

Derivatives: Artesunate, arteether, artemether

Acts against all forms of schizonts of all parasites.

Can cause cytopenia and gastrointestinal disturbance.

Preparations and dosage

Tab artesunate: 50 mg tablets

Dose: 100 mg 2 tablets: 1st day and then 50 mg 1-0-1 = 5–7 days

Inj. artesunate: 2.4 mg/kg 1st day and then 1.2 mg/kg into 5 days.

Quinine

Derived from the bark of cinchona tree.

Actions

- Schizonticidal antimalarial
- Can cause local irritation
- Nausea, vomiting and bitter taste.
- Myocardial depression
- Hypoglycemia due to release of insulin

Adverse reactions

- Pruritis and angioedema
- Cardiac arrest
- Hypoglycemia
- Black water fever
- Cinchonism: Ringing in the ear, nausea, headache, vertigo and visual impairment.
- Intravenous quinine can cause convulsions.

ANALGESICS AND ANTIPYRETICS

Paracetamol (Acetaminophen)

Belongs to paraminophenol derivative

Uses

Very good antipyretic and analgesic. Not a very good anti-inflammatory agent.

Adverse reactions

- Hepatic and renal toxicity (after 7–10 gr of consumption)
- Rarely neutropenia, thrombocytopenia and hemolysis.

Dosage

500 mg 3 or 4 times/day should not exceed 2.5 gr/day.

Mechanism of action

Inhibit prostaglandin synthesis and inactivation of cyclogenase.

Aspirin

- Salicylate analgesic
- Mechanism of action

  Inhibit prostaglandin synthesis and inactivates cyclogenase.

Uses

- Analgesic and antipyretic and anti-inflammatory
- Acute rheumatic fever
- Ant platelet activity

Adverse reactions

- GIT: Erosive gastritis
- Allergic rashes and angioneurotic edema
- In children with viral infection it can cause Reye's syndrome
- Salicylism—high dose causes tinnitus and dizziness
- Acute salicylate intoxication

Dosage

- Analgesic and antipyretic (325 mg to 1 gr/day)
- Anti-rheumatic: 60–100 mg/kg/day
- Anti-platelet: 75 to 150 mg/day
- Local application as ointment

Indomethacin

Indole acetic acid derivative. Potent anti-inflammatory agent.

Uses

- Acute attack of gout
- Arthritic disorders

Adverse reactions

- Erosive gastritis and peptic ulcer
- Headache dizziness and confusion
- Blood dyscrasia

Diclofenac Sodium

- A heterocyclic arylacetic acid derivative
- A very potent analgesic and anti-inflammatory agent.

Dosage

- 75 mg to 100 mg/day
- Available as oral and parenteral preparations.

Uses

In the treatment of:

- Rheumatoid arthritis
- Osteoarthritis
- Postoperative pain
- Ankylosing spondylitis

Ibuprofen

- Propionic acid derivative
- Analgesic, antipyretic and anti-inflammatory agent

  Dosage: 400 to 1200 mg/day

Piroxicam

- An oxicam derivative
- Analgesic and anti-inflammatory agent
- Can cause peptic ulceration and CNS side effects.

Dosage: 20–40 mg/day

ANTIHYPERTENSIVE DRUGS

Beta-blockers

Classification

Cardioselective β-blockers (blocks β_1–receptors), e.g. atenolol (25 to 100 mg/day), metaprolol (100 to 200 mg/day) and bisoprolol (10 mg/day).

Noncardioselective β-blockers (blocks both β_1 and β_2 receptors), e.g. propranalol 80–240 mg/day.

Uses of β-blockers

- Cardiovascular:
  - Tachyarrhythmias
  - Hypertension
  - Obstructive cardiomyopathy
  - Pheochromocytoma along with α-blockers.

Other Uses

- Portal hypertension
- Thyrotoxicosis
- Anxiety neurosis
- Chronic simple glaucoma (timolol drops)
- Migrainous headache

Side Effects of β-blockers

- Bradycardia
- Worsening of cardiac failure
- Bronchospasm
- Masking of hypoglycemia
- Fatigue

Contraindications for the Use of β-blockers

- Bronchial asthma
- Congestive cardiac failure
- Bradycardia and cardiac conduction defect
- Depression
- Peripheral vascular disease and Raynaud's phenomenon.

Note

- β-blockers alone should not be used in pheochromocytoma.
- Carvedilol which has got non-selective beta-adrenergic effect with selective alpha blocking effect is used in patients with CCF.
- Labetalol which has got both beta and alpha blocking effects is used in patients with hypertensive emergency.

Diuretics

Frusemide (Lasix)

Potent loop diuretic (acts on loop of Henle)

Uses

- In treating edema states
- Pulmonary edema and cardiac failure
- Acute and chronic renal failure
- Antihypertensive
- Hypercalcemia
- Forced alkaline diuresis, e.g. barbiturate poisoning.

Side effects

- Hypotension, hyponatremia and hypokalemia
- Hyperglycemia and hyperuricemia
- Allergic rashes and bone marrow suppression

Large dose: Transient hearing loss

Dosage: 40 to 100 mg/day

Other loop diuretics

- Bumetanide
- Ethacrinic acid

Thiazides

Belong to benzothiadiazines. Primarily acts on the renal tubules by inhibiting sodium reabsorption.

Uses

- As a diuretic
- Antihypertensive
- In nephrogenic diabetes insipidus
- In recurrent renal calculi due to idiopathic hypercalciuria.

Adverse effects

- Hypokalemia and hyponatremia
- Hyperglycemia and hyperuricemia
- Allergic reactions
- Blood dyscrasias, e.g. hydrochlorothiazide 25 to 50 mg/day.

Spironolactone

- An aldosterone antagonist
- Potassium sparing diuretic
- Structurally similar to aldosterone
- It prevents potassium excretion and sodium reabsorption in the renal tubules.

Indications and Uses of Spironolactone

a. Cirrhotic edema
b. CCF
c. Conn's syndrome
d. In the treatment of hypertension
e. Lethargy and drowsiness

Dosage: 100 to 200 mg/day, up to 400 mg/day

Note: Eplerenone is a specific aldosterone antagonist with least endocrine effects which is specifically used in CCF.

Other potassium sparing diuretics: Triamterene and amiloride.

Calcium Channel Blockers

Classification

Dihydropyridines: Nifedipine and amlodipine benzothiazepines, e.g. diltiazem. Phenylalkalylamines, e.g. verapamil.

Uses

Nifedipine and amlodipine

- Hypertension
- Peripheral vascular disease
- Coronary artery disease (Prinzmetal's angina)

Verapamil is mainly used in the treatment of SVT (supraventricular tachycardia).

Diltiazem

In treating hypertension and coronary artery disease.

Adverse reactions

- Nifedipine and amlodipine
  - Headache, tachycardia, gum hyperplasia and peripheral edema.
  - Verapamil and diltiazem: Bradycardia

Contraindications for the Use of Calcium Channel Blockers

- Hypertension
- CCF
- Severe aortic stenosis

Dosage

- Nifedipine 30–60 mg/day–longer acting preparations are preferred
- Amlodipine: 2.5 to 10 mg/day
- Verapamil: 120 to 240 mg/day
- Diltiazem: 120 to 360 mg/day

Angiotensin Converting Enzyme Inhibitors

Example: Captopril, lisinopril, enalapril and ramipril.

Mechanism of action: Completely inhibit the conversion of angiotensin I to angiotensin II leading to vasodilatation.

Uses: Treatment of

- Hypertension
- Diabetic nephropathy
- CCF
- Proteinurias
- Acute myocardial infarction

Dosage

- Captopril: 12.5 to 50 mg/day
- Enalapril: 5 to 20 mg/day

- Ramipril: 2.5 to 20 mg/day
- Lisinopril: 5 to 40 mg/day

Contraindications for ACE Inhibitors

- Severe aortic stenosis
- Bilateral renal artery stenosis
- Pregnancy

Adverse reactions

- Allergic reactions
- Intractable cough
- Ist dose hypotension

ANGIOTENSIN RECEPTOR BLOCKERS

Losartan

- A selective angiotensin receptor blocker (ARB)
- Decrease peripheral vascular resistance

Dosage: 25 to 100 mg/day

Use: In the treatment of hypertension especially in patients with ACE inhibitor induced cough.

Other angiotensin receptor blockers, e.g. irbesartan and valsartan.

Clonidine

Centrally acting antihypertensive agent.

Site of action: Activates postsynaptic α_2 receptors leading on to decrease sympathetic out flow and decrease of release of noradrenaline from nerve terminals.

Uses: Treatment of hypertension, diabetic diarrhea.

Adverse reactions

- Dry mouth
- Drowsiness

Note: Sudden stoppage of clonidine causes rebound rise of blood pressure.

Dosage: 100 to 900 mg/day.

ALPHA BLOCKERS

Prazosin

Selective α_1 adrenergic receptor blockers.

Dose: 2.5 to 7.5 mg/day

Uses: In the treatment of hypertension especially in patients with hyperlipidemia, renal failure and benign prostatic hypertrophy.

Adverse reactions

Drowsiness and postural hypotension.

Other analogues of prazosin: Doxazosin, terazosin and afluzosin.

Other alpha receptor blockers: Phentolamine and phenoxybenzamine.

Alpha Methyl Dopa

Centrally acting antihypertensive drug.

Action: Similar to clonidine at the vasomotor centre.

Adverse reactions

- Drowsiness
- Skin rashes
- Cholestatic jaundice
- Coombs positive hemolytic anemia

  Dosage: 250 mg tablets

  Dose: 250–500 mg 8th hrly.

Drugs Used in Hypertensive Crisis and Emergencies

- Inj. labetalol IV
- IV sodium nitroprusside
- IV nitroglycerin
- Inj. enalapril

Note: Nifedipine 10 mg can be tried sublingually in hypertensive emergencies.
Captopril 12.5 to 25 mg can also be tried sublingually.
Injectable diuretics can be used in patients with acute LVF induced by hypertension.

CARDIAC GLYCOSIDES

Digoxin

A cardiac glycoside acts by inhibiting membrane bound ATPase enzyme.

Uses of digoxin

- In congestive cardiac failure especially with atrial fibrillation with rapid ventricular rate.

- Low output cardiac failure in hypertensive, valvular, ischemic and congenital heart disease.
- In high output cardiac failure like thyrotoxicosis.

Contraindications for the Use of Digoxin

- AV block
- Hypertrophic cardiomyopathy HOCM

Adverse reactions

- GIT: Nausea, vomiting
- Cardiac conduction defects—bradycardia multiple ectopics, various atrial and ventricular arrhythmias.
- Gynaecomastia
- Neurological–vertigo and hallucinations.

Digitalis toxicity is more common in following situations

- Elderly
- Hypokalemia
- Hypercalcemia
- Corpulmonale
- Impaired renal function
- Recent myocardial infarction

Treatment of Digoxin Toxicity

- Stop tablet digoxin
- Correct hypokalemia
- Anti digoxin antibodies
- Treatment of cardiac arrhythmia—for supraventricular tachycardia—IV propranalol
- For ventricular tachycardia: IV lignocaine/ phenytoin IV

DRUGS USED IN THE TREATMENT OF ANGINA PECTORIS

Nitrates

For example, isosorbide dinitrate, isosorbide mononitrate.

Mechanism of Action

- Coronary vasodilatation
- Direct relaxation of smooth muscle mediated through nitric oxide (NO)

Uses of Nitrates

- Angina pectoris
- Acute myocardial infarction
- Refractory cardiac failure
- Cyanide poisoning

Adverse reactions

- Throbbing headache
- Hypotension
- Development of tolerance after repeated administration
- Abrupt stoppage of drug can precipitate an attack of angina.

Different Formulations of Nitrate

- Glyceryl trinitrate: Tablets
- Sustained release preparations
- Sublingual spray
- 2% skin ointment
- Transdermal patches
- Intravenous preparations.

Drugs Used in the Treatment of Angina Pectoris

1. Organic nitrates, e.g. isosorbide nitrates
2. β-blockers
3. Calcium channel blockers
4. Potassium channel activators, e.g. nicorandil.

Statins

For example, atorvastatin, simvastatin, A HMG–CoA reductase inhibitor.

Uses

- In the treatment of primary hyperlipidemia
- In prevention of atherosclerotic progression
- In patients with acute MI
- In the treatment of coronary artery disease.

Non-lipid lowering effects of statins

- Repairs endothelial function
- Decrease arterial smooth muscle proliferation
- Decreases in the hypertrophy of muscle
- Decreases platelet aggregation and fibrinogen level.

Adverse reactions

- Raise in the hepatic enzymes
- Myositis
- CNS dysfunction

Dosage: Atorvastatin 10–20 mg/day

Other Drugs Used in Hyperlipidemias

- Cholesterol absorption inhibitor: Ezetimibe
- Bile acid sequestrants: Cholestyramine
- Nicotinic acid
- Fibric acid derivatives: Gemfibrozil

DRUGS USED IN THE TREATMENT OF BRONCHIAL ASTHMA

Aminophylline

- Melthylxanthine derivative
- Phosphodiesterase inhibitor–inhibits conversion of cAMP–leads on to increase tissue concentration of cAMP

Uses

- Acute attack of asthma, e.g. IV aminophylline
- Chronic persistent asthma, e.g. slow release theophylline tablets.

Route of administration of amiophylline

a. Intravenous–slowly
b. Tablets and injections of theophylline.

Adverse reactions

- GIT—nausea and vomiting
- Cardiac—tachycardia and cardiac arrhythmias
- CNS—confusion and tremors

Salbutamol

Selective β_2 receptor agonist causes bronchodilatation.

Methods of administration: Tablets/syrups/injections/inhalation/nebulisation.

Other β_2-Agonists

Short acting: Terbutaline

Longer acting: Salmeterol, formoterol

Therapeutic Uses of β_2-Agonists

a. Acute attack of asthma
b. Chronic persistent asthma
c. Uterine relaxation

Side effects

- Tremor
- Tachycardia
- Hypokalemia

Ipratropium Bromide

- Atropine derivatives cause parasympathetic blockage resulting in bronchodilatation
- Used as inhalation and nebulisation
- Useful in patient with bronchial asthma and COPD.

Other Bronchodilators

- Mast cell stabilisers: Sodium chromoglycate
- Corticosteroids: Inhalers (fluticasone betamethasone oral tablets and injections.
- Antileukotriens: Montelukast

DRUGS USED IN THE TREATMENT OF PEPTIC ULCER

Antacids

Types of Antacids

a. Systemic antacids: e.g. sodium bicarbonate can get absorbed and causes systemic alkalosis.
b. Non systemic antacids: e.g. aluminium hydroxide and maganesium hydroxide.

Antacids are administered at one and three hours after each meal and at bed time and if needed extra dose for pain.

Aluminium hydroxide gel: 4–8 ml can cause constipation.

Magnesium hydroxide (milk of maganesia) 4–8 ml

Magnesium trisilicate: 2–4 gr 1–4 hrs

Magnesium salts cause diarrhea.

H_2 Receptor Antagonists

Competitively block parietal cell H_2 receptors, e.g. cimetidine 400 mg 2 or 3 times/day
Ranitidine 150 mg to 300 mg/day
Famotidine 20 mg to 40 mg/day

Therapeutic Uses of H_2 Receptor Blockers

- Duodenal and gastric ulcer
- NSAID induced ulcer
- Gastroesophageal reflux disease
- Erosive gastritis
- Zollinger-Ellison syndrome

Side effects

- Allergic reaction
- Fatigue
- Mental confusion, delirium and hallucination
- Hepatotoxicity
- Gynaecomastia

Proton Pump Inhibitors

Inhibit gastric H^+, K^+, ATPase proton pump—Final common pathway for acid secretion, e.g.

- Omeprazole 20–40 mg/day
- Lansoprazole 30 mg/day
- Pantoprazole 40 mg/day
- Rabeprazole 20–40 mg/day

Side effects

- Drowsiness and dizziness
- Prolonged use can cause achlorhydria.

Indication: Same as for H_2 receptor blockers.

Sucralfate

Complex of sulfated sucrose and aluminium hydroxide. Has no antisecretory activity. It coats the ulcer forming a gel over the ulcer and becoming impermeable to hydrogen ion of gastric acid.

Bismuth Salts

- Commonly used are: Colloidal bismuth subcitrate and bismuth subsalicylate.
- Coats the ulcer crater with bismuth glycoprotein complex.
- Impermeable to gastric acid
- Also acts against *H. pylori*.

Treatment of Helicobacter Pylori Infection

- Regime (1)—following drugs for 14 days
  Metronidazole 250 mg QID + tetracycline 500 mg QID + Omeprazole 20 mg/day + Bismuth subsalicylate 2 tab QID.
- Regime (2)—following drugs for 14 days
  Amoxycillin 1 gr BID or metronidazole 500 mg BD + clarithromycin 250/500 mg BD + omeprazole 20 mg 1-0-1.

INOTROPIC AGENTS

Adrenaline

Uses

- In acute severe asthma
- Anaphylaxis
- Cardiopulmonary resuscitation
- Along with local anesthetic to prolong the action of anesthetic.
- Control of bleeding in concentration of 1: 1000 for topical application, e.g. epistaxis.

Noradrenaline: Mainly used in patients with shock to elevate the blood pressure.

Adverse Reaction Adrenaline and Noradrenaline

- Palpitation, tremor and headache
- Sudden raise of blood pressure and precipitate subarachnoid hemorrhage.
- Can precipitate ventricular tachycardia and fibrillation.
- Precipitation of anginal pain
- Extravasations of noradrenaline can cause vasospasm and sloughing

Preparation and dosage: injection adrenaline 0.2 to 0.5 ml of 1: 1000 adrenaline in water.

Route of administration: Subcutaneous/intramuscular.

Noradrenaline: IV infusion 4 μg/ml

DRUGS USED IN THE TREATMENT OF CEREBRAL EDEMA

- IV mannitol
- IV frusemide
- Inj. dexamethasone
- Oral glycerol
- Magnesium sulphate rectal administration.

Other measures to decrease cerebral edema

- Mechanical hyperventilation to achieve PCO_2 of 25 to 30 mm of Hg.
- Surgical decompression of the cranium.

Mannitol

Polyhydroxyaliphatic alcohol.

Causes osmotic diuresis.

Preparation and dosage: IV mannitol 20% 100 ml 8th hrly.

Indications

- Raised intracranial tension
- Increased intraocular pressure
- Barbiturate poisoning

Contraindications

- Acute renal failure with anuria
- Right-and left-sided cardiac failure
- In some cases of intracranial bleeding.

Adverse reactions

- Can precipitate cardiac failure in patients with borderline cardiac dysfunction
- Hyponatremia

H_1 Receptor Antagonists

Example

- Chlorpheniramine maleate (zeet)
- Pheniramine maleate
- Cetrizine

Uses

- Allergic disorders
- Antitussive effect
- Antiemetic effect
- In motion sickness and vertigo
- Mastocytosis

Adverse reactions

- Nausea and epigastric distress
- Sedation and fatigue
- Dry mouth and blurring of vision.

DRUGS USED IN ENDOCRINE DISORDERS

Somatostatin

- Peptide containing 14 amino acids
- It decreases secretion of gastric acid
- It inhibits splanchnic blood flow.

Octreotide

Synthetic longer action analogue of somatostatin.

Useful in the treatment of

- Insulinomas
- Severe diarrhea caused by carcinoid syndrome
- Dumping syndrome
- Bleeding esophageal varies.

DRUGS USED IN THE TREATMENT OF THYROID DYSFUNCTION

Hypothyroidism

Thyroxine (Eltroxin and thyronorm)

Contains thyroxine sodium

Dose: 25 ugr, 50 ugr, 100 ugr, 200 ugr— to be administered on empty stomach in the morning.

Uses of Thyroxine

- In cretinism
- In adult hypothyroidism
- In certain cases of thyroid carcinomas.

> *Note:* Thyroxine treatment in cases of hypothyroidism is lifelong.

Hyperthyroidism

Carbimazole and Methimazole

They inhibit thyroid peroxidase enzymes decreasing the synthesis of thyroid hormones.

Preparations and dosage: Carbimazole (neomercazole): 5, 10, 20 mg tablets

Dose: 30–60 mg/day

Side effects

- Drug fever and rash
- Agranulocytosis and thrombocytopenia
- Drug induced hypothyroidism

Uses: Treatment of hyperthyroidism

Propyl Thyouracil

Tabs—50 mg. Dosage: 300 to 600 mg

Used in the treatment of hyperthyroidism (safer in pregnancy).

TREATMENT OF DIABETES MELLITUS

Antidiabetic Drugs

Oral Antidiabetic Drugs

- Sulphonyl ureas: 2nd generation drugs:
- *Glybenclamide*
  - 5–10 mg/day acts 12–24 hrs
  - *Glyclazide*: 40–80 mg/day acts 12–24 hrs
  - *Glymepride*: 1 to 2 mg tablets acts 16–24 hrs

Mechanism of Action

- Stimulation of insulin release by pancreatic beta cells.
- Inhibit hepatic neoglucogenesis and glycogenolysis

Side effects

- Hypoglycemia
- Weight gain
- Skin rashes
- Cytopenias

Indications

Obese type 2 diabetes mellitus without acute complications.

Contraindications

- Type I diabetes mellitus
- Acute complications of diabetes mellitus
- Pregnancy
- Severe liver and kidney disease

Ist generation sulphonylureas like tolbutamide and chlorpropamide are not much in use in clinical practice.

Biguanides

Metformin

- Increases the peripheral utilization of glucose
- Decreases hepatic neoglucogenesis
- Insulin sensitizer at the level of muscle and adipose tissue
- Decreases appetite and delays glucose absorption.

Dosage: Tablets of 500 and 1000 mg maximum dose up to 2.5 gr/day.

Indications

- Obese type 2 diabetes mellitus
- Sulphonylurea failure disease
- Nonalcoholic steatohepatitis

Contraindications

- Renal and hepatic dysfunction
- Congestive cardiac failure
- Chronic alcoholism

Adverse reactions

- Nausea, vomiting, bitter/metallic taste.
- Severe weight loss
- Lactic acidosis

> *Note:* Metformin as such does not produce hypoglycemia in a diabetic but can potentiate the action of insulin and sulphonylureas.

Repaglinide

- Belongs to meglitinide group of antidiabetic drug
- Not a sulphonylurea but acts like sulphonylureas
- Causes less hypoglycemia and can be used in patients with renal dysfunction.

Indications

Used in the control of post prandial hyperglycemia in type 2 diabetes mellitus.

Dosage and preparation: 0.5 mg tablets can be administered up to 4 mg/day.

Administration

- Just before intake of meal
- Acts only up to 4 hrs.

Acarbose

An oligosaccharide

Mechanism of Action

Binds to alpha-glucosidase enzyme in the brush border jejunum and inhibits carbohydrate absorption.

Indications and Usages

Type 2 diabetes mellitus to control postprandial hyperglycemia.

Dosage

25 to 50 mg chewed and swallowed along with food, can be combined with other antidiabetic drugs.

Adverse reactions

Abdominal discomfort, loose stools and flatulence.

Contraindications: Inflammatory bowel disease, intestinal obstruction and chronic intestinal disease.

Pioglitazone

Belongs to thiazolidinediones (glitazones).

Mechanism of Action

- Increase the insulin sensitivity at adipose tissue level
- Reduce the production of proinflammatory cytokines
- Lowers hepatic fat content and dyslipidemia
- Decreases hepatic production of glucose
- Preserves and enhances beta–cell function.

Dosages and Preparations

15 to 45 mg/day

Other glitazones: Rosiglitazone 4 to 8 mg/day

Side effects

- Elevation of hepatic enzymes
- Weight gain
- Fluid retention and cardiac failure.

Indications

- Type 2 diabetes mellitus
- Polycystic ovarian syndrome
- Nonalcoholic steatohepatitis

Sweetening Agents Used in Patients with Diabetes

- Saccharin
- Aspartame
- Neotame
- Sucralose

INSULIN

Effects of Insulin

- Increases cellular uptake of glucose and potassium
- Decreases lipolysis, decreases hepatic glycogenolysis and increases protein synthesis
- Has got anti-inflammatory action
- Decreases fibrinolysis
- Causes vasodilatation
- Increases growth

Different Preparations of Insulin

- Short acting–regular—clear fluid
  - Starts acting within half an hour and acts up to 5 to 8 hrs.
- Intermediate acting
  - NPH/lente (insulin zinc)
  - Acts within 2 hours and acts up to 18–24 hours.

Presently Available Insulins

- *Human insulin*: Rapid, short acting–regular insulin, e.g. actrapid
- *Intermediate acting:* NPH (insulatard)
- *Human insulin analogues:* Very rapid acting: Lispro, aspart—acts within 5 to 15 minutes and acts for 4 to 6 hrs.
- *Longer acting,* e.g. glargine, detemir, starts acting within 2 to 4 hours and action lasts up to 20 to 24 hrs.

Inhaled insulin: Inhalation of aerosolized dry powder. Effective as regular insulin—can cause mild cough and decrease in the pulmonary function after prolonged use. Inhaled insulin is contraindicated in patients with COPD/bronchial asthma.

Adverse reactions of insulin

- Hypoglycemia
- Insulin lipodystrophy—2 types–lipodystrophy and lipohypertrophy
- Insulin presbyopia
- Insulin neuropathy
- Weight gain
- Edema

Indications of Insulin Use

- Patients with type 1 diabetes mellitus
- Patients with type 2 diabetes mellitus. After primary/secondary failures to oral hypoglycemic agents.
- All acute complications of diabetes mellitus (ketoacidosis and infection)
- Chronic complications of diabetes mellitus like retinopathy, renal involvement and CCF.
- Surgical procedures in a diabetes especially with general anesthesia
- Pregnant diabetic

CORTICOSTEROIDS

Use of Corticosteroids

- In acute and chromic adrenal insufficiency
- Anti-inflammatory agent, e.g. rheumatic and rheumatoid arthritis
- Collagen vascular disease
- Vasculitic syndromes
- Immune suppressive therapy, e.g. ITP
- ARDS, septic shock, hypocalcemia and anaphylaxis.

Local Applications

Ocular, ear and dermatological conditions.

Adverse reactions

- Suppression of hypothalamopituitary axis after prolonged therapy
- Retardation of linear growth children
- Hyperglycemia and hypertension
- Cushingoid features
- Proximal myopathy and osteoporosis
- Glaucoma and cataract formations
- Steroid psychosis
- Erosive gastritis and GI hemorrhage
- Immune suppression predisposes to bacterial, fungal and TB infection.

Different Types of Corticosteroids

- *Short acting,* e.g. hydrocortisone—half-life: 8–12 hrs
- *Intermediate acting,* e.g. prednisolone, methyl prednisolone half-life 12–36 hrs.
- *Longer acting:* Dexamethasone 36–54 hrs and betamethasone 36–54 hrs.

Note: Highest mineralocorticoid activity occurs with hydrocortisone and prednisolone.

Highest glucocorticoid activity occurs with dexamethasone and betamethasone.

Precautions during glucocorticoid therapy

Check and rule out following disorders before starting corticosteroids.

- Diabetes mellitus
- Cataract
- Tuberculosis
- Myopathy
- Peptic ulceration
- Osteoporosis
- Septic foci

Guidelines to be followed during steroid therapy.

- Administer the drug with food
- Restrict the intake of sodium and increase potassium intake
- Monitor body weigh, blood pressure, blood sugar, infection, GI bleed, potassium level and eye changes
- Growth monitoring in pediatric age
- Steroid should not be stopped abruptly and to be tapered and stopped

- In acute stress conditions like infection, surgery further increase in the dose of corticosteroid is required in patient on long-term steroid replacement therapy (e.g. Addison's disease)
- For long-term steroid therapy supplement calcium, vit D_3 and bisphosphonates to prevent steroid induced osteoporosis.

SEDATIVES, HYPNOTICS AND ANTICONVULSANT DRUGS

Diazepam

Belongs to benzodiazepines

Actions

- Anticonvulsant
- Muscle relaxant
- Anxiolytic
- Sedative hypnotic
- Dose: 5, 10 mg tablets up to 10 mg/day

Adverse reactions

- Lethargy, ataxia and drowsiness
- Amnesia
- Drug allergy

Phenobarbitone

- Derivative of barbituric acid
- Acts for more than 8 hours

Actions

- Sedative hypnotic effect
- Anti consultant effect
- Depression of respiration
- Minimal decrease of blood pressure
- Decrease GFR
- Hepatic microsomal enzyme induction.

Therapeutic Uses

- In the treatment of epilepsy
- In status epileptics
- In neonatal jaundice

Dosage: Tablets of 30 mg. 30 to 60 to 120 mg/day

Adverse reactions

- Allergic reactions
- Megaloblastic anemia
- Precipitation of acute porphyria
- Drug automatism, tolerance and dependence.

Principle in the Management of Barbiturate Overdosage

- Admission to the ICU
- Gastric lavage
- Care of breathing and airway and circulation
- Forced alkaline diuresis
- Maintenance of fluid and electrolyte balance
- Dialysis–peritoneal/hemodialysis
- Adequate nutrition and administration of antibiotics.

Diphenyl Hydantoin (Phenytoin sodium)

Uses

- In tonic clonic and partial seizures
- In status epilepticus
- Cardiac arrhythmias

Neuralgias: In trigeminal, glossopharyngeal and diabetic neuropathy.

Side effects

- Gum hyperplasia
- Drug allergy and Stevens-Johnson syndrome
- Cerebellar dysfunction
- Peripheral neuropathy
- Megaloblastic anemia
- Generalized lymphadenopathy and pseudolymphoma syndrome
- Hypertrichosis

Carbamazepine

Antiepileptic

Uses

- Tonic clonic and partial seizures
- Trigeminal neuralgia
- Central diabetes insipidus

Adverse reactions

- Allergic rashes
- Ataxia

- Obstructive jaundice
- Cytopenia

Sodium Valproate

- Antiepileptic drug
- Chemically, it is sodium dipropyl acetate

Uses

- Partial and tonic clonic seizures
- Status epileptics
- Manic depressive psychosis
- Migrainous headache

Side effects

- Allergic rashes
- Serum ammonia increase
- Thrombocytopenia

Dosage: 500 mg to 1500 mg/day

Chlorpromazine (Largactil)

Uses

- Manic depressive psychosis
- Senile psychosis
- Behavioral disorder in children
- Schizophrenia
- Antiemetic and anti-hiccup treatment

Side effects

- Photosensitivity and contact dermatitis
- Extrapyramidal symptoms, e.g. Parkinsonian tremor
- Behavioral abnormalities: Like restlessness and excitement
- Autonomic disturbance
- Cholestatic jaundice
- Cytopenia
- Neuroleptic malignant syndrome

Dose: 25 to 50 mg

Drugs Used in the Treatment of Helminthiasis

Mebendazole

- A benzimidazole derivative
- Useful in the treatment of:
  - Ascariasis
  - Ancylostoma infection
  - Enterobiasis (pinworm)
  - Trichuriasis
  - *Strongyoloides stercoralis*
  - *Trichenella spiralis*
  - *Echinococcus granulosus*

Dose: Enterobial infection: 100 mg single dose, repeat the dose after 1 week.

Hookworm and roundworm infection: 100 mg 1-0-1 × 3 days.

Adverse reactions

- Vertigo and dizziness
- To be avoided in pregnancy

Albendazole

Broad spectrum benzimidazole derivative

Use: As for mebendazole

Dosage: Most of the helminthic infection—400 mg of single dose, can be repeated after 1 week.

For hydatid disease 400 mg 1-0-1 × 1 month

For cysticercosis 400 mg 1-0-1 × 3 weeks.

Piperazine

- Useful in ascariasis and enterobiasis
- Causes flaccid paralysis of worms
- Can cause nausea, vomiting diarrhea and neurotoxicity

Dose: 300 mg tablets

Adults: 4 gr—single dose

Pyrantel Pamoate

- Tetrahydropyrimidine derivative
- Very effective against roundworms and enterobiasis.

Dosage: 10 mg/kg up to 1 gram–single dose cause gastrointestinal disturbance and drowsiness.

Ivermectin

- Effective against microfilariae and onchocerciasis
- Effective as single dose

Uses

- Onchocerciasis
- Lymphatic filariasis
- Scabies and head lice infestation

Levamisole

- Is a tetramisole
- Has got immunostimulant activity
- Effective against hookworm and ascariasis

Dose: 150 mg—single dose

Thiabendazole

- Benzimidazole derivative
- Acts against roundworms, hookworms, pinworms and strongyloidosis can cause GI disturbance, fever, hypoglycemia, disturbance of color vision

Dosage: 25 mg/kg body weight in adults.

Drugs Used in the Treatment of Amoebiasis

Drugs used in the treatment of intestinal amoebiasis (luminal amoebicides)

- Diloxanide furoate
- Antibiotics–tetracyclines and paramomycin
- Drugs used in extraintestinal amoebiasis only: Chloroquine

Drugs Used in Both Intestinal and Extraintestinal Amoebiasis

- Metronidazole
- Tinidazole
- Secnidazole
- Emetine hydrochloride

Metronidazole

- Imidazole derivative
- Drug of choice in intestinal and extra-intestinal amoebiasis
- Ineffective against asymptomatic cyst passers
- Less toxic

Dosage: 400 to 800 mg 8th hrly × 5 to 7 days, available as oral and intravenous preparations.

Uses

- Intestinal and hepatic amoebiasis
- Trichomoniasis
- Anaerobic infection
- Giardiasis and ulcerative gingivitis

Adverse reactions

- Nausea, anorexia, headache
- Peripheral neuropathy
- Antabuse like reaction

Tinidazole

600 to 800 mg 8th hrly 5–7 days useful in resistant amoebiasis. Idochlorohydroxy quinoline:

- A quinoline derivative
- More useful in amoebic cyst passers

Dose: 750 mg × 10 days.

Can cause peripheral neuropathy and SMON (subacute myelooptic neuropathy).

Diloxanide Furoate

- Effective in chronic intestinal amoebiasis
- In chronic amoebic cyst passers
- Not effective in extraintestinal amoebiasis

Dose: 500 mg 8th hrly 5 to 10 days

Other drugs used in the treatment of amoebiasis.

DRUGS USED IN THE TREATMENT FILARIASIS

Diethylcarbamazine

- A piperazine derivative
- Kills microfilariae and adult worms of *Wuchereria bancrofti*
- Sensitises microfilariae as they become susceptible to phagocytosis.

Dose: 6 mg/kg/day into 10–14 days

Uses

- Treatment of filariasis
- Tropical pulmonary eosinophilia.

Side effects

Nausea, vomiting, allergic reactions, drowsiness and convulsions.

DRUGS USED IN THE TREATMENT OF VIRAL INFECTIONS

Acyclovir

Contains virus specific thymidine kinase

Dose: Oral 200 to 400 mg 4 to 5 times day and IV 10 mg/kg 8th orally.

Adverse reactions

- Renal dysfunction
- Tremors
- Thrombophlebitis

Uses

- Herpes simplex infection
- Varicella zoster infection

Antiviral drugs related to acyclovir

- Famcyclovir
- Gancyclovir
- Valcyclovir

Other antiviral drugs

- Amantadine
- Forscarnet
- Ribavirin

DRUGS USED IN THE TREATMENT OF ANEMIA

Iron Therapy

Daily iron requirement

- Children: 8–15 mg/day
- Adult men: 10–15 mg/day
- Adult women: 15–20 mg/day
- Pregnancy and lactation: 20–25 mg/day

Preparation and dosage

- Oral iron
  - Tab ferrous sulphate 200 mg 8th hrly
  - Tab ferrous fumerate 200 mg 8th hrly.

Parenteral iron

- Iron dextran (imferon IM/IV)
- Iron sorbital (jectofer)
- Iron carbohydrate complex (uniferon)

Indication for Iron Therapy

Therapeutic

- Nutritional iron deficiency
- Anemia of blood loss
- Anemia of pregnancy and lactation.

Causes of Failure of Oral Iron Therapy

- Noncompliance
- Improper diagnosis
- Iron malabsorption
- Continuous blood loss
- Underlying chronic disease
- Underlying malignancy

Indication for Parenteral Iron Therapy

- Noncompliance
- Failure to tolerate oral iron
- Extensive bowel resection
- Malabsorption of iron

Formula for total dose parenteral iron therapy

15 – patient's Hb in gram/dl × 2.3 × patient's weight in kg = mg of iron required + 500 mg to 1000 mg for iron stores.

Vitamin B_{12} (Cyanocobalamin)

Indication for vitamin B_{12} replacement

- Malabsorption of vitamin B_{12}
- Inadequate utilization (inherited deficiency of enzymes)
- Fish tapeworm infestation
- Deficient intake of vitamin B_{12}

Preparation available

- Oral vitamin B_{12} tablets
- Injectable cyanocobalamin 1000 ug/ml

Folic Acid (Pteroylmonoglutamic acid)

Indication of folic acid supplementation:

- Deficient intake of folic acid
- Malabsorption
- Increased requirement
  - Pregnancy
  - Hemolytic anemias
  - Chronic infection
- Impaired utilization:
  - *For example:* Phenytoin/phenobarbitone therapy
  - Chronic alcoholism
  - Liver disease
  - Prevention of fetal neural tube defect.

Preparation: Tab folic acid 5 mg

Dosage: 1–5 mg/day.

16 Medical Emergencies

CHECKLIST FOR GENERAL PHYSICAL EXAMINATION

- Acute pulmonary edema
- Anaphylaxis and anaphylactic shock
- Shock
- Status epileptics
- Sudden cardiac death
- Management of acute myocardial infarction
- Drowning
- Acute severe asthma
- Organophosphorous poisoning
- Myxedema coma
- Thyrotoxic crises
- Addisonian crises
- Hypoglycemia

ACUTE PULMONARY EDEMA

Acute Pulmonary Edema
(Acute left heart/left ventricular failure)

Causes

- Acute myocardial infarction
- Acute myocarditis
- Acute MR/AR
- Atrial fibrillation in previously diseased heart
- Accelerated hypertension.

Clinical features

- Dyspnea and orthopnea
- Pulsus alternans
- Central cyanosis
- Left sided 3rd heart sound
- Bilateral basal crepitations in the lung

Management

Steps in the management:

- Oxygen administration
- Diuretics
- Digitalis
- Dilators–vasodilators
- Treatment of the cause

Positioning the patient: Keeping the leg downwards when the patient is sitting, reduces the venous return decreasing the pulmonary edema.

Oxygen administration

- 100% oxygen administration is essential for adequate oxygenation of tissues.
- If patient cannot maintain adequate oxygenation it is ideal to start:
  - Noninvasive ventilation via mask
  - Endotracheal intubation and ventilation with positive end expiratory pressure.

Other Measures

Nitrates: In severe pulmonary edema without hypotension has got systemic venodilator and coronary dilator effect, e.g. sublingual nitrates:

- IV nitroglycerin 5–10 micrograms/min
- IV sodium nitroprusside 0.1 to 5 micrograms/kg/min (systemic vasodilator)
  Useful in patients with sever hypertension.

ACE Inhibitors

- Arteriolar dilators

- Useful in patients with pulmonary edema, e.g. ramipril 1.25 to 2.5 mg/day

Special circumstances: In patients with severe left ventricular dysfunction with pulmonary edema with hypotension.

Intravenous dopamine and intravenous dobutamine have got positive inotropic effect.

Diuretics

IV furosemide 0.5 mg/kg–rapid relief of symptoms–dose can be repeated.

It is also a venodilator.

In patients with renal insufficiency– intravenous furosemide 1 mg/kg may be required. Bumetanide/torsemide can also be used as alternatives to furosemide.

Digitalis

Beneficial in patients with left ventricular dysfunction with rapid heart rate due to atrial flutter/fibrillation can cause side effects in patients with hypokalemia.

Dose: Tab digoxin 0.25 mg/day

Morphine

In anxious patients, can decrease breathlessness due to pulmonary edema, decreases anxiety, tachycardia and catecholamine release.

Dose: 2–4 mg IV and can be repeated

Amrinone and Milrinone

These drugs increase myocardial contractility and can cause vasodilatation of peripheral and pulmonary vasculature.

In patients with acute pulmonary edema due to acute severe mitral regurgitation/ventricular rupture: Intracardiac balloon pump/LV assist device can be used.

Above measures can also be used in patients before cardiac transplantation in patients with severe pulmonary edema due to myocarditis/cardiomyopathy.

Treatment of primary disorders like tachyrhythmia and hypertension require treatment in patients with pulmonary edema.

ANAPHYLAXIS AND ANAPHYLACTIC SHOCK

Definition and clinical features: Rapid appearance of allergic reactions to specific antigen in a susceptible individual.

Manifestations

- Urticarial rash with intense itching
- Breathlessness due to laryngeal edema or bronchospasm
- Hypotension and shock (anaphylactic shock)
- Cardiac arrhythmias.

Usual Predisposing Factors

Drugs

- Beta-lactam antibiotics (penicillins and cephalosporins)
- Lignocaine and procaine
- Vitamin preparations
- Radiographic contrast
- Vaccines, serums and insulin
- Food materials, fish, milk and egg.

Treatment

- For urticarial rashes: IM/IV diphenylhydramine 50–100 mg
- For bronchospasm: 250 to 500 mg IV aminophylline
- For severe anaphylaxis: Subcutaneous/intramuscular adrenaline 0.3 to 0.5 ml 1:1000 dose can be repeated at 20 to 30 minutes intervals.

In Case of Bite/Stings

- Removal of the insect stings if present
- Tourniquet application proximal to the site of bite/reaction.
- Subcutaneous injection of 1:1000–0.2 ml of adrenaline into the reaction site.

In Case of Hypotension/Shock

IV fluids–normal saline several liters and Inotropic agents IV dopamine.

If severe hypoxia, bronchospasm and cardiac arrhythmias:

- Nebulised β_2 agonist
- Oxygen administration by nasal prongs/ mask
- Intermittent positive pressure breathing
- Endotracheal intubation/tracheostomy

Corticosteroids: IV hydrocortisone 100 mg. Prevents further development of urticaria, angioedema, shock and laryngospasm.

SHOCK

Shock (circulatory failure): A state wherein there is hypoperfusion of the tissues despite normal oxygen content of the blood.

Different Types of Shock

1. *Hypovolemic shock*: Condition associated with significant reduction in the circulating blood volume, e.g.
   - Internal bleeding
   - Burns
   - Severe dehydration
2. *Anaphylactic shock*: Due to allergic reaction, e.g. penicillin administration.
3. *Cardiogenic*: Due to severe myocardial dysfunction and cardiac failure, e.g. acute MI severe mitral regurgitation, myocarditis.
4. *Neurogenic*: Due to disruption of neurogenic vasomotor control and brain stem abnormality, e.g. severe brain/injury the spinal cord.
5. *Obstructive*: Due to obstruction to the circulation, e.g. massive pulmonary embolism, tension pneumothorax, cardiac tamponade.
6. *Septic shock*: Due to bacterial endotoxins with gram-negative bacterial infections.

Clinical Features of Shock

- Cold clammy extremities
- Tachycardia (HR > 100/min)
- Hypotension (systolic BP < 90 mm of Hg)
- Breathing–tachypnea, may be rapid and shallow.
- Altered sensorium and urine output decreased < 30 ml/hr
- JVP central venous pressure reduced (in hypotension)/elevated (in cardiac failure)
- Multiple organ dysfunction.

Treatment of Shock

- Early recognition of state of shock
- Treatment of initiating event
  - Correction of blood volume—IV fluids, blood transfusion, plasma and plasma transfusion
  - Hemostasis
  - Defibrillation
  - Antibiotics
  - Removal of necrotic tissue.
- Treatment of secondary effect of shock
  - Correcting hypoxemia
  - Metabolic acidosis
  - Renal failure
- Maintenance of cardiac output, blood pressure and urine output (by volume replacement, inotropic support–by dopamine, dobutamine and vasopressin.

Treatment of Specific Conditions

- Like anaphylaxis, pulmonary embolism, acute MI and sepsis
- Neurogenic shock to be treated as hypovolemic shock
- Glucocorticoids–in anaphylaxis, sepsis and adrenal insufficiency.

STATUS EPILEPTICUS

Status epilepticus is a clinical condition characterized by continuous attack of seizures without regaining consciousness in between. Usual duration of attack for definition of status epilepticus is 15–20 mins. But drug therapy is to be administered if the seizure lasts for more of 5 minutes.

Types of Status Epilepticus

- Generalized tonic clonic status
- Absence seizure status

- Partial seizure status (epileptia partialis continua)
- A state of confusion/coma.

Precipitating Factors for Status Epilepticus

- Head injury
- CNS infection
- CNS tumors
- Abrupt withdrawal of antiepileptic drugs.
- Metabolic abnormalities
- *Drugs and toxins:* Quinalones/theophylline.

Management of Status Epilepticus

Medical emergency requires urgent medical attention.

Immediate Measures

- Maintenance of airway
- Attention to acute cardiorespiratory disturbance
- Treatment of hyperthermia
- Take blood samples for blood sugar, RFT, LFT, electrolytes, etc.
- Start drug therapy

Drug Therapy of Status Epilepticus

- *1st step:* Intravenous 25 to 50 ml of 50% dextrose before drawing blood samples for investigations.
- *2nd step:* IV lorazepam 4 mg or 0.1 mg/kg and repeat after 10 minutes if required or IV diazepam 10 mg over 2 minutes.
- *3rd step:* If seizures continue to occur–IV phenytoin/phosphenytoin–20 mg/kg in IV normal saline. Alternative to phenytion–IV sodium valproate 25 mg/kg.
- *4th step:* If seizures continue to occur. Try repeat dose of phenytoin 10 mg/kg–50 mg/min or IV phosphenytoin 10 mg/kg–150 mg/min or alternative IV sodium valproate 25 mg/kg.
- *5th step:* If seizures continue to occur. IV phenobarbitone–20 mg/kg–60 mg/min and continuous administration 10 mg/kg if required.
- *6th step:* If seizures are not controlled with the above measures:
  - Try general anaesthesia with propofol/pentobarbitone with ventilatory assistance
  - Neuromuscular blockade

Note: Phosphenytoin can be converted to phenytoin after IV administration.

Advantages of Phosphenytoin Over Phenytoin

- No dosing adjustment required in renal insufficiency
- Less likely to cause reaction at the infusion site.
- Can be given with all common solutions
- Can be administered at a faster rate—150 mg/min, phosphenytoin is expensive.

While administering IV phenobarbitone/diazepam respiratory depression can occur and it is preferred to be administered in ICU.

IV midazolam can control the seizures in refractory epilepsy.

Dose: Loading dose: 0.2 mg/kg and later 0.05 mg to 0.2 mg/kg maintenance dose.

Complications of Status Epilepticus

- Metabolic abnormalities
- Hyperthermia
- Cardiorespiratory disturbances
- Irreversible injury to the neurons.

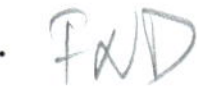

SUDDEN CARDIAC DEATH

Cardiac Arrest

Sudden stopping of pumping of blood from the heart, can result in sudden death but death can be prevented by immediate measures.

Common Causes of Cardiac Arrest

- Ischemic heart disease, e.g. acute MI
- Obstructive/dilated cardiomyopathy
- Valvular heart disease, e.g. severe aortic stenosis

Rare causes

- Myocarditis
- Electrophysiological abnormalities, e.g. WPW syndrome
- Congenital QT prolongation.

Precipitating Causes of Cardiac Arrest

- Hypo/hyperkalemia
- Hypoxia
- Heart failure
- Autonomic dysfunction
- Acidosis
- *Drugs:* Digoxin, antiarrhythmic drugs.

Cardiovascular Collapse

Sudden onset of cardiac dysfunction or dysfunction of peripheral vascular system resulting in losing effective blood flow, e.g. vasovagal syncope, neurogenic syncope and cardiogenic syncope.

Cardiovascular collapse may reverse spontaneously or with intervention.

Management of Cardiac Arrest

Suspect/confirm cardiac arrest.

Following observations are essential in a patient of cardiac arrest

- Examination of carotid and femoral pulse.
- Respiratory movement.
- Level of consciousness.

Absence of pulse, respiratory movement and unconsciousness suggest cardiac arrest.

Following immediate measures are essential in a suspected patient of cardiac arrest

- Immediate precordial thump
- Precordial thump is delivered at the junction of middle and lower part of the sternum forcibly by a clenched first.

It the pulse is felt and patient has got evidence of upper airway obstruction/aspiration is suspected and immediate hemlich maneuver is performed to dislodge the secretions to visualize the pharynx and clear the airway.

The head is held backwards and lift the chin upwards making the airway and pharynx visible.

Clearing the airway

- Clear the secretions in the oral cavity.
- Clear the foreign body and artificial dentures if present.

Cardiopulmonary Resuscitation (CPR)

Basic Life Support (BLS)

Purpose of CPR: To maintain the perfusion and oxygenation to vital organs till definitive measures are available.

Maintenance of circulation: Compress and depress the sternum (about 5 cm) at the level of lower part of the sternum around 100/minute.

Place the lower part of the palm of one hand over the dorsum of the other hand which is placed over the lower part of the sternum and administer the compression.

After compressing the sternum with abrupt relaxation, circulation is maintained by pumping action of the heart which is facilitated by chest compression.

Maintenance of respiration: Perform mouth to mouth breathing. Special instruments can be used like Ambubag and oropharyngeal airways.

For every 30 chest compression inflate the lung two times in succession. 30/2

Advanced Cardiac Life Support (ACLS)

Purpose of advanced life support

- To maintain/restore vital organ perfusion
- Maintain of cardiac output and blood pressure stabilization
- Adequate ventilation
- To control the rhythm abnormalities of the heart.

Requirements for advanced cardiac life support

- Intravenous line
- Endotracheal intubation
- Electrical cardioversion/pacing.

Drugs–antiarrhythmics, adrenaline, atropine, vasopressin, sodium bicarbonate.

If the diagnosis of ventricular tachycardia (VT)/ ventricular fibrillation (VF) (with absence of pulse)

- Defibrillate it within 5 minutes of onset of VT/VF
- If there is a delay of more than 5 minutes perform CPR.

If there is no response to above measures endotracheal intubation, obtain IV line and continue the CPR.

If patient is not responding administer intravenous adrenaline, can be repeated after 3–5 minutes. Vasopressin 40 units IV can be tried.

If there is no response immediate administration of defibrillation 360 joules.

If there is no response readminister adrenaline and IV sodabicarbonate (1 mEq/ kg), consider antiarrhythmic drugs.

If patients condition is not responding repeated cycles of defibrillation and drugs can be tried.

Antiarrhythmic drugs which can be tried: Amiodarone 150 mg–1 mg/min or lidocaine –1.5 mg/kg or magnesium sulphate 1–2 gr IV or procainamide 30 mg/IM.

Causes of Bradycardia Asystole

Cardiovascular

- Acute MI
- Massive pulmonary embolism
- Hypovolemia

Respiratory

- Tension pneumothorax
- Hypoxia

Electrolytes and metabolic abnormalities hypokalemia, hyperkalemia, acidosis and hypothermia.

Management of Bradycardiac Asystole

- Immediate CPR
- Obtain intravenous line
- Endotracheal intubation
- IV adrenaline 1 mg IV
- IV atropine 1 mg IV
- IV sodabicarbonate 1 mg/kg
- Above drugs can be repeated
- Identify and treat the cause
- Pacemaker implantation external or with pacing wire may be required.

MANAGEMENT OF ACUTE MYOCARDIAL INFARCTION (MI)

Steps in the Management of Acute (MI) Admission to the ICU

Relief of chest pain

- Sublingual nitroglycerine 0.4 mg till pain is relieved (maximum 3 doses) and IV nitroglycerin if pain persists.
- IV morphine 4 to 10 mg + IV metoclopramide (antiemetic)
- Administer O_2 inhalation
- Aspirin 325 mg to be chewed.

General measures

- Bed rest
- ACE inhibitors
- IV beta-blockers
- Thrombolysis and anticoagulation
- Treatment of complications

Other measures: Soft diet and sedation.

Discharge and Rehabilitation

- Graded increase in physical activity
- To continue aspirin, beta-blockers and ACE inhibitors.
- Treatment of risk factors:
  - Diabetes mellitus
  - Hypertension
  - Hyperlipidemia
  - Obesity
  - Abstinence from smoking and alcohol.

DROWNING

- Common cause of accidental death
- Death occurs due to asphyxiation due to immersion in water.

After water inhalation there will be

- Ventilation perfusion imbalance
- Hypoxemia
- Diffuse pulmonary edema

Fresh Water Drowning (Hypotonic fluid)

- Can cause hemolysis
- Alveolar edema due to impaired surfactant action.

Salt Water Drowning (Hypertonic fluid)

- Can cause pulmonary edema
- Secondary infection occurs due to inhalation of water.

Clinical Features

- Hypotension
- Dehydration
- Acidosis
- Cardiac arrhythmias
- ARDS
- Hypoxic cerebral damage
- External injury to the body.

Treatment

- Remove the person from water in horizontal position
- Standard cardiopulmonary resuscitation
- Administration of oxygen
- Continuous positive airway pressure to maintain the arterial oxygenation
- Antibiotics if secondary infection.

Near Drowning

Victims of drowning in water are alive (unconscious and usually not breathing).

Dry Drowning

Death occurs in a person of drowning due to laryngospasm (no water enters into the lungs). Cardiac arrest can occur if a person jumps into extremely cold water.

ACUTE SEVERE ASTHMA

Definition: Severe attack of breathlessness with wheeze which is not responding to usual medications which the patient is taking.

Precipitating factors

- Respiratory infection
- Abrupt stopping of ant asthmatic drugs like corticosteroids
- Exposure to allergens, β-blockers and NASIDs
- Anxiety and stress

Clinical Features

- Symptoms of severe wheezing, chest tightness and dyspnea
- Unable to speak in sentences
- Tachypnea
- Tachycardia
- Central cyanosis
- Pulsus paradoxus
- *Chest:* Hyperinflated, breath sounds severely reduced (silent chest)
- *Pulmonary function tests:* Severely reduced spirometric values
- *ABG:* Decreased PaO_2 with reduced $PaCO_2$ (initially due to hyperventilation) and later increased $PaCO_2$

Steps in the Management

Initial management

- 100% oxygen administration
- Nebulised β_2-agonists and ipratropium bromide
- Correction of dehydration
- Intravenous corticosteroids
- Monitor peak exploratory flow rate and arterial blood gas.

If there is no response within 15 minutes for the above measures

- Repeat nebulised β_2-agonists
- Repeat nebulised ipratropium
- Intravenous infusion of aminophylline

- Injectable β_2-agonists like terbutaline
- Continuation of corticosteroids

Rule out: Chest infection, pneumothorax and monitor serum potassium.

If bronchospasm and hypoxia persist, intensive care management with endotracheal intubation and ventilatory support is required.

ORGANOPHOSPHORUS POISONING

Clinical Features

Muscarinic Effects

- *Gastrointestinal:* Nausea, vomiting and diarrhea
- *Respiratory*: Bronchospasm pulmonary edema
- *Nicotinic effects*: Generalised muscle weakness, fasciculations, muscle paralysis and bradycardia.
- *Central effects*: Confusion, hypotension, convulsions and coma.

Treatment Guidelines

- Washing the skin and eyes
- Removal of clothes
- Cleaning the mouth and throat
- Maintenance of airways if necessary endotracheal intubation
- Gastric lavage

Specific Treatment

- Inj Pralidoxime (cholinesterase activator) 1–2 gm/day; 2–3 days.
- Inj. atropine 0.6 mg/ml till atropination and maintained for 2–3 weeks.
- Treatment of shock, hypoxia (ventilation) and treatment of convulsions.
- Continuous monitoring till 2–4 weeks for delayed effect of the poison.

MYXEDEMA COMA

Serious complication of untreated hypothyroidism.

Precipitating factors

- Elderly who are exposed to cold temperatures.
- Inadequate treatment of hypothyroidism
- Infection
- Trauma

Features

- Usually known case of hypothyroidism with features of myxedema
- Bradycardia
- Hypotension
- Hypothermia
- Altered sensorium

Additional Features

- Hypoglycemia
- Hyponatremia
- Hypoventilation
- Lactic acidosis
- Carbon dioxide retention

Management

- Admission to the ICU
- Levothyroxine in large doses if not orally through Ryle's tube
- Triiodothyronine injectable is available
- Injectable corticosteroids
- Antibiotics
- IV dextrose
- Management of hyponatremia and other electorate disturbances.

THYROTOXIC CRISES

Thyrotoxic crises occurs in patients with severe untreated hypothyroidism.

Precipitating Factors

- Infection
- Trauma
- Non-thyroid surgery in a patient of inadequately treated hyperthyroidism
- In a patient who has undergone thyroidectomy without adequate preparation.

Manifestations

- Tachycardia
- Hyperpyrexia
- Nausea, vomiting, diarrhea
- Irritability and altered sensorium.

Management

- Hospital admission into the ICU
- Treatment of the precipitating cause.

Supportive Measures

- O_2 administration
- IV dextrose, vitamins and minerals
- Antibiotics if required
- Treatment of hyperpyrexia with aspirin/ice packs and cooling blankets
- Digoxin if CCF present

Definitive Measures

IV propranolol 2–10 mg every 4 hrs.

Anti-thyroid drugs: Large dose of propylthiouracil 200 mg (prevents the conversion of T_4 to T_3 peripherally) or carbimazole 20 mg every 4 hrs.

Iodine

IV sodium iodide 1 gr IV infusion or through Ryle's tube 8th hrly.

ADDISONIAN CRISES (ACUTE ADRENAL INSUFFICIENCY)

Cause

- Sudden stopping of steroids from a person who is on long term steroid therapy
- Infection surgery trauma in a known case of Addison's disease
- Fulminant menigococcal sepsis.

Features

- Nausea, vomiting and abdominal pain
- Presence of fever
- Altered sensorium
- Hypotension and shock

Treatment

- IV fluids—dextrose saline infusion
- In hydrocortisone—100 mg bolus and then either IV infusion or 6th hrly administration
- Vasopressor drugs it required
- Treatment of the precipitating cause
- Once the patient is better he can be maintained with adequate dose of oral glucocorticoids and if required fluorocortisone.

HYPOGLYCEMIA

Symptoms appear when the plasma glucose level reaches less than 55 mg/dl.

Whipple Triad

1. Symptoms of hypoglycemia
2. Accurately measured low plasma glucose
3. Abolition of symptoms of hypoglycemia after raising plasma glucose.

Causes

Fasting hypoglycemia

- *Drug introduced:* Insulin, sulphonylureas and quinine
- *Endocrine deficiency:* Decrease of growth hormone and cortisol
- Endogenous increase of insulin, e.g. insulinoma
- *Systemic illness:* Severe renal and hepatic disease and severe sepsis.

Postprandial Hypoglycemia

Postgastrectomy, hereditary—fructose intolerance.

Causes of Hypoglycemia in a Diabetic

- Extradose of medication
- Inadequate food intake
- Unusual exercise
- Alcohol intake

Clinical Features

Autonomic symptoms

- Sweating
- Palpitation
- Anxiety
- Hunger
- Tremors

Neuroglycopenic Symptoms

- Headache
- Behavioural changes
- Confusion
- Coma
- Convulsions
- Death

Management

- If the patient is conscious and able to take orally: Oral glucose (carbohydrate intake).
- If the patient is not able to take orally: IV glucose 25% or 50%–100 ml and can be repeated. Continuous parenteral glucose administration if required.
- 1 mg glucagon SC or IM (if IV access not possible), useful in type 1 diabetes.
- Glucagon is not useful in type 2 diabetes mellitus (because glucagon increases insulin secretion).
- Glucagon is not useful in alcohol induced hypoglycemia (because of depleted glycogen).

17 Instruments

CHECKLIST FOR GENERAL PHYSICAL EXAMINATION

- Stomach tube
- Foley's catheter
- Malecot's catheter
- Ambubag
- Ryle's tube
- Endotracheal tube
- Tracheostomy tube
- Sengstaken-Blakemore tube
- Disposable syringe
- BD syringe and needle
- Insulin syringe

STOMACH TUBE

Indications for the use of stomach tube

- In patients with drug over dosage or consumption of poison—for giving stomach wash.

Description of the Tube

Length of the tube: 30 inches.

Marking on the tube

- Presence of a black ring at a point 18 inches from the tip of the tube. The black ring corresponds to the distance between the incisor teeth and cardiac end of the stomach
- A funnel can be attached to the proximal end of the stomach tube.

Administration of Stomach Tube (Fig. 17.1)

- Attach a funnel to the proximal end of a stomach tube and keep the funnel above the level of the stomach.
- Administer fluid-plane water through the funnel and the tube into the stomach. Lower the funnel below the level of stomach and fluid will be starting coming out through the tube. Repeat the procedure till the stomach contents are clear.

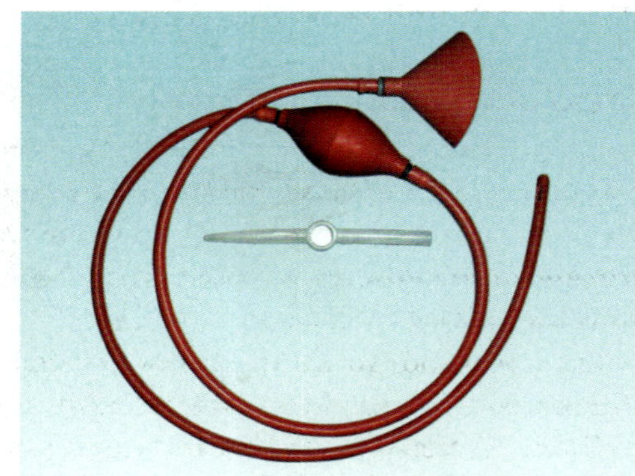

Fig. 17.1: Stomach tube

Foley's Catheter (Fig. 17.2)

Self-retaining flexible tubes which can be passed through the urethra to drain urine from the urinary bladder for prolonged duration.

Parts of Foley's Catheter

- Urinary drainage tip
- Inflatable balloon

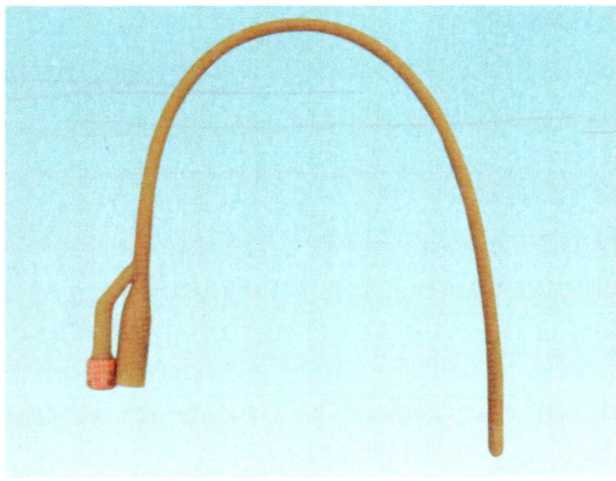

Fig. 17.2: Foley's catheter

- *Balloon sizes:* 5 cc and 30 cc
- *Material used for the catheter:* Silicon or natural rubber
- *Most common size of the catheter:* 10 f or 28 f (F = French unit reflecting diameter).

Method of Introduction of Foley's Catheter

- After aseptic precautions with lubrication, catheter is introduced through the penial part of urethra. Urine starts draining through the catheter as the catheter enters into the urinary bladder.
- Inject about 30–40 ml of sterile water into the small rubber side tube to inflate the balloon. When the balloon is adequately distended, catheter cannot be withdrawn from the urinary bladder.

Note: Balloon should not be inflated with air, as in case of rupture of balloon escaped air can infect the bladder.

Removal of Catheter

Remove the fluid from the balloon and deflate it and then withdraw the catheter from the bladder.

Indications for Foley's Catheter

- Unconscious patients
- Patients with urinary incontinence
- Patients who are sedated, anaesthetized or undergone surgery
- Acute retention/obstructive uropathy.
- Urethral surgeries

Rarer Indications

- In neuronal bladder dysfunctions
- While monitoring urine output
- After furosemide administration

Potential Complications while Using Foley's Catheter

Common: Urinary tract infection

Less common

- Urethral damage
- Hematuria
- Hypersensitivity/allergic reaction to latex

Change of catheter is required if the catheter is clogged, infected or becoming painful.

Care of Foley's Catheter

- Clean with soap and water catheter itself and exit area of the catheter from the body.
- It is mandatory to thoroughly clean the area after every bowel movement.
- In patients with suprapubic cystostomy use soap and water and clean the area over the abdomen around the catheter and cover the area with dry gauze.
- Washing the hand before and after handling the drainage tube can prevent the infection.

Causes of Leakage of Urine around the Foley's Catheter

- Urinary tract infection
- Spasm of urinary bladder
- Smaller sized catheter
- Improper balloon size
- Severe constipation

Care of the Drainage Tube and Bag

- Empty the urinary bag which is full or at least once in 8 hrs.
- Keep the drainage bag lower than the bladder level as it will prevent the urine from flowing backwards into the bladder.

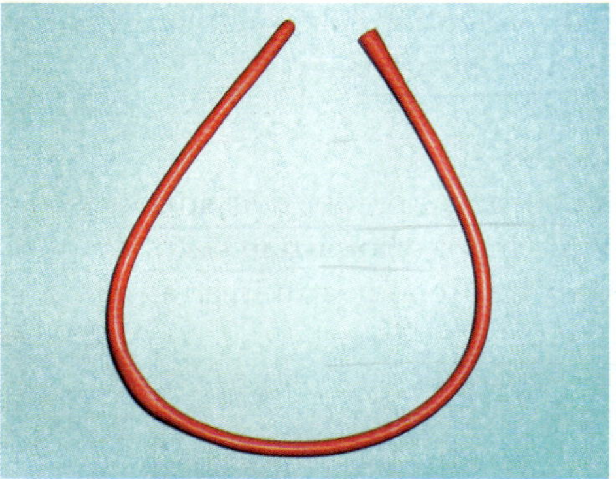

Fig. 17.3: Simple rubber catheter

- Vinegar/chlorine bleach can be used to clean deodorize the drainage bag.

Simple Rubber Catheter (Fig. 17.3)

- Simple rubber catheter is usually 16 inches long with an opening at its end.
- Use to drain the urine from the bladder momentarily. Urine can be easily drained into a bedpan.
- Continuous drainage of urine is not possible with the simple rubber catheter.

Oxygen administration can also be done by simple thinner rubber catheter.

Malecot's Catheter (Fig. 17.4)

Flower tipped (winged) catheter

Wings when introduced into the body cavity stabilises the catheter.

Uses of Malecot's catheter

- Drainage of urine from the bladder
- Drainage of empyema thoracis
- Drainage of urine from nephrostomy.

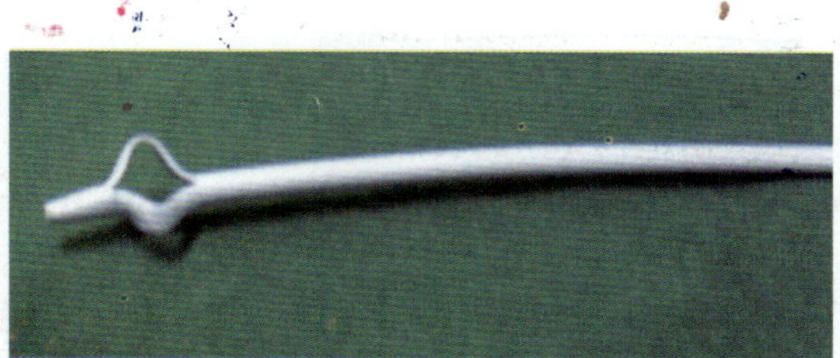

Fig. 17.4: Malecot's catheter

Ambubag (Fig. 17.5)

Technically called–bag valve mask resuscitator.

Parts of Ambubag

Ambubag consists of

- One way valve and an adapter
- Bag is the main part of the apparatus. Bag can be connected to the endotracheal tube directly or using the adapter. It can be attached to the mask.
- One way valve
- Allows the flowing of oxygen to the patients and prevents exhaled air to be breathed in from the patient.

Functioning of ambubag

- Helps in artificial respiration
- By squeezing the bag (manually inflated) air can be administered to the lungs
- When the squeezing pressure is released bag gets automatically inflated
- Due to the elastic recoiling of the chest air comes out of the lung
- Bag can be squeezed up to a rate of 20 breaths/minute

Indications

In all persons with respiratory difficulties either during resuscitation and or before connecting to the ventilator.

Risks Associated with Using Ambubag

- Hyperventilation resulting in respiratory alkalosis may occur due to too fast squeezing of the bag.

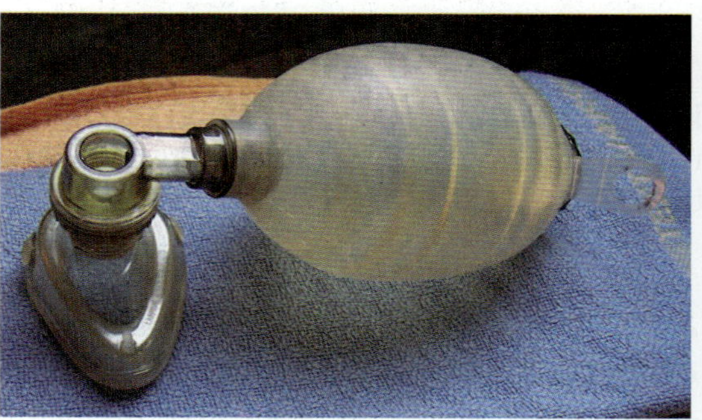

Fig. 17.5: Ambubag

- Gaseous distention of the abdomen may occur due to escape of some amount to air in to the stomach. This can interfere with breathing.

Ryle's Tube (Fig. 17.6)

A device which helps in administration of nutritious fluids, medications and removal of secretions from stomach/duodenum.

Features of Ryle's Tube

- Standard length of the tube: 105 cm
- Consists of a radio-opaque line which can be visualized by X-ray.
- Distal end of the tube is closed and contains metallic balls which are sealed into the tube. These metallic balls help in introduction of the tube.
- There are markings on the tube at 50, 60 and 70 cm from the tip of the tube which help in accurate placement of the tube.
- There are lateral holes in the tube at the distal end which help in administration of substances and aspiration of stomach contents.
- Ryle's tubes which are made of PVC material can remain for 2 weeks in the gastrointestinal tract.
- Feeding tubes made up of silicon/poly urethane can remain for a longer time in the gastrointestinal tract.

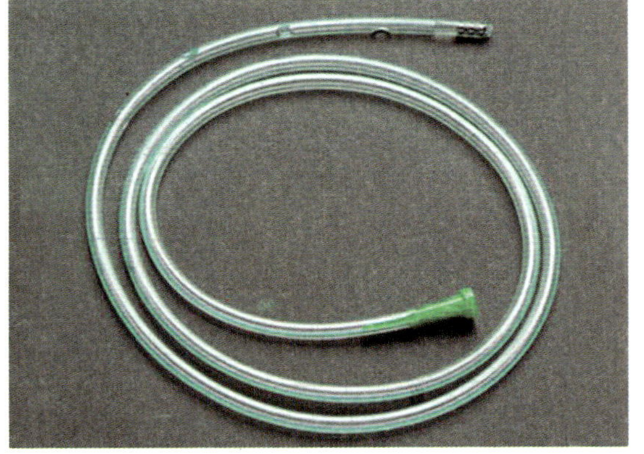

Fig. 17.6: Ryle's tube

Indications for RT Insertion

Diagnostic indications

- For detection of bleeding from the upper GI tract.
- To detect consumption of poison/drugs and to give stomach wash in such conditions.
- For analysis of gastric fluid in cases of peptic ulcer disease.

Therapeutic indications

- Administration of fluids and medications
- Removal of stomach contents in patients with upper GI bleed, GI perforation and GI obstruction.

Methods of Insertion RT

- Clean the tube properly and dip the tube in 1% xylocaine.
- Apply glycerine/liquid paraffin to make the tube lubricated.
- Pass the bulbous end of the tube via the nostril till to the pharynx and ask the patient to swallow (may be helped–if the patient has already asked to hold the water in the mouth and asked to swallow). When the tube enters into the stomach, stomach contents will start coming out of the tube. Positioning of black ring of the tube should be opposite the nose.

Taking Care of RT

- Keep the RT with its outer surface adhere to the side of the nose with the plaster.
- Withdraw the tube daily for about 2 inches and smear it with antiseptics and insert back the tube.

Nasogastric feeding through the RT is not suitable under following circumstances

- Gastric stasis
- Gastrooesophageal reflux
- Nasal injuries
- Stricture of upper GIT
- In patients with high-risk of aspiration.

Endotracheal Tube (Fig. 17.7)

Endotracheal tube is a device which is introduced into the trachea to keep the airway

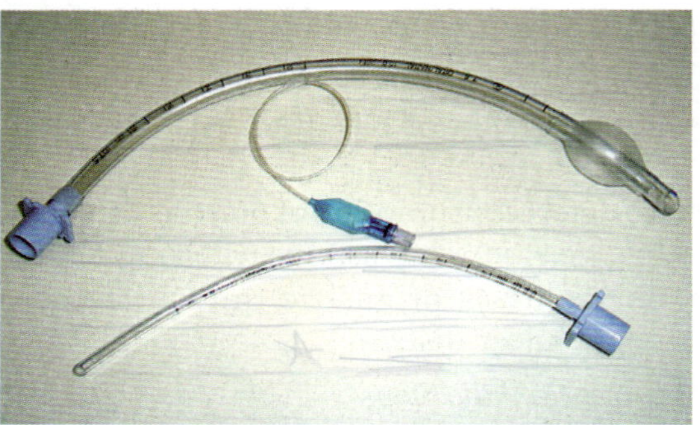

Fig. 17.7: Endotracheal tube

patent and air is able to reach the lungs. Endotracheal tube is the best device to protect the patient's airway.

Indications for ET Tube Insertion

- For artificial ventilation
- For administration of general anesthesia
- For protection of airways:
  - In unconscious patients
  - In patients with cardiac arrest
  - Patients with areflexia of pharynx
- In patients with obstruction to the airflow—tumor/trauma.

Description of Tube

- Cuffed or uncuffed ET tube
- Oral/nasal tubes
- Double lumen tubes/tracheostomy tubes

Material Used in Endotracheal Tubes: Portex/Rubber Tube

Cuffed tube

A cuff is attached to the lower edge of the tube.

Significance of the cuff

Cuff helps in securing the position of the tube in the trachea and prevents aspiration.

Size of the tube

Size of the tube depends on the internal diameter.

Usual size of the tube for males—7.5 to 8 mm

For females: 7.5 mm

Double lumen endotracheal tube

- Useful in patients with intrathoracic surgery
- Single lung ventilation is possible with double lumen endotracheal tube allowing the other lung to collapse to make the surgery easier.

Tracheostomy Tube

- Shortened form of endotracheal tube
- Tracheotomy tube can be introduced into the trachea through tracheotomy stoma in the neck. Patient can permanently live with the tracheostomy tube.

Method of Introduction of Endotracheal Tube

- Keep the patient's mouth open and introduce the endotracheal tube through the mouth guided by laryngoscope (deflate the cuff before introducing the tube).
- Endotracheal tube is passed through the vocal cords into the trachea. Cuff is inflated while injecting air into the cuff.

Note: While inflating the cuff— fluid should not be used as it can be aspirated with the cuff rupture. Portex type of ET tube cam be kept in position for a period up to 1 week.

Sengstaken-Blackemore Tube (Fig. 17.8)

Indication: To stop bleeding from gastric and esophageal varices in patients with portal hypertension.

Parts of Sengstaken tube

- Gastric balloon
- Esophageal balloon
- Holes for gastric aspiration
- Holes for esophageal aspiration.

Method of introduction of Sengstaken tube

- Insert the tube through the nasal cavity
- Inflate the esophageal and gastric balloon once the tube is in the stomach.
- Inflation of the balloon is carried out by the introduction of air
- Tube is made to be kept in position and inflation of the balloon produces hemostasis by its pressure effect

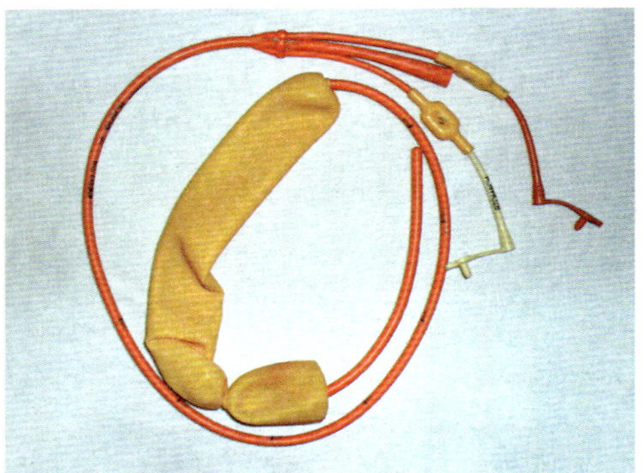

Fig. 17.8: Sengstaken-Blackemore tube

- Tube is usually kept for a maximum duration of 2–3 days
- Minnesota modification of Sengstaken tubes are more frequently used.

Complications of using Sengstaken tube

- Rupture of balloon and escape of air and air embolism
- Pressure effect of the balloon on the respiratory tract.

Disposable Syringe (Fig. 17.9)

- Disposable syringes are useful for prevention of transmission of hepatitis B and C and HIV infection.
- Disposable syringes are made of plastic material.
- These are effective because of their availability in sterilized conditions, ready to use, cost effective and for single use. They are available in the sizes of 1 ml, 2 ml, 5 ml and 10 ml.

BD Syringe and Needle

- B and D is the name of the manufacturers
- B and D is the short form of Becton and Dickinson
- BD syringe is a all glass syringe and sterilized with autoclaving
- It is available in 2 ml, 5 ml, 10 ml and 50 ml syringe.

Uses of BD Syringe

- For intravenous administration and collection of blood samples

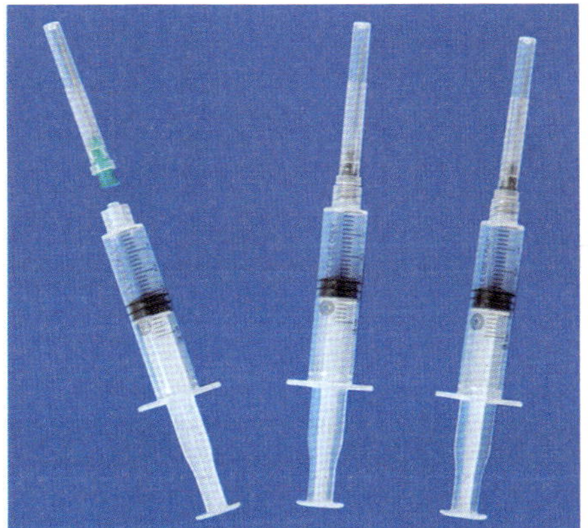

Fig. 17.9: Disposable syringe

- For intramuscular injections
- For aspiration of fluids from body cavity.

Record Syringe and Needle

Record syringe consist of partly metal and partly made-up of glass.

Parts of the Syringe

- Body of the syringe–made-up of glass
- Piston of the syringe–made-up of metal

Syringe cannot be autoclaved because it is made-up of partly glass and partly metal. Syringes are available in different sizes of 2 ml, 5 ml, 10 ml and 20 ml. Syringe is useful for injections.

Insulin Syringe (Fig. 17.10)

It is a 1 ml syringe

1 ml is graduated as 40 units/ml or 100 units/ml depending on the availability of insulin, e.g. 1 ml contains 40 units or 100 units. It can be administered as required by the patient. Piston of the syringe is white in color in contrast to tuberculin syringe (piston is blue in color).

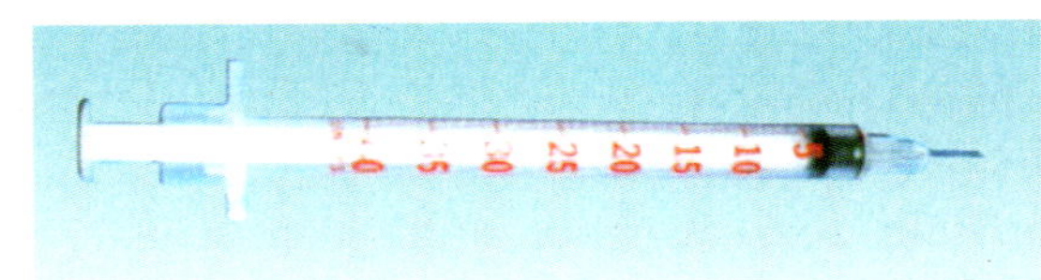

Fig. 17.10: Insulin syringe

18 ECG and Common ECG Abnormalities

CHECKLIST FOR GENERAL PHYSICAL EXAMINATION

- Normal ECG waves and intervals
- Determination of heart rate and electrical axis
- Chamber enlargements and hypertrophy
- Rhythm disorders
- Ischemic heart disease
- Drugs and electrolytes and ECG
- Miscellaneous disorders

Electrocardiogram

Normal ECG waves: P, Q, R, S, T and U waves (Figs 18.1a to c).

P Wave

- First wave to be noticed in the ECG tracing.
- Best recorded in leads II and chest lead V_1
- Normal P wave amplitude is 2.5 mm and normal duration of P wave is 0.11 secs.
- It indirectly indicates the time taken by the electrical impulse to spread from sinoatrial node (SA node) to atrioventricular node (AV node).
- Depolarisation of right and left atrium is represented by the P wave in the ECG (indicates atrial contraction).

QRS Complex

QRS complex consists of:

- Q wave—negative wave preceding R wave
- R wave—positive wave after Q wave
- S wave—negative wave after the R wave

QRS complex represents depolarization of the ventricles (contraction of ventricles).

T Wave

T wave appears after the R wave. T wave indicates repolarization of the ventricles.

U Wave

Occasionally, seen in normal ECG tracing following the T wave. Papillary muscle and Purkinje fibre repolarization results in U wave.

U wave becomes prominent in hypokalemia.

P-R Interval

Represents the time taken by the electrical impulse to spread from atria to ventricle. It is the interval measured from beginning of P wave to the starting of QRS complex. Normal duration of P-R interval is 0.12 to 0.2 secs.

QRS Interval

Normal duration 0.05 to 0.12 secs. QRS interval is measured from beginning of Q wave to the end of S wave.

P-P Interval

P-P interval is measured as interval between two consecutive P waves.

P-P interval is regular in sinus rhythm. It indicates atrial rate.

R-R Interval

R-R interval is measured as interval between two consecutive R waves.

R-R interval indicates ventricular rate.

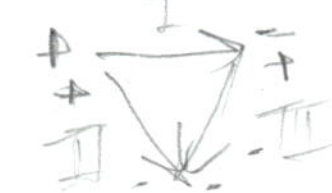

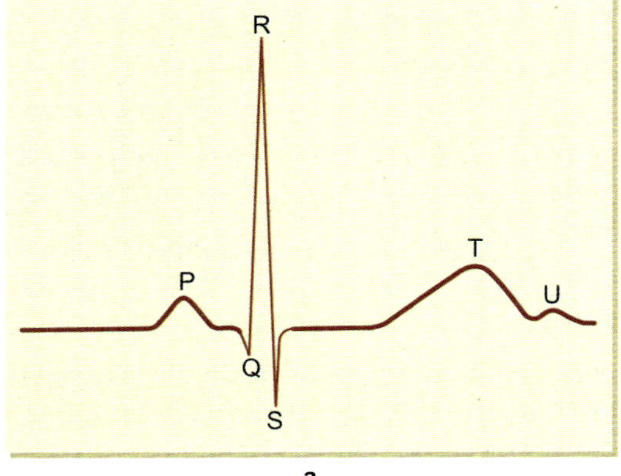

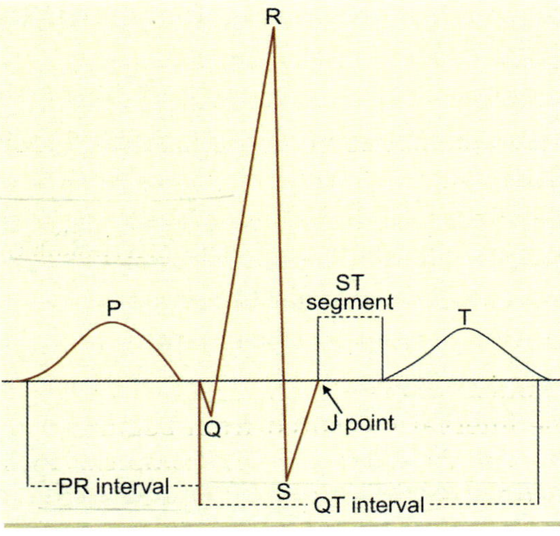

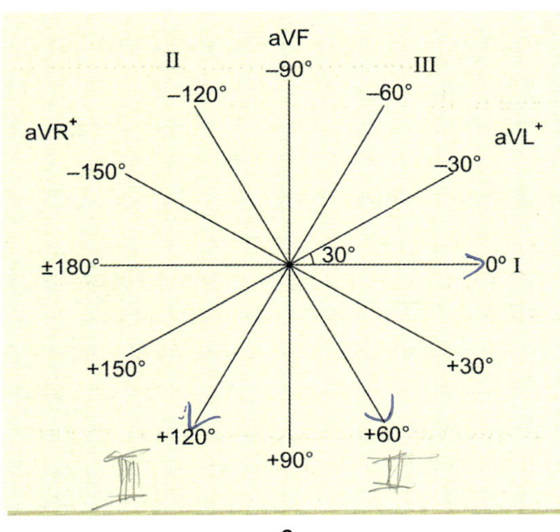

Figs. 18.1a to c: Normal ECG

Q-T Interval

Normal upper limit of Q-T interval is 0.43 secs.

Q-T interval is measured from beginning of QRS complex to the end of T wave.

Total duration of electrical systole is represented by Q-T interval.

Increased heart rate decreases the Q-T interval.

Ventricular Activation Time (VAT)

Normal duration 0.03 to 0.05 secs.

It is measured from beginning of QRS complex to the peak of R wave.

It represents the time taken by the electrical impulse to travel from endocardium to epicardium through the entire myocardium.

S-T Segment

It is the segment in the ECG which is measured from the end of QRS deflection and up to the beginning of T wave. It is usually isoelectric.

P-R Segment

Normally isoelectric.

It is the segment measured from the end of the P wave up to the beginning of QRS complex.

J Point (Junction of R-S and S-T segment)

J point represents the point at which QRS complex ends and at which S-T segment begins. Elevation or depression of T segment occurs in ischemic heart disease.

Calculation of Heart Rate

Calculation of heart rate when the rhythm is regular:

1st Method

- Calculate the number of small squares (1 mm or 0.04 secs) between two consecutive R waves and divide 1500 by the number of small squares counted.
- For example, if number of squares in between two consecutive R waves is 25 squares then the heart rate is 1500/25 = 60/min

2nd Method

Count the number of R waves in 3 seconds (25 small squares =1 sec) and multiply it by 20 = then the product is heart rate/minute.

Calculation of heart rate when the rhythm is irregular

Count the number of R waves in 6 seconds (25 small squares = 1 second) and multiply them by 10.

Determination of Electrical Axis in the ECG

- Determine the lead with smallest or most equiphasic deflection
- Determine also the lead perpendicular to the leads showing minimal or equiphasic deflection like
  - For lead I-perpendicular lead is aVF or vice versa
  - For lead II–perpendicular lead is aVL
  - For lead III–perpendicular lead is aVR

Electrical axis corresponding to the leads

- Lead I (0° to 180° +/–)
- Lead II (+60° to –120°)
- Lead III (–60° to +120°)
- aVR (+30° to –150°)
- aVL (–30° to +150°)
- aVF (–90° to +90°)
- If the QRS complex of the perpendicular lead indicates positive deflection the axis is indicated towards the positive pole of the lead.
- If QRS complex indicates a negative deflection then the axis is towards the negative pole, e.g.: If the lead II shows QRS with most equiphasic deflection the perpendicular lead will be aVL. If aVL lead shows QRS with positive deflection, then the axis is positive + 150°. If the QRS in aVL shows negative deflection then axis is –30°.

Rapid Calculation of Electrical Axis

- Look at only lead I and aVF

1. If lead I and aVF–QRS is in the same direction—axis is normal (Fig. 18.2a).

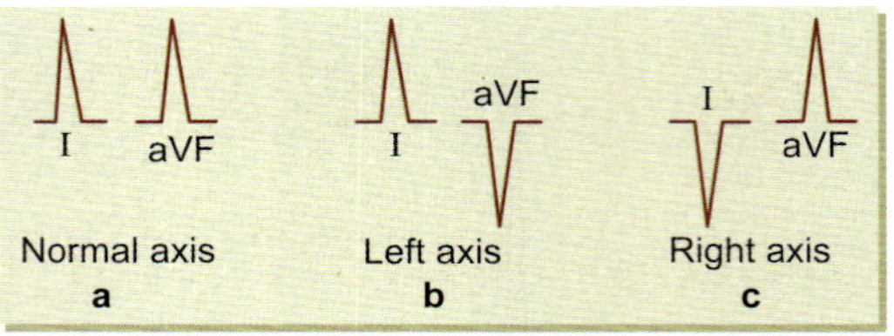

Fig. 18.2: Calculation of electrical axis

2. If lead I QRS is positive and QRS is negative in lead aVF it is indicative of left axis deviation (Fig. 18.2b).
3. If ORS is negative in lead I and positive in aVF it represents right axis deviation (Fig. 18.2c).

Normal QRS axis is between –30° and + 90°

Left axis deviation: Axis is between –30° and –90°

Causes of left axis deviation

- LBBB (left buddle branch block)
- LVH (left ventricular hypertrophy)
- LAHB (left anterior hemi block)
- Hyperkalemia

Right Axis Deviation

Electrical axis is between + 90° and +180°

Causes of right axis deviation

- Right ventricular hypertrophy (RVH)
- Right bundle branch block (RBBB)
- COPD
- Pulmonary embolism: Normal variant.

Left Atrial Enlargement

ECG characteristics

- Broad and notched P wave in lead II (P-mitrale)—duration between the peaks of P wave notches will be more than 0.04 secs.
- Maximum P wave duration will be more than 0.11 secs.
- Biphasic P wave with delayed and deep terminal (negative component) in lead V_1.

Causes of left atiral enlargement: Mitral valve disease and aortic valve disease.

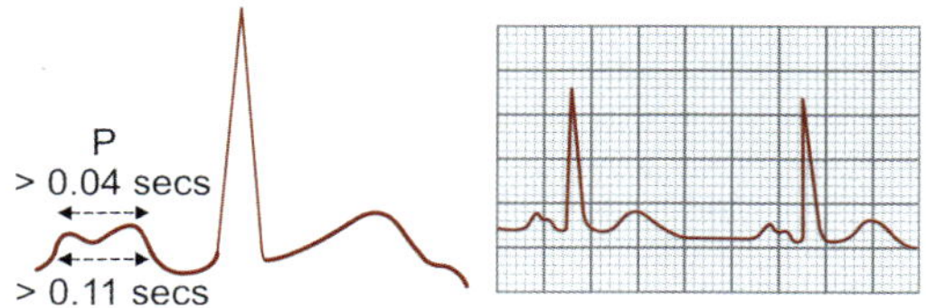

Fig. 18.3: P-Mitrale

Right Atrial Enlargement

ECG characteristics

Causes tall and peaked P waves (> 2.5 mm) in lead I and lead II (P-pulmonale)

Causes

- COPD
- Pulmonary stenosis
- Tricuspid valve disease

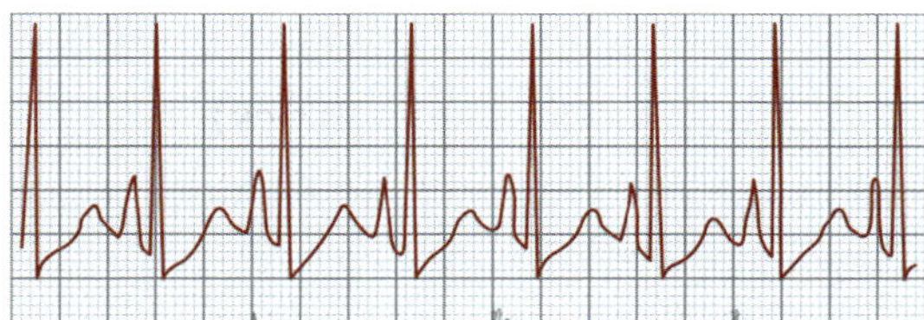

Fig. 18.4: P-Pulmonale

Left Ventricular Hypertrophy (LVH) (Fig. 18.5)

ECG characteristics of LVH

- Increased voltage of QRS
- S-T and T changes (S-T depression and T inversion)
- Left axis deviation
- Left atrial enlargement
- Increase in the ventricular activation time

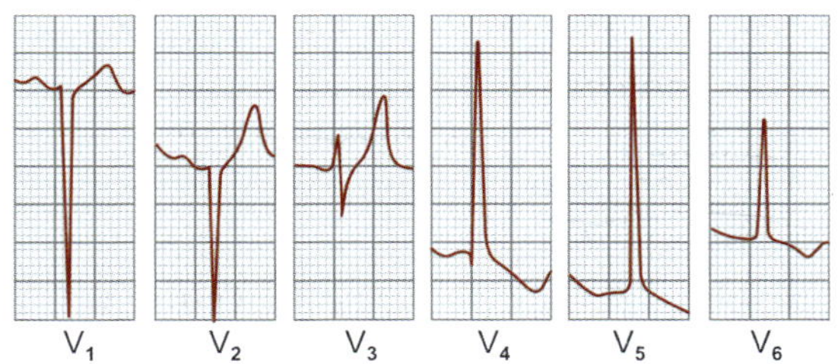

Fig. 18.5: Left ventricular hypertrophy

Voltage criteria of QRS

- R Wave in lead V_5 or V_6 > 25 mm
- S in V_1+R in V_5 Or V_6 > 35 mm

Causes of LVH

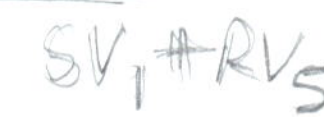

- Systemic hypertension
- Aortic stenosis
- Mitral regurgitation
- VSD
- PDA
- Coarctation of aorta

Right Ventricular Hypertrophy (RVH) (Fig. 18.6)

RVH: Dominant R wave in V_1 (R/S ratio in V_1 is more than one)

- Deep S wave in V_5 and V_6
- Right axis deviation
- S-T segment depression and T inversion in right ventricular leads.

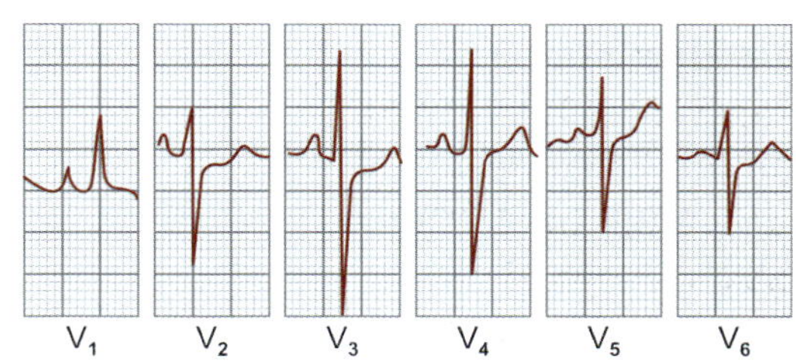

Fig. 18.6: Right ventricular hypertrophy

Causes of RVH

- All causes of pulmonary hypertension
- Pulmonary stenosis

Biventricular Enlargement

Large R wave in V_5 or V_6 (LVH)

Equiphasic QRS in V_5 and V_6 (Katz-Wachtel Phenomenon)

R/S ratio greater than one in V_1

ECG CHANGES IN RHYTHM DISORDERS

Sinus Bradycardia (Fig. 18.7)

Sinus rate is less than 60/min

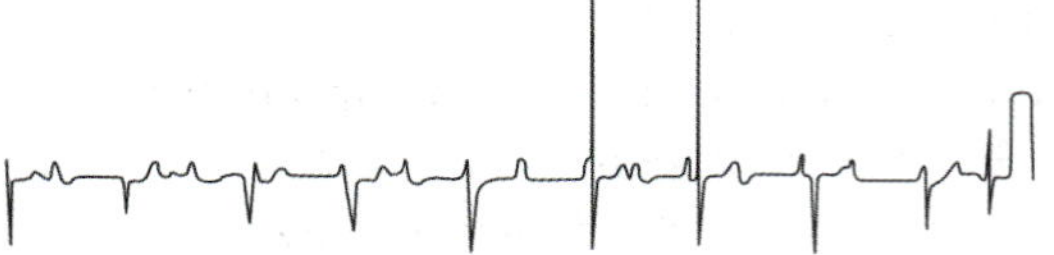

Fig. 18.7: Sinus bradycardia

Causes

- *Physiological*
  - Athlets
  - Sleep
- *Pathological*
  - Inferior wall
  - Myocardial infarction
  - Hypothyroidism
  - Obstructive jaundice
  - Raised intracranial tension

Drugs: Digitalis, beta-blockers, diltiazem

ECG pattern: Normal PQRST at regular intervals.

Sinus P wave precedes QRST with rate less than 60/minute.

Sinus Tachycardia (Fig. 18.8)

ECG: Sinus rate exceeds more than 100/minute.

Causes

- Exercise
- Anemia
- Fever
- Thyrotoxicosis
- CCF
- Drugs: Adrenaline, atropine and vasodilators.

ECG pattern: Normal PQRST complexes at regular intervals.

Sinus P wave preceding QRST with rate more than 100/minute.

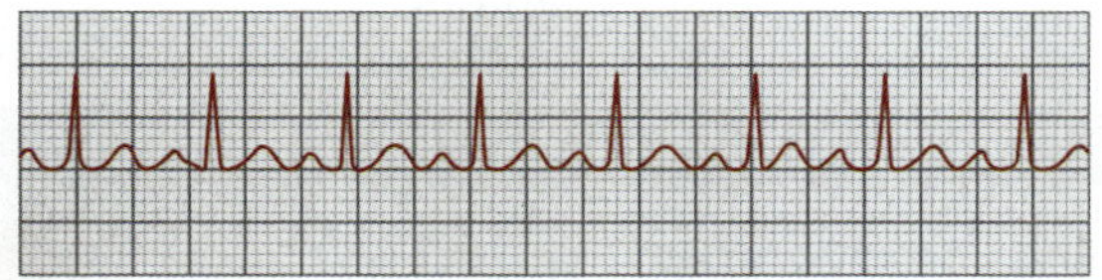

Fig. 18.8: Sinus tachycardia

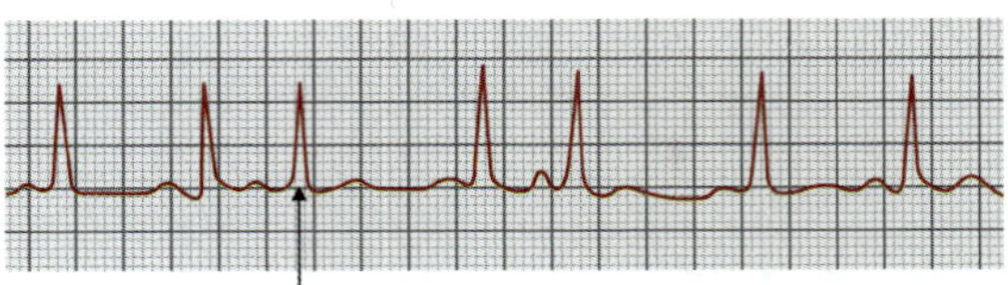

Fig. 18.9: Atrial ectopics

Sinus Arrhythmia

Physiological phenomenon: Waxing and waning of heart rate due to irregular discharge of SA node impulse.

ECG pattern: Normal PQRST with gradual shorting of R-R interval during inspiration and R-R interval lengthens during expiration.

Atrial Extra-asystole (Atrial ectopic and atrial premature beat) (Fig. 18.9)

ECG pattern

- Premature P wave (configuration of P′ wave is different from normal sinus P wave)
- Abnormal P′ wave is upright or inverted
- Normal QRST complex
- Incomplete compensatory pause

> *Note:* Compensatory pause: Atrial ectopic beat as it spreads across the atrium causes premature discharge of SA node.

After premature discharge, SA node undergoes complete cycle of recovery so as to discharge again. This results in compensatory pause meaning a pause following an ectopic beat.

Incomplete Compensatory Pause

Sum of the pre and post extra systolic internal is less than the 2 times the regular R-R interval (*see* under ventricular ectopics).

Causes of atrial ectopics

- Alcohol
- Excessive consumption of tea and coffee
- RHD
- IHD
- Thyrotoxicosis
- Hypertension

Paroxysmal Supraventricular Tachycardia (Fig. 18.10)

Occurs due to atrial rapid ectopic activity.

ECG features

- Rate 160–220/min and regular QRS complexes
- Normal S-T and T wave changes
- Preceding the QRS complex there will be a preceding P′ wave.
- P′ wave may not be made out as it is hidden in the QRST complex.

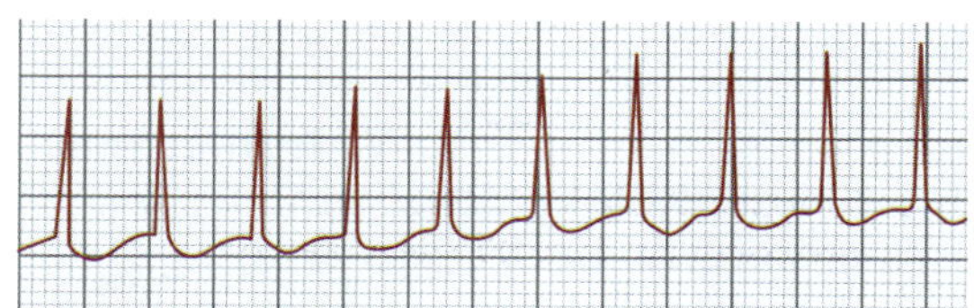

Fig. 18.10: Paroxysmal supraventricular tachycardia

ECG causes

- Rheumatic heart disease
- IHD
- Mitral valve prolapse
- Thyrotoxicosis
- WPW syndrome

Atrial Fibrillation (AF) (Fig. 18.11)

AF occurs due to completely disorganized atrial depolarization without effective contraction. P waves are not occurring and are replaced by small irregular or coarse undulations.

Ventricular response is irregular due to varying refractory period of the AV node conducting atrial impulses irregularly to the ventricles.

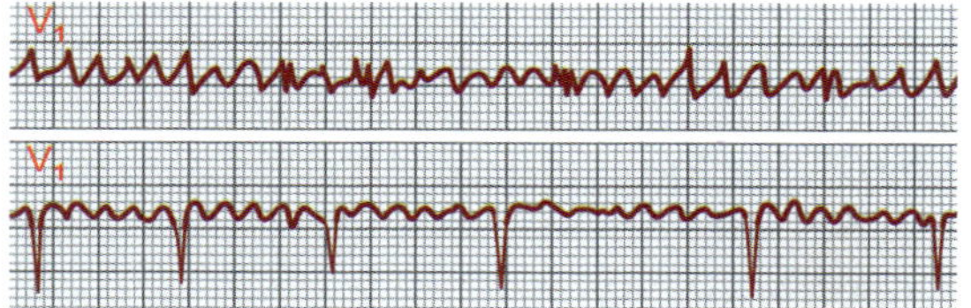

Fig. 18.11: Atrial fibrillation

Causes atrial fibrillation

Remembered with the mnemonic thrill

- T–Thyrotoxicosis
- H–Hypertensive heart disease
- R–Rheumatic heart disease
- I–Ischemic heart disease
- L–Lone atrial fibrillation

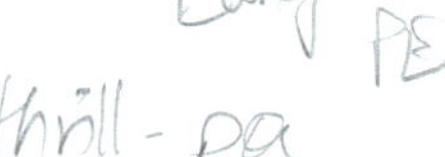

Other causes: Pericarditis and ASD

ECG characteristics

- Irregularly irregular rhythm
- Varying R-R interval
- Normal QRST complex
- Atrial rate is around 300–600/min with ventricular rate of 100–160/min
- No definite P wave preceding QRS and is replaced by fibrillatory F waves with undulating base line.

Atrial Flutter (Fig. 18.12)

- Atrial flutter indicates organic heart disease
- Reentry mechanism and atrial ectopic activity are the responsible mechanisms
- Atrial flutter is characterized by rapid atrial rate varying from 250–350/min.

Due to rapid atrial activity there will be block in the AV conduction usually in the ratio of 2:1 or 4:1.

Causes

- Mitral valve disease
- Coronary artery disease
- Corpulmonale
- Cardiomyopathy

ECG pattern

- Rapid atrial rate: Regular 250–350 beats/minute
- Normal QRST with regular ventricular rhythm

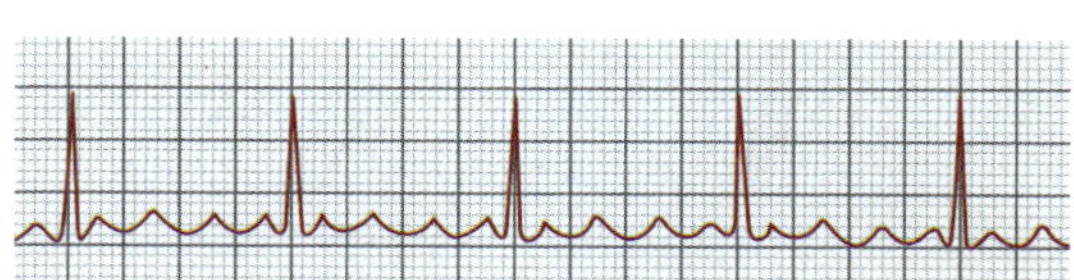

Fig. 18.12: Atrial flutter (Note: 4:1 AV block)

- There will be flutter F waves replacing P waves with saw tooth appearance.

Best seen in leads aVF, V_1, II and III

- Ventricular rate depends on the AV conduction block (2:1 or 4:1). If atrial rate is 300/min then ventricular rate will be 150/min with 2:1 block.

Ventricular Extra-systoles (Ventricular premature contraction–VPC–Ventricular ectopic) (Fig. 18.13)

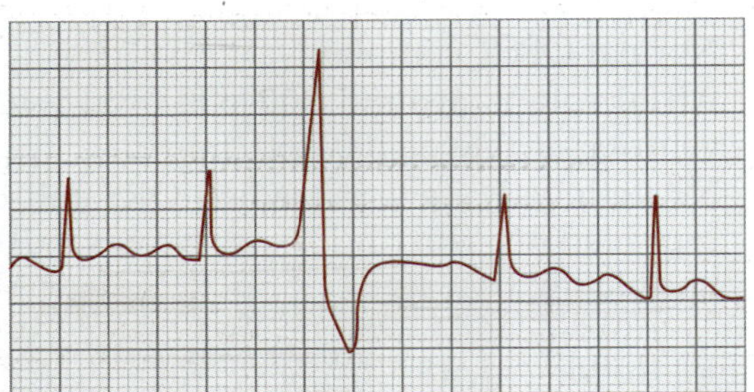

Fig. 18.13: Ventricular extra-systoles

Ventricular Ectopic with Full Compensatory Pause (Fig. 18.14)

Causes: Physiological, fatigue/emotional stress

Organic causes

- IHD/myocardial infarction
- RHD
- MVP
- Hypertensive heart disease
- Hypokalemia
- Hypoxia
- Digitalis toxicity

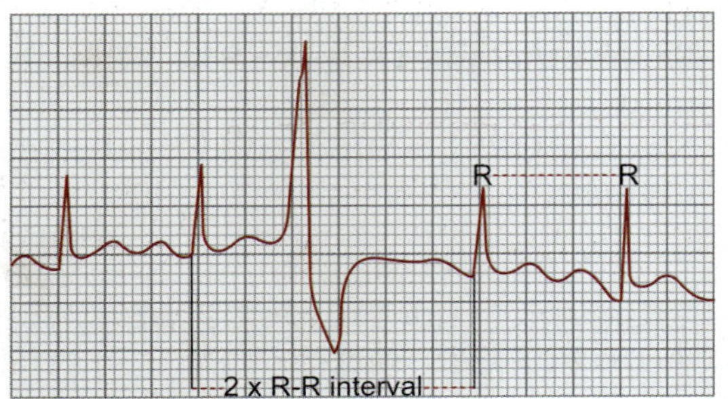

Fig. 18.14: Ventricular extra-systoles with full compensatory pause (note pre and post extra-systolic interval is twice the normal R-R interval)

Ventricular premature complexes occur due to ventricular etopic focus (distal to the bifurcation of bundle of His) discharging prematurely.

ECG

- P wave—absent
- QRS complex wide (> 0.12 secs) and bizarre
- S-T and T waves: S-T depression
- T wave—opposite to QRS complex
- Compensatory pause complete

> *Note:* Complete compensatory pause: Sum of pre and post extrasystolic interval is two times the normal R-R interval.

Left ventricular ectopic: In V_1 lead ectopic is upright with RBBB pattern.

Right ventricular ectopic: In V_1 lead ecopic is downwards with LBBB pattern.

Couplet: A pair of two ventricular ectopics is called couplet.

Ventricular bigeminy: Runs of ventricular ectopics with each ectopic is preceded by a sinus beat, e.g. digitalis toxicity.

Ventricular trigeminy: Each ventricular ectopic is preceded by 2 sinus beats.

Interpolated ectopic: Ventricular ectopic which occurs in between two sinus beats without with compensatory pause.

Multifocal ventricular ectopics: Ventricular ectopic of varying morphology and direction occurring in a single lead.

Multifocal ventricular ectopics occurs due to activation of ventricle due to different ectopic foci.

RONT phenomenon: Occurring of ventricular ectopic which will be falling on the T wave of the preceding sinus beat. It may precipitate VT/VF.

Ventricular Tachycardia (VT) (Fig. 18.15)

Characteristics: At least 3 consecutive ventricular extra systoles occurring in rapid succession (rate exceeds >100/min).

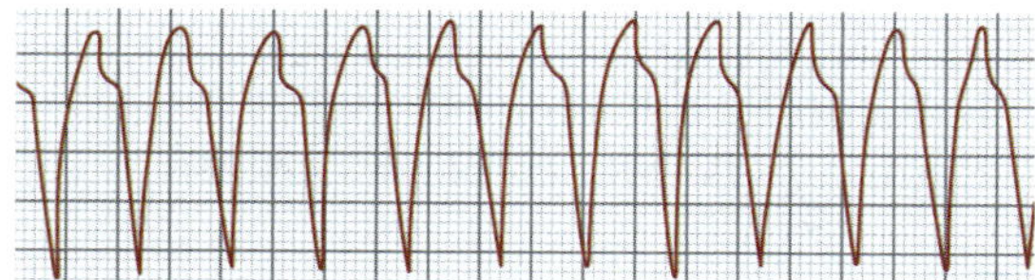

Fig. 18.15: Ventricular tachycardia

Sustained VT: VT lasting for more than 30 seconds.

Causes of sustained VT

- Myocardial infarction
- Cardiomyopathy
- Sustained VT can terminate into ventricular flutter and ventricular fibrillation

Mechanism of ventricular tachycardia

a. Enhanced automaticity resulting in ectopic rhythm
b. Reentry Mechanism

ECG Pattern: 3 or more wide bizarre QRS complex is in succession (> 0.12 secs) with S-T and T changes (direction of T wave is opposite to QRS)

- Rate is 100–200/minute
- AV dissociation
- Presence of capture and fusion beats (dressler beat).

Ventricular Fibrillation (VF) (Fig. 18.16)

Usually a terminal event unless reverted.

Causes

- Acute myocardial infarction
- Digoxin toxicity
- Hyperkalemia

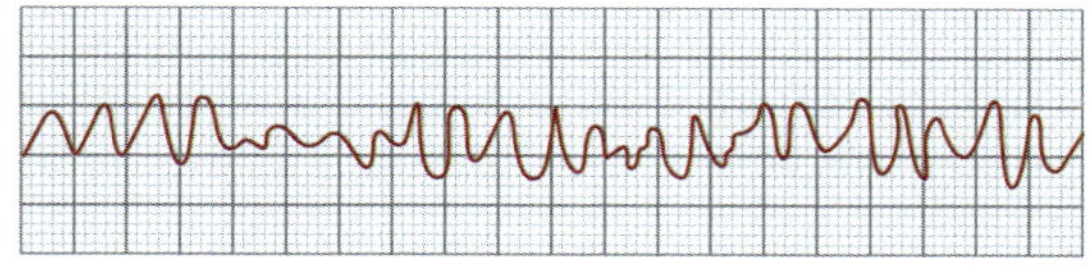

Fig. 18.16: Ventricular fibrillation

ECG: VF is an irregular and chaotic ventricular rhythm. QRST morphology cannot be made out.

ECG pattern

- Definite wave pattern cannot be made out
- Complexes are of varying height, shape and width.

CARDIAC CONDUCTION DEFECTS

Atrioventricular (AV) Blocks

Types

- First degree AV block
- Second degree AV block
- Third degree AV block (complete AV block).

First Degree Block (Fig. 18.17)

Delay in the conduction of impulse from atria to ventricle through AV node.

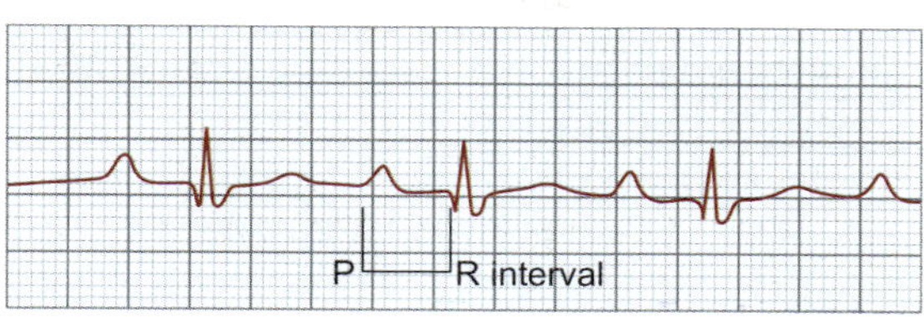

Fig. 18.17: First degree block (prolonged P-R interval)

ECG characteristics: Prolonged P-R interval (>0.20 seconds).

Causes

- Drugs: Beta blockers, digitalis
- Acute rheumatic fever
- Myocardial infarction
- Acute infection

2nd Degree AV Block

2 types: Mobitz type I block (Wenckebach's type) and Mobitz type II block.

Mobitz Type I Block (Fig. 18.18a)

There will be gradual prolongation of P-R interval in successive beats till P wave is completely blocked and a dropped beat occurs (Wenckebach's phenomenon). P wave is not followed by a QRS complex.

Causes

- *Drugs*
  - Beta blockers

- – Digitalis
- – Verapamil
- Rheumatic carditis
- Acute myocardial infarction

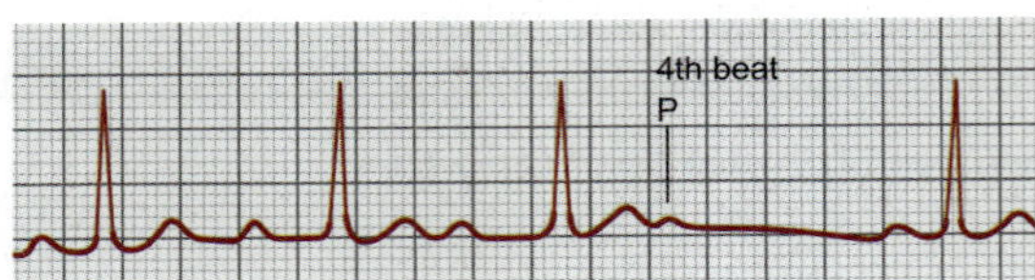

Fig. 18.18a: Mobitz type I block (Wenckebach's phenomenon) progressive increase in P-R interval and dropped 4th beat

Mobitz Type II Block (Fig. 18.18b)

ECG characteristics: Intermittent drops of beats with constant P-R interval. P-P and P-R interval remain constant, e.g. 4 atrial impulses can excite 3 times the ventricles causing 4:3 second degree AV block.

Causes: Acute myocardial infarction

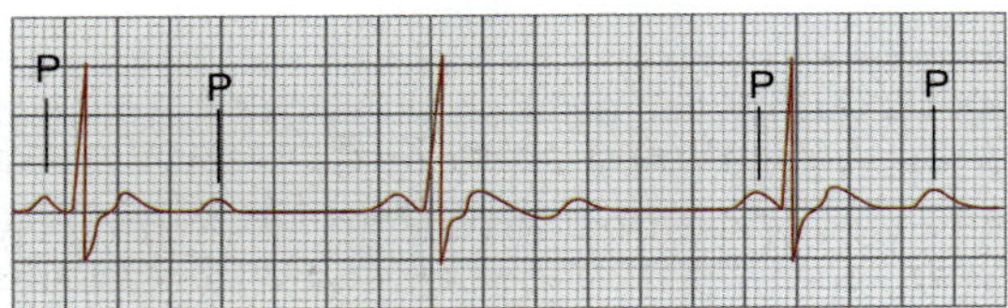

Fig. 18.18b: Mobitz type II block (2nd degree AV block beats are intermittently dropped)

Complete Heart Block (Fig. 18.19)

- Atrial impulse is not conducted to the ventricles
- Ventricles is excited by lower junctional rhythm/ventricular rhythm.

ECG pattern

- Bradycardia (HR < 50/min)
- P-P interval remains constant
- Wide QRS complex
- Complete AV dissociation (QRS is not preceded by P wave) atria and ventricle contract independent of each other

Causes

- Acute myocardial infarction
- Digitalis toxicity
- Congenital AV block

Bundle Branch Block

- Left bundle branch block (LBBB)
- Right bundle branch block (RBBB)

Hemi Blocks

- Left anterior hemi block
- Left posterior hemi block

Fascicular Blocks

- Bifascicular block
- Trifascicular block

Right Bundle Branch Block (Fig. 18.20)

Causes

- Normal variant
- Pulmonary embolism
- IHD
- All causes of RVH

ECG pattern

- RSR′ in lead V_1
- QRS duration of less than 0.12 secs (in complete) or more than 0.12 secs (complete) RBBB
- Deep and wide S waves in lead I, aVL, V_5 and V_6
- S-T depression and T wave inversion in right ventricular lead.

Left Bundle Branch Block (Fig. 18.21)

Causes

- IHD
- Hypertensive heart disease
- Cardiomyopathy

ECG pattern

- Wide and notched R waves (M Pattern) in lead I, aVL, V_5 and V_6
- QRS duration > 0.12 secs. S-T depression and T inversion in LV leads.

Left Anterior Hemi Blocks (LAHBs)

- Left ventricle is activated by posterior fascicle of the bundle
- Impulse is not passing through the anterior fascicle.

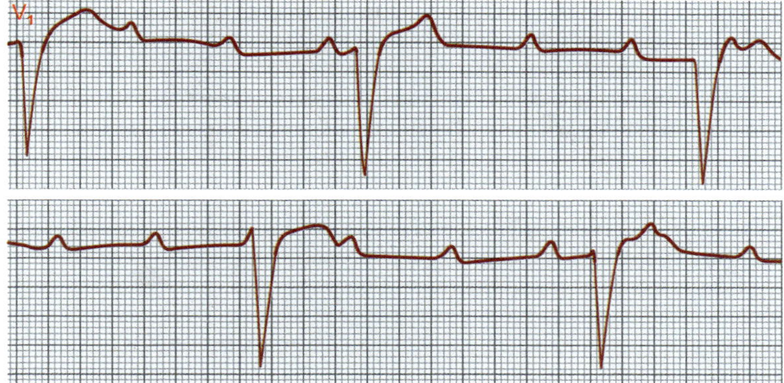

Fig. 18.19: Complete heart block (3rd degree AV block)

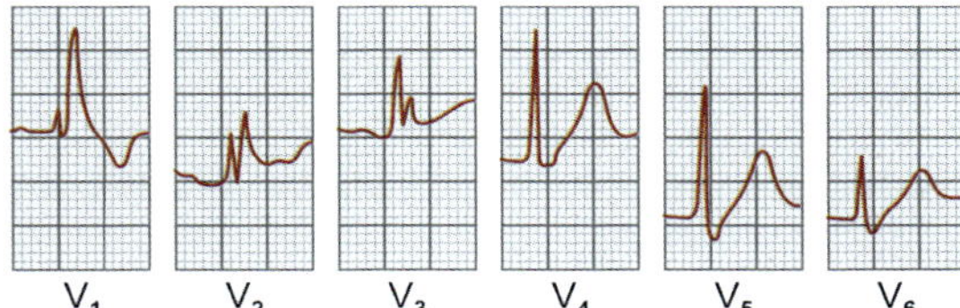

Fig. 18.20: Right bundle branch block

ECG characteristics

- Normal duration of QRS complex
- Left axis deviation
- Q wave in lead I
- R wave in lead II, III, aVF

Left Posterior Hemi Blocks (LPHBs)

- Left ventricle is activated by anterior fascicle of the conducting system
- Impulse is not passing through the posterior fascicle.

ECG pattern

- Normal duration of QRS
- Right axis deviation (+120° or more)
- R wave in lead I
- Q wave in lead II, III and aVF

Bifascicular Block

RBBB is combined with left anterior hemi block or left posterior hemi block. When bifascicular block is present QRS duration is prolonged to be at least 0.12 secs.

Trifascicular Block

Complete or incomplete block of three fascicles, e.g: RBBB + LAHB + Ist degree AV blocks (right bundle branch block + left anterior hemi block + Ist degree AV block).

Myocardial Ischemia and Infarction

ECG characteristics of myocardial ischemia:

- S-T depression
- T wave inversion

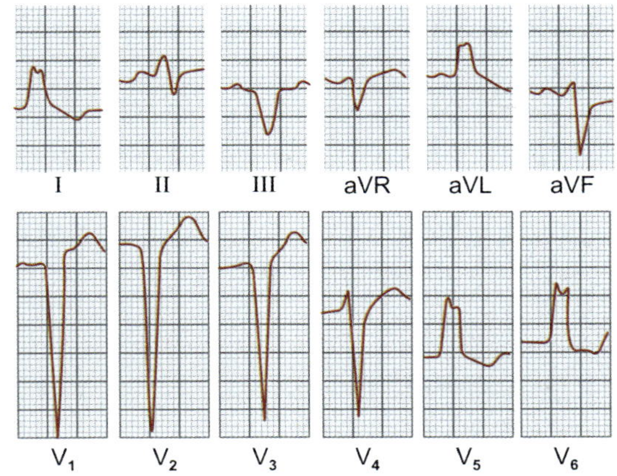

Fig. 18.21: Left bundle branch block

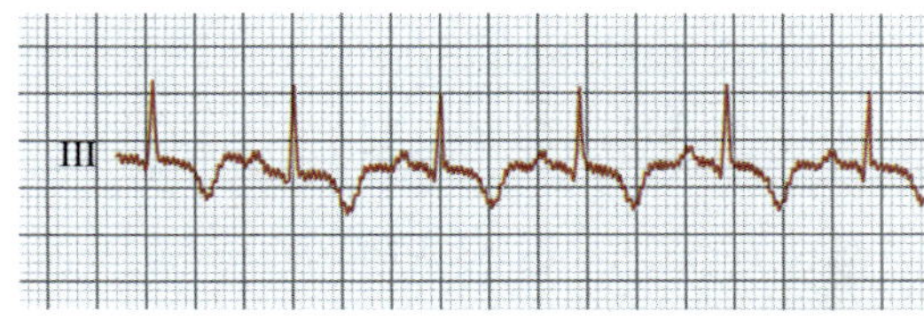

Fig. 18.22: Ischemic S-T depression

ECG Charecteristics of Ischemic S-T Depression

- Horizontal or downward sloping towards the end of the S-T segment at its junction with the T wave.
- J point depression of 1 mm (0.1 millivolt)

Myocardial infarction: ECG characteristics of different zone of myocardial infarction.

Myocardial Ischemia

Inverted symmetrical T waves

Myocardial injury: Elevation of S-T segment with convexity upwards.

Myocardial necrosis: Presence of abnormal/ pathological Q waves.

Characteristics of Pathological Q Waves

- Q wave > 2 mm depth
- Q wave duration of > 0.04 seconds
- Q wave depth of more than 25% of following R wave height.

Note: Pathological Q wave in lead III is associated with abnormal Q wave in lead II aVF, non-pathological Q waves in lead III /aVF disappears on deep inspiration.

ECG Typical of Myocardial Infarction (Transmural)

ECG pattern reveals pathological Q waves, S-T segment elevation and T wave inversion and Reciprocal changes (S-T depression) in opposite leads.

Evolution of myocardial infarction (ECG changes)

- Earliest abnormality: S-T elevation
- Within hours to days: Q wave appears
- Later stage: T wave becomes symmetrically inverted.

Presence of only Q wave suggests old myocardial infarction.

Localisation of Myocardial Infarction

Anterior Wall Infarction (Fig. 18.23)

ECG changes occur in the following leads

- Anteroseptal: Leads V_1 to V_4
- Anterolateral: I, aVL, V_5 and V_6
- Apical or localized anterior: V_3 and V_4

There will be reciprocal changes in inferior leads ECG (II, III, aVF).

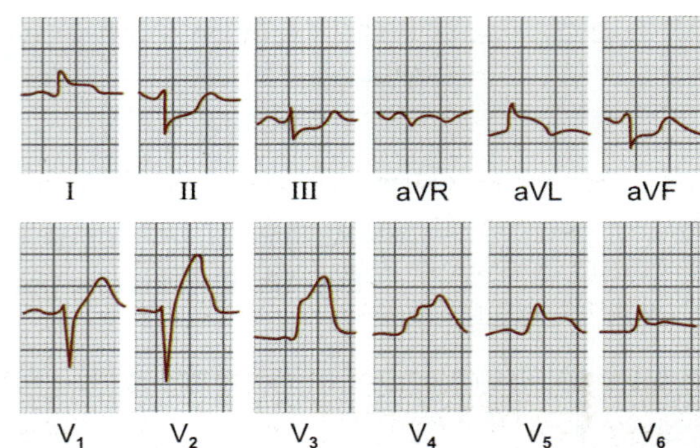

Fig. 18.23: Acute anterior wall infarction (lead I, avL, V_1–V_4 S-T elevation)

Inferior Wall Infarction (Fig. 18.24)

- Changes occur in lead II, III and aVF
- Reciprocal changes in anterior leads (I, aVL, V_1–V_4).

Posterior Wall Infarction

ECG pattern: Tall R waves in lead V_1 and V_2 tall symmetrical T waves in V_1 and V_2

Sub-endocardial Infarction (Fig. 18.25)

Nontransmural or non Q wave infarction

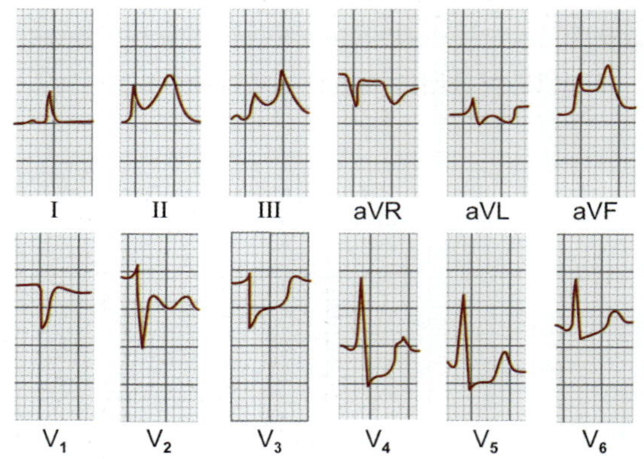

Fig. 18.24: Acute Inferior wall infarction (lead II, III, aVF) S-T elevation

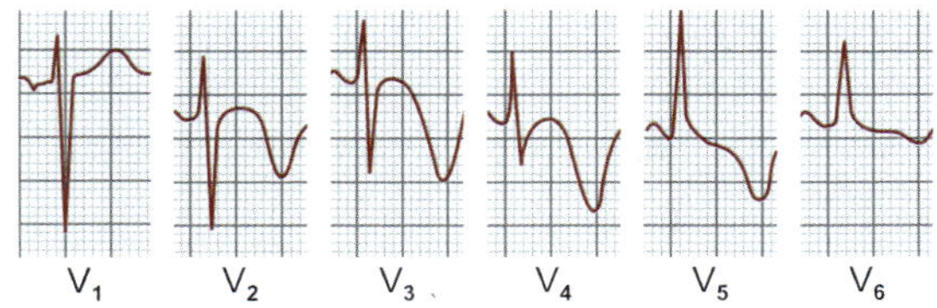

Fig. 18.25: Subendocardial infarction (symmetrical arrow head T inversion)

ECG changes of subendocardial infarction: S-T segment depression with symmetrical T wave inversion in the overlying leads. Changes are persistant compared to ischemia.

ECG CHANGES IN DRUGS AND ELECTROLYTE ABNORMALITIES

Hyperkalemia (Fig. 18.26)

ECG changes: peaked or tented tall T wave

- Decrease in the height of P waves and then P waves disappear
- Decrease in the amplitude of R wave
- Gradual widening of QRS with sine wave pattern.

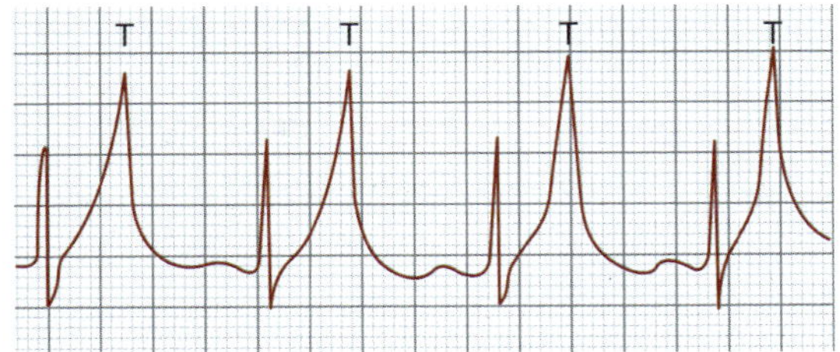

Fig. 18.26: Hyperkalemia–tall tented T waves

Hypokalemia (Fig. 18.27)

ECG characteristics

- Prominent U wave
- S-T depression with T wave changes.

Hypercalcemia (Fig. 18.28)

Acute hypercalcemia causes shortening of Q-T interval.

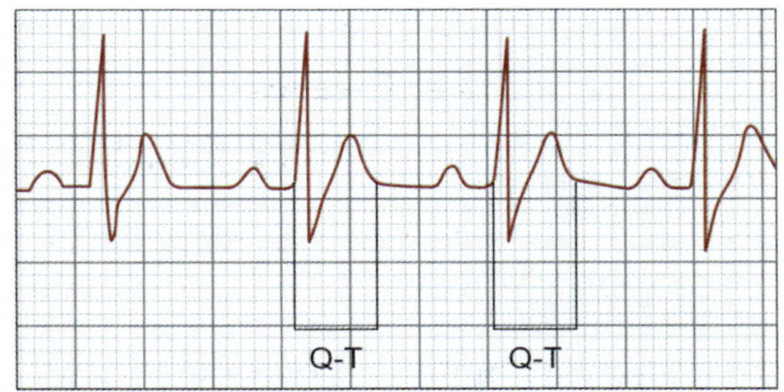

Fig. 18.28: Hypercalcemia (shortening of Q-T interval)

Hypocalcemia (Fig. 18.29)

Hypocalcemia cuases prolonged Q-T interval

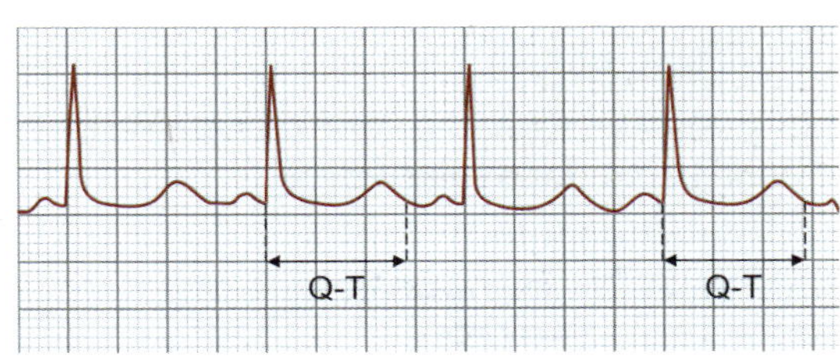

Fig. 18.29: Hypocalcemia (prolonged Q-T interval)

Effect of Digitalis on the ECG (Fig. 18.30)

Digitalis causes S-T depression with T wave inversion causing reversed tick mark (√) in leads with prominent R waves.

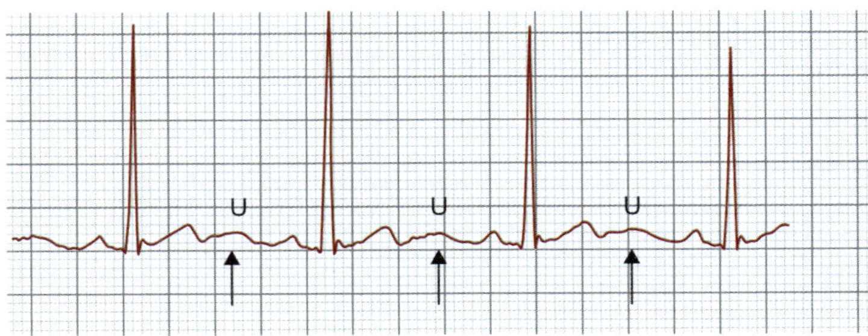

Fig. 18.27: Hypokalemia (notice U wave)

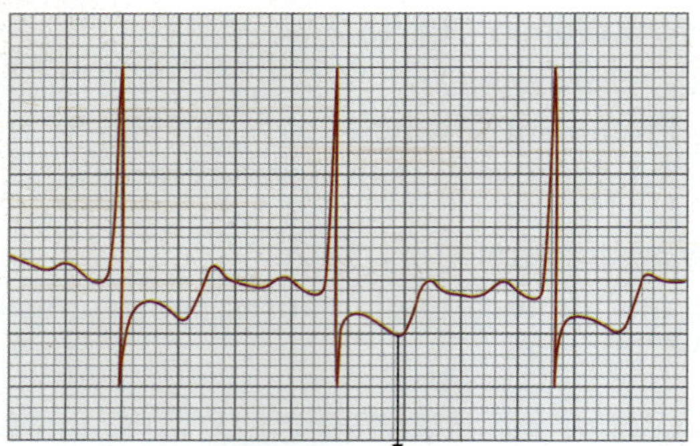

Fig. 18.30: Digitalis effects (S-T depression—reversed tick mark)

Digitalis Toxicity

Can cause any type of arrhythmia except mobitz type II block. Hypokalemia exacerbates digitalis toxicity.

Common ECG manifestations of digitalis toxicity:

- Sinus bradycardia
- Sinoatrial blocks
- Paroxysmal atrial tachycardia with block
- Ventricular tachyarrhythmias
- AV junctional tachycardia
- AV block (except mobitz type II)

Quinidine Toxicity

ECG changes

- Widening of QRS
- AV block
- Atrial asystole
- Ventricular rhythm abnormalities.

ECG Abnormalities in Miscellaneous Cardiac Abnormalities

Early repolarisation syndrome

- Occurs in young adults
- Normal physiological variant

ECG features

- S-T elevation with concavity upwards
- Changes are present in precordial leads V_4 to V_6
- There are no reciprocal charges in other leads

Dextrocardia

ECG features

- Tall R wave in lead V_1
- Gradual decrease of R wave height from leads V_1 to V_6
- P wave inversion in lead I
- P wave upright in lead aVR

Pulmonary Embolism

ECG features : Transient RBBB (right bundle branch block)

S_1 Q_3 T_3 Pattern–S wave in lead I, Q waves in lead III and T inversion in lead III

Acute Pericarditis

ECG features

- S-T elevation (concavity upright)
- T wave upright
- No Q Waves
- No reciprocal changes (unlike acute MI)

Chronic Cor Pulmonale

- Right ventricular hypertrophy
- P—Pulmonale
- Right axis derivation
- Poor progression of R wave

Pericardial Effusion

ECG features pericardial effusion

- Generalised low voltage of all ECG complexes
- S-T segment may be elevated
- Electrical alternans–(beat-to-beat alternate variation of PQRS complexes)

Normal Laboratory Data

19

URINE ANALYSIS

- Volume: 800–2500 ml/day
- Specific gravity: 1.002–1.025
- Titrable acidity: 20–40 mEq/day
- Amylase: 40–400 U/day
- Protein: Less than 150 mg/day
- Potassium: 25–100 mEq/24 hrs
- Sodium: 100–260 mEq/24 hrs

CELLULAR COMPONENTS

Urinary Sediments

Normal cellular constituents

- Epithelial cells: 3–5/HPF
- RBCs: 3–5/HPF
- WBCs: 5/HPF

Urinary Casts

- Casts are formed when the tubular glycoprotein Tomm-Horsfall protein is precipitated in the tubular lumen.
- Cells, cellular debris, crystals get into the precipitated Tomm-Horsfall protein (cast matrix) to form different types of casts.

Hyaline Casts

- Formed of only Tomm-Horsfall protein.
- Does not contain any cellular material.
- Fever, dehydration, exercise can cause small increase in the hyaline casts.
- Broad, long hyaline casts suggest underlying renal disease.

Broad Casts

Represent tubules of hypertrophied nephrons/large collecting ducts–indicate advanced renal disease.

Granular Casts

Formed due to aggregation of tubular cell debris. Large numbers of coarsely granular casts are found in patients with acute tubular necrosis.

Waxy Casts

May represent terminal phase of degeneration of granular casts–suggest advanced renal disease.

Fatty Casts/Lipiduria

Usually present in patients with nephrotic syndrome/in patients with fat embolism.

RBC Casts

Suggest glomerular source of bleeding.

WBC Casts

Usually suggests acute/chronic pyelonephritis.

Bacterial Casts

Seen in acute pyelonephritis.

Bacteriuria

Significant bacteriuria is indicated by the presence of more than 1,00,000 (10^5) organisms/ml of mid-stream sample of urine.

STOOL ANALYSIS

- Protein content–nil
- Stool nitrogen < 1.7 gr/day
- *Fat:* < 6 gm/day (measured on a 3 days stool collection—on a diet containing at least 50 gm of fat).

CEREBROSPINAL FLUID

- CSF pressure: 50–180 mm of water
- Total protein: 20–50 mg/dl
- Chloride: 116–122 mEq/L
- Glucose: 40–70 mg/dl
- Cells: Up to 5 cells/mm (all mononuclear cells).

TUMOR MARKERS

Tumors	*Markers*
Breast carcinoma	Ca 15.3
Colonic carcinoma	Carcinoembryonic antigen
Hepatocellular carcinoma	Alpha-fetoprotein
Medullary carcinoma of thyroid	Calcitonin
Ovarian malignancy	Ca 125
Carcinoma prostate	Prostate specific antigen Acid phosphatase
Multiple myeloma	Bence-Jones protein
Testicular malignancy	
Choriocarcinoma	hCG (human
Gonadotrophin)	chorionic
Pancreatic carcinoma	Ca 19.9

HEMATOLOGICAL INDICES

- *Hemoglobin concentration*
  - Males: 13–18 gm/dl
  - Females: 12–16 gm/dl
- *Haematocrit (PCV)*
  - Males: 0.42–0.52 (42–52%)
  - Females: 0.37–0.48 (37–48%)
- *RBC counts*
  - In males: 4.1 to 4.9 × 10^6 cells/cubic mm
  - In females: 5.4 × 10^6 cells/microlitre
- Reticulocyte count (%) < 2%
- *Erythrocyte sedimentation rate (ESR)*
  - Males: 0–15 mm/hr
  - Females: 0–20 mm/hr
- *Mean corpuscular hemoglobin (MCH)*: 28–33 pg/cell
- *Mean corpuscular hemoglobin concentration (MCHC)*: 32–36 gr/dl
  - *Lifespan of RBCs*: 120 days
  - *Total WBC count*: 4 to 11 × 10^3/mm^3
- *Differential count*

  Neutrophils: 40–75%
  Eosinophils: 0–7%
  Basophils: 0–2%
  Lymphocytes: 20–45%
  Monocytes: 4–10%

Platelet count: 1.3 lakhs–4 lakhs/cmm
Bleeding time (Ivy): 2–8 minutes
Prothrombin time: 10.5–14.5 seconds
Vitamin B_{12} level: 200–600 pg/ml
Serum folate: 3–16 ng/ml cells
Serum iron: 50–150 micrograms/dl
Total iron-binding capacity: 250–370 micrograms/dl
Ferritin: 150–400 ng/ml

CHEMICAL CONSTITUENTS OF BLOOD

Albumin	: 3.5–5.5 gr/dl
Alkaline phosphatase	: 40–125 u/L
Amylase	: 60–180 u/L
AST and ALT	: 0–35 u/L
Bicarbonate	: 23–28 mEq/L
Total bilirubin	: 0.3–1.0 mg/dl
Direct	: 0.1–0.3 mg/dl
Indirect	: 0.2–0.7 mg/dl
Calcium	: 9–10.5 mg/dl
Calcium ionize	: 4.5–5.6 mg/dl
Chloride	: 98–106 mEq/L
Copper	: 70–140 micrograms/dl
Magnesium	: 1.8–3 mg/dl
Osmolality	: 282–295 mOsmol/kg

FSH and LH levels

	FSH	*LH*
Adult women	1.4–9.6 mIU/ml	0.8–26 mIU/ml
At ovulation	2.3–21 mIU/ml	25–57 mIU/ml
Postmenopausal	34–96 IU/ml	40–104 mIU/ml
Men	0.9–15 mIU/ml	1.3–13 mIU/ml

Potassium : 3.5–5.0 meq/L
Sodium : 136–145 mEq/L
Uric acid : 2.5–8 mg/dl
Urea : 10–20 mg/dl
Creatinine : Less than 1.5 mg/dl
Cholesterol : Total cholesterol < 200 mg/dl
  LDL : < 130 mg/dl
  HDL : > 60 mg/dl
Triglycerides :< 160 mg/dl

Glucose

- Fasting (plasma): 70–110 mg/dl (plasma)
- Postprandial (2 hrs after food): 140 mg/dl (plasma)

Impaired glucose tolerance

- Fasting: 110–125 mg/dl
- Postprandial: 140–199 mg/dl

Diabetes mellitus

- Fasting sugar equal to or more than 126 mg/dl
- Postprandial sugar: Equal to or more than 200 mg/dl

HORMONE LEVELS

Thyroid Hormones

- TSH : 0.4–5 micro units/ml
- T_4 : 5–12 microgram/dl
- T_3 : 70–190 ng/dl

Adrenal Hormones

- Cortisol 8 am: 5–25 micrograms/dl
- 4 pm: 3–12 micrograms/dl
- ACTH at 8 am: 10 to 50 pg/ml
- Parathyroid hormones: 10 to 60 pg/ml
- Insulin: Fasting serum levels 6–26 micro units/ml
- Growth hormone: Usually less than 2 ng/ml (varies with stress)
- Prolactin: 2–15 ng/ml

Gonadotrophins and Gonadal Steroids

Estradiol

- Men < 50 pg/ml
- Women 20–60 pg/ml (higher level at ovulation)

Testosterone

- Males: 3–10 ng/ml
- Females: < 1 ng/ml

Progesterone

- Males < 2 ng/ml
- Females (luteal phase): 2–20 ng/ml

Index

Abdominal
- distension 118
- jugular reflux 47
- paradox 90
- wall edema of 134

Abducens nerve palsy 214
Abnormal ophthalmic fundal
- appearance 283
- patterns and rhythm of respiration 90

Abnormalities of
- different parts of the eye 280
- height 1
- knee joint 248
- lips 16

Abscess 21
Abulia 268
Acanthosis nigricans 264
Acarbose 326
Accelerated hypertension 45
Accommodation reflex 167
ACE inhibitors 332
Acromegaly 262, 263
Action
- of extraocular muscles 164
- tremor 184

Acute
- herpetic gingivostomatitis 130
- lymphoblastic leukemia (ALL) 226
- myocardial infarction 337
- myeloblastic leukemia (AML) 226
- nephritic syndrome 236
- renal failure 237
- rheumatic fever 76

Acyanotic Fallot (pink Fallot) 75
Addisonian crises 340
Addison's disease 264
Adenoma sebaceum 157
Adrenal hormones 363
Adrenaline 323
Adventitious sounds 104
Aegophony 105
Agranulocytosis 226
Akinetic mutism 268
Albendazole 329
Albuminocytological dissociation 304
Allergic oedema 12
Alpha
- blockers 320
- methyl dopa 320

Alteration
- in body size and shape 255
- of skin colour 22

Altered
- bowel habit 120
- sensorium degree of 271

Ambubag 344
Amenorrhea 259
Aminoglycosides 310
Aminophylline 322
Anacrotic pulse 42
Anal canal and rectum, bleeding from 118
Anal reflex 196
Analgesics and antipyretics 317
- acetaminophen 317
- aspirin 317
- diclofenac sodium 317
- ibuprofen 318
- indomethacin 317

Anaphylactic shock 334
Anasarca 12
Anemia 3
Anemic patient examination of 3
Aneurysm of aorta 72
Angina
- decubitus 28
- differential diagnosis 29
- equivalents 28
- pectoris description of 27

Angioedema 22
Angiotensin receptor blockers 320
Anisocoria 281
Ankle
- clonus 194
- jerk 194

Ankylosing spondylitis 243
Anomie aphasia 159
Antacids 322
Anterior cerebral artery occlusion 206
Anterior wall MI 358
Anti
- fungal drugs 311
- retroviral drugs 312
- TB drugs 314
- viral drugs 331

Anuria 231
Aorta, coarctation of 75
Aortic
- combined AS and AR 72
- complications 72
- regurgitation severe 72

Aortic
- severe 71
- stenosis–complications 72

Aphasia
- anomic aphasia 164
- aphemia 160
- aphrosodia 159
- conduction aphasia 159
- isolation aphasia 160
- subcortical aphasia 160
- transcortical aphasia 160

Apical impulse 49
Aplastic anemia (primary) 225
Apnea 85
Apneustic breathing 271
Apraxic gait 201
Aprosodia 159
Arcus senilis 281
Argyl Robertson pupil 167
Arm span 1
Arterial
- bruit 65
- system 77

Arteries, corkscrew 37
Arteriosclerotic retinopathy 286
Arthritis
- associated with HLA-B27
- positivity 252
- non-inflammatory 239
- psoriatic 252
- rheumatoid 243, 252

Ascitic
- indications 297
- procedure 297
- tap analysis 297

Assessment of
- exophthalmos 263
- joint pain 238
- nutritional status 2

Asterixis 128
Astigmatism 280
Ataxia
- manifestations of 199
- telengiectasia 157

Athetosis 185
Atrial
- ectopics 352
- fibrillation 76, 353
- flutter 353
- septal defect (ASD) 74

Atrophy, testicular 127
Attitude of
- a hemiplegic 176
- limbs 176, 268

Austin flint murmur 64
Autoimmune hemolysis 225
AV nipping 284
Avoiding response 195
Axillary lymphadenopathy 9

BD syringe 347
Bacterial casts 361
Bacteriuria 361
Bad breath (halitosis) 122
Balint's syndrome 208
Bedside tests for myasthenia 184
Beevor's sign 180
Behçet's syndrome, skin changes in 245
Bell's phenomenon 171
Beta
- blockers 318
- lactamase inhibitor 309

Biceps 181
Biceps jerk 192
Bifascicular block 357
Bilateral UMN facial palsy 170
Biot's breathing 271
Bisferiens pulse 42
Bitot's spots 281
Bladder and bowel dysfunction
- symptoms of 151

Bleeding from the anal canal and rectum 118
Blepharitis (inflammation of eyelids) 280
Blood chemical constituents of 362
Blood
  diastolic 44
  measurement of 44
  normal 45
  pressure 44
  recording of by cuff method 44
  supply of internal capsule 204
Blue bloater 110
Body
  hair, loss of 21
  mass index 3
  size and shape, alteration in 255
  weight and body mass index (Quatelet's index) 3
Bone marrow examination 298
  indications 298
  needles 299
  procedure 299
Bony pain and muscle cramps 260
  tenderness 222
Borderline hypertension 45
Bouchard's nodes 243
Bovine cough 81
Bowel habit, altered 120
Bradycardia 30
Bradypnea 90
Brain death 276
  demonstration of apnea before declaring 276
  diagnostic tests for 276
  evidences for 276
Brainstem lesion 202
Brassy cough 81
Breast
  abscess 18
  atrophy in females 128
  examination of 18
Broad casts 361
Broca's (motor) aphasia 159
Bronchial
  asthma 108
  carcinoma 110
Bronchiectasis 109
Bronchophony 105
Bronchovesicular breathing 103
Brudzinski's sign 200
Bubo 8
Bulbocavernous reflex 196
Bulla 21

Café au lait spots 157
Calcification, corneal 262
Calcium channel blockers 319
Calculation of heart rate 349
Caloric test 275
Caput medusa 132
Carbimazole 324
Carboxy hemoglobin 6
Carcinoma breast 18
Card test 216
Cardiac anomalies malformations associated 78
Cardiac asthma 26
Cardiopulmonary resuscitation 336
Cardiovascular disease symptoms of 152
Cardiovascular system
  examination of 35, 206
Carey-Coombs' murmur 65
Carotids examination of 201
Casts, bacterial 361
Cataract 262, 282
Causes of
  delayed puberty 259
  excessive hair growth 21
  facial puffiness 12
  hemiplegia 201
  hepatosplenomegaly 139
  intra-abdominal lymphadenopathy 11
  jaundice 4
  paraplegia 202
  peripheral vascular disease 7
  rhonchi 104
  splenomegaly 139
  yellowish discoloration apart from jaundice 4
Cavity in the lung 109
Cellular components 361
Central and peripheral cyanosis
  differences 6
  cyanosis 5
  neurogenic hyperventilation 271
  speech defects (aphasia/dysphasias) 159
Cephalosporins 310
Cerebellar dysfunction symptoms of 151
Cerebellar gait 201
Cerebral embolism, features of 204
  hemorrhage, features of 204
  thrombosis, features of 204
Cerebrovascular
  accidents examples 204
  types 204
Cerebrospinal fluid 362
Cervical
  lymphadenopathy 8
  lymph nodes, examination of 8
Charcot's joint 244
Chemical constituents of blood 362
Chemosis (conjunctival edema) 12, 281
Chest pain 27, 85
  respiratory causes of 85
Chest X-ray
  air crescent (meniscus) sign 292
  bronchiectasis 295
  chronic bronchitis 294
  congenital heart disease 293
  emphysema 294
  ground glass appearance 290
  hydropneumothorax 293
Cheyne-Stokes breathing 271
Chickenpox 129
Chloasma 22
Chloramphenicol 311
Chlorpromazine 329
Chorea (dance) 185
Choroid tubercle 286
Chronic
  cor pulmonale 353
  lymphocytic leukemia 226
  myeloid leukemia 226
  renal failure 237
Circumduction gait (hemiplegic gait) 201
Cirrhosis
  anemia in cirrhosis 145
  causes 145
  diagnosis 145
  fever in cirrhosis 145
  hepatocellular carcinoma in a cirrhotic 145
  hepatic encephalopathy 145
Clasp knife spasticity 177
Claw hand 216
Clinical
  aspects of cyanosis 6
  evaluation of expectoration 82
  signs associated with Marfan's syndrome 1
Clonidine 320
Clonus 185
Clubbing
  differential diagnosis 6
  grades of 6
  pathogenesis of 7
Coarctation of aorta 75
Cog wheel rigidity 178
Coin test 106
Collapsing pulse 41
Colonic obstruction 133
Colour
  vision 280
  defects of 280
Coma 268
Coma vigil (vigilant coma) 268
Common
  causes of haemoptysis 83
  hypertrophic osteoarthropathy 7
Compensatory emphysema 110
Complete
  heart block 356
  ptosis 166
Completed stroke 204
Concentric hypertrophy 52
Concomitant squint 166
Conduction aphasia 159
Conjunctival
  oedema (chemosis) 12
  conjunctivitis 281
Constipation 120
Constrictive pericarditis 76
Continuous murmurs 65
Conus medullaris lesions 204
Convulsion 152
COPD 109
Corkscrew arteries 37
Cornea, severe damage to 281
Corneal calcification 262
Corrigan's or waterhammer pulse 41
Cortical lesion 202
Cortical
  examination of 190
  sensation 190
Corticosteroids 327
Cotrimoxazole 308
Cough 80
  associated with hoarseness of voice 81
  types and nature of 81
Crackling sensation of joint 240
Cranial nerve dysfunction symptoms of 151
Cranial nerves examination of 161
Crepitations (crackles) 104
Cullen's sign 132
Cushing's disease 262
Cushing's syndrome 264
Cutaneous vasculitic lesions 244
Cyanosis, and clubbing 157
  clinical aspects of 6
  peripheral 5
  types of 5
Cyanotic spells 34

Dacryoadenitis 279
Dacryocystitis 279
Day blindness (hemaralopia) 279
Decerebration (decerebrate state) 268

Decortication 268
Decreased pigmentation of skin 23
Deep
reflexes 192
vein thrombosis 77
Defects of color vision 280
Deformities
and contractures 243
of feet 243
of hand and wrist 243
Degree of altered sensorium 271
Delayed
causes of 259
puberty 259
Demonstration of apnea before declaring brain death 276
Dermatomyositis, skin rash of 244
Description of
an attack of PND 26
angina pectoris 27
D'Espine's sign 106
Detection of exophthalmos 263
Determination of electrical axis in the ECG 350
Dextrocardia 360
Diabetes mellitus 257, 264
Diabetic retinopathy 285
Diagnosis of cardiovascular disease 67
Diagnostic tests for brain death 276
Diarrhoea 120
Diastolic blood pressure 44
Diastolic murmurs 64
Diazepam 328
Dicrotic pulse 42
Diethylcarbamazine 330
Differences
between central and peripheral cyanosis 5
different types of jaundice 5
Different CNS disorders 305
Different types of dysarthrias 160
facial appearances 14
gait abnormalities 201
refractory defects 280
rhonchi 104
tremors 184
xanthomas and their clinical significance 3
Differential
clubbing 6
diagnosis of angina pectoris 29
haemoptysis 83
syncope 31
Digitalis effect on ECG 359
Digoxin 320
Diloxanide furoate 330
Diphenyl hydantoin 328
Diphtheria 129
Diplopia (double vision) 166
Discharge from nipples 18
Discolouration of skin 132
Disposable syringe 347
Distension of abdomen 131
Disturbance in
sweating 255
sexual maturation 259
Diuretics 333
Diurnal variation, cough with 81
Divarication of rectus abdominis 132
Diverticulosis 117
Doll's head movement 274
Double vision 166
Down's syndrome 78
Drowning 337
Drowsiness 268
Drugs in leprosy 315
clofazamine 315
dapsone 315
Drugs in
chloroquine 315
malaria 315
mefloquine 315
primaquine 315
proguanil 316
quinine 317
Dryness of mouth 122
Dupuytren's contracture 19, 128
Dwarfism (short stature) 2
Dysarthrias 160
Dyschezia 120
Dyskinetic segment 50
Dyspepsia 117
Dysphagia 119
Dysphonia 161
Dyspnoea 25, 84
in a patient of cardiac failure
mechanism of 25
slowly progressive 26
Dystonia 185

Ear
examination of 17
low set 17
Early background retinopathy (nonproliferative) 285
Early
diastolic murmur 64
repolarisation syndrome 360
Ebstein's anomaly 75
Eccentric hypertrophy 52
Ecchymoses 22
Ectropion 281
Edema 12
and puffiness of face 86
conjunctival (chemosis) 12
generalised (anasarca) 12
localised 12
non-pitting 12, 222, 262
of abdominal wall 134
periorbital 280
Ejection (midsystolic) murmur 62
Electrocardiogram 348
Empyema necessities 107
Endotracheal tube 345
Enlargement of
lacrimal gland 16, 279
tongue 130
Enophthalmos 16, 167
Entropion 280
Epididymis 236
Epididymitis 236
Episcleritis 282
Epistaxis 17
Eruptions, fixed drug 23
Erythema ab igne 21
Erythema nodosum 22
Evidences for brain death 276
Ewart's sign 76
Examination of
anemic patient 3
breast 18
cardiovascular system 35
carotids 201
cervical lymph nodes 8
cortical sensations 190
cranial nerves 161
different parts of eye 15
ear 17
face and oral cavity 222
face, head and neck 14
facial nerve 169
feet 20
genitalia 267
hair 20
hands and feet 18, 263
hands, lower limbs and spine 234
head and neck 16
lacrimal gland 279
lips, cheeks and glands of the face 16
nails 19
neck 17
nervous system 155
nose 17
peripheral vascular system 77
precordium 36, 49
reflexes 190
respiratory system 89
sensory system 186
skin 21
skull and spine 201
spine 250
Excessive
causes of 21
hair growth (hypertrichosis) 21
Excessive salivation 122
Exophthalmos 15
assessment of 263
detection of 263
measurement of 263
of Graves' disease 263
Expectoration
clinical evaluation of 82
cough with 82
Extramedullary intradural compression 203
Extradural extramedullary compression 203
Extraocular muscles, action of 164
Exudates in the retina 285
Eye discharge 278
Eyeball, inward displacement of 279
Eyes
examination of different parts of 15
movements of 164
pain in 278

Facial
appearances, different types 14
expression, muscles of 169
oedema 12
palsy, types of 169
puffiness, causes of 12
(7th) nerve 169
Fallot's tetralogy 75
Fasciculation 185
Fat distribution and its abnormalities 2
Fatty casts/lipiduria 361
Features of
cerebral embolism 204
cerebral hemorrhage 205
cerebral thrombosis 205
Marfan's syndrome 36
neurogenic claudication 78
Feet
deformities of 243
examination of 20
swelling of 33
Females, puberty in 259
Fever 13
with chills and rigors 14
with rigors and skin eruption 123
Fibrillation 186

Fibroadenoma 18
Fibrocystic disease 18
Finger
flexion reflex 196
nose test 199
First degree AV block 355
Fixed drug eruptions 21
Flag sign 21
Flapping tremors (asterixis) 128, 184
Flatulence 117
Flow murmurs 64
Foetal alcohol syndrome 78
Foley's catheter 342
Folic acid 331
deficiency 224
Freidrich's ataxia 158
Froment's sign 216
Frontal bossing 17
FSH and LH levels 363
Fundoscopic examination 274

Gag reflex 174
Gait
abnormalities different types 201
high stepping 201
stamping 201
Galactorrhea 258
Gall bladder 137
Gallavardin phenomenon 71
Gegenhalten, phenomenon of 178
Generalised
lymphadenopathy 11
oedema (anasarca) 12
Genesis of pulsus alternans 42
Genitalia, examination of 267
Gingivitis 130
Glabellar tap reflex (Myerson's sign) 195
Glasgow
coma scale 272
significance of 272
Glaucoma 280
Global aphasia 159
Globus hystericus 119
Glossopharyngeal nerve 174
Gonadotrophins and gonadal steroids 363
Gottron's sign 213
Gout 252
Gower's sign 180
Grades
murmurs 63
of clubbing 6
reflexes 194
Granular casts 361
Graphesthesia 190
Grasping response 195
Graves' disease 264
Gums, hypertrophy of 130
Gynaecomastia 127
physiological 258

H_1-Receptor antagonists 324
H_2-Receptor antagonists 323
HAART (highly active anti-retroviral therapy) 313
Haemoptysis 32, 83
common causes of 83
differential diagnosis 83
Hair
examination of 20
loss of 260
Hair growth, phases of 20
Hamman's sign 106
Hamstrings 183
Hands and feet, examination of 18, 263
Hands and wrist, deformities of 243
Hands, lower limbs and spine examination of 234
Hard exudates 285
Harrison's sulcus 94
Head and neck examination of 16
Hearing, tests of 173
Heart failure
left-sided 76
right-sided 76
Heartburn (pyrosis) 116
indigestion and flatulence 116

Heaving apex 51
Heberden's nodes 243
Heel pad thickness 2
Helicobacter pylori treatment 323
Heliotroph rash 213
Hemaralopia 279
Hematochezia 118
Hematological indices 362
Hematoma 22
Hematuria 230
Hemetemesis 117
Hemianopias 280
Hemiballism 185
Hemiplegia, causes of 201
Hemolytic anemia 225
Hepatic
encephalopathy 128
outflow obstruction 133
Hepatojugular reflux 47
Hepatomegaly 136
Hepatosplenomegaly, causes of 139
Hereditary spherocytosis 225
Hernial orifices 133, 140
Herpes zoster 129
Herpetic gingivostomatitis, acute 130
Hiccups 122
High stepping gait 201
Hippocratic splash 106
Hirsutism 21, 260
Hoarseness of voice, cough associated with 81
Hodgkin's lymphoma 227
Hoffman's sign 195
Holt Oram's syndrome 37, 78
Homan's sign 77
Homonymous hemianopia 162
Hoover's sign 96
Hormone levels 363
Hormones, adrenal 363
Horner's
syndrome 15, 167, 217
with miosis 273
Horner's syndrome—different sites of lesion 217
Hung up reflex 194
Hutchinson's teeth 130
Hyaline casts 361
Hydrocephalus 16
Hydrocoele 235
Hydropneumothorax 108, 293
Hypercalcemia 359
Hypercarotenemia 4
Hyperdynamic apex 51
Hyperkalemia 359
Hypermetropia 280
Hyperpigmentation of skin 23
Hyperpyrexia 13
Hyperresonant note 100
Hypertelorism 16
Hypertension
accelerated 45
malignant 45
pulmonary 85
systolic 45
white coat 45
Hypertensive retinopathy 284
Hyperthermia 13
Hyperthyroidism 257, 324
Hypertonia 177
Hypertrichosis 21
Hypertrophic obstructive cardiomyopathy (HOCM) 75
Hypertrophic osteoarthropathy 7
Hypertrophic osteoarthropathy, common causes of 7
Hypertrophy
concentric 52
eccentric 52
of gums 130
of muscles 176
Hypocalcemia 359
Hypoglossal nerve 175
Hypokalemia 359
Hypoplastic teeth 130
Hypotension, postural 265
Hypothermia 13
Hypothyroidism 256, 324
Hypotonia 178, 198
Hysterical hyperventilation 26

Ibuprofen 318
Icterus 4, 91, 126
Idochlorohydroxy quinoline 330
Impairment of movement 240
Importance
of handedness 161
shaking hands with the patient 20
Impotence 257
and loss of libido 257
and sexual dysfunction 123
Improper coordination (ataxia) manifestations of 199
Inclusion body myositis 212
Incomplete compensatory pause 352
Incontinence 229
Increased frequency of micturition 229
Inequality in size of pupil 166
Infectious mononucleosis 129
Infective
arthritis 252
endocarditis 34
Inferior
vena caval obstruction 133
wall MI 358
Infertility 258
Inflammatory arthritis 239
Infraspinatus 180
Inguinoscrotal swellings 235
Innocent murmurs 63
Insulin 326
syringe 347
Integrity of diaphragm tests for 98
Intention tremor (ataxic) 184
Intermittent claudication (vascular) 77
Internal capsular lesion 202
Internuclear ophthalmoplegia 164
Interossei 180
cannonball shadow 291
interpretation 287
miliary mottling 290
multiple punched out lesions in the skull 295
nodular lesions 290
pancreatic calcification 296
pericardial effusion 76, 295

pleural thickening 293
pneumothorax 294
pulmonary cavity 291
pulmonary collapse 291
pulmonary fibrosis 294
pulmonary nodule 290
recticulonodular shadows 293
rheumatic mitral valve disease 394
salt and pepper/pepper pot skull 295
solitary pulmonary nodule 291
Intra-abdominal lymphadenopathy, causes of 11
Intramedullary lesions 203
Intraocular pressure 282
Inverted supinator jerk 193
Involuntary movements 184
Ipratropium bromide 322
Iridocyclitis 282
Iritis 282
Iron
deficiency anemia 224
therapy 331
Ischemic penumbra 204

J point 349
Jaccoud's arthritis 243
Jaundice 38, 121
causes of 4
different types of differences 4
latent 4
sites to look for 4
Jaw jerk 169, 192
Joint
crackling sensation of 240
pain, assessment of 239
swelling 239
tenderness 242
Joint crepitus 243
Jugular venous pulse and pressure (JVP) 46
Juvenile mitral stenosis 69

Keratitis (inflammation of cornea) 281
Kernig's sign 200
Knee
heel in coordination 199
jerk 193
Koplik's spots 129
Kussmaul breathing 271
Kussmaul's sign 48
Kyphoscoliosis, and pes cavus 158

Lacrimal
gland enlargement of 279
examination of 279
Lacunar
infarct 204
syndrome 207
Lasegue's sign 251
Late systolic murmur 63
Latent jaundice 4
Lateral medullary syndrome 208
Latissimus dorsi 181
Lead poisoning 130
Left
anterior hemi block 356
axis deviation 350
bundle branch block 356
posterior hemi block 357
ventricular hypertrophy 351
Left-sided heart failure 76
Lepromatous leprosy 23

Leprosy
lepromatous 23
skin lesions of 23
Lesions
conus medullaris 204
cortical 202
cutaneous vasculitis 244
internal capsular 202
medial nerve 246
of nipple 18
ulnar nerve 246
Levamisole 330
Levine's sign 28
Libido, loss of 257
Light reflex 166
Limbs
attitude of 176
of a hemiplegic attitude of 176
Lipiduria 361
Lipomastia 258
Lips, cheeks and glands of face, examination of 16
Litten's sign 96
Livedoreticularis 21
Liver
biopsy 300
indications 300
needle 300
procedure 301
Liver cell failure, signs of 127
Localised lymphadenopathy 8
Localised
oedema 12
pigmentation of skin 21
Locked in state 268
Locking of joint 240
Loss of
body hair 21
hair 260
libido 257
sexual hair 21
vision 279
Low set ears 17
Lower
gastrointestinal bleed 117
motor neuron (LMN) 175
segment 1
Lumbar puncture 302
Lumbricals 180
Lung
abscess 108
apex, percussion of 100
Lymphadenopathy 7, 126, 157, 222
generalised 11
localised 8
Lymphatic oedema 12
Lymphatic system 77
Lymphoma, non-Hodgkin's 227

Macrolides
Erythromycin 311
Azithromycin 311
Macule 21
Malecot's catheter 344
Malena 117
Males, puberty in 259
Malformations associated cardiac anomalies 78
Malignant hypertension 45
Mammary souffle 66
Manifestations of improper coordination (ataxia) 199
Mannitol 324

Marcus gun pupil 167
Marfan's habitus 36
Marfan's syndrome 34
clinical signs associated with 1
features of 36
Mass reflex 196
Mean blood pressure 45
Measles 129
Measurement of
blood pressure 44
exophthalmos 263
skeletal height 1
Mebendazole 329
Mechanism of
dyspnoea in a patient of cardiac failure 25
PND 26
Medial
medullary syndrome 208
nerve lesions 247
Median nerve 216
Metacarpal index 1
Method of examination of thyroid 264
Metronidazole 330
Microalbuminuria 237
Micturition, increased frequency of 229
Mid-diastolic
flow murmurs 64
murmur 64
Milroy's disease 13
Mimitic type of UMN facial palsy 170
Mini mental scale examination 161
Minipolymyoclonus 185
Mitral
regurgitation 70
regurgitation (MR) 70
severe 70
Mitral stenosis 68
Mobitz
type I block 355
type II block 356
Moniliasis 129
Moses sign 77
Motor system 175
Mouth, dryness of 122
Movements
impairment of 240
involuntary 184
of eyes 164
Multiple myeloma 226
Murmurs 62
Austin flint 64
Carey-Coombs' 65
continuous 65
diastolic 67
early diastolic 64
ejection (midsystolic) 62
flow 64
grading of 63
innocent 63
late systolic 63
pan (holosystolic) 63
systolic 62
to and fro 64
Murphy's sign 137
Muscle bulk 2
Muscle cramps, and bony pain 260
Muscle disease symptoms and signs 209
Muscle
causes 209
ocular 210
types 209
weakness 209

Muscles
- hypertrophy of 176
- of facial expression 169
- of mastication, testing 168
- wasting and hypertrophy of 176

Muscular
- amyotrophy 209
- atrophy 209
- dystrophy 209
- myopathy 209

Muscular dystrophy of Becker 212
- Duchenne 211
- fascioscapulo humeral 212
- limb girdle 212
- myotonic dystrophy 212

Myasthenia 184
- bedside tests for 184

Myerson's sign 195
Myocardial infarction 358
Myoclonus 185
Myopia 280
Myotonia 178, 211
Myotonic pupil of Adie 167
Myxedema, pretibial 264
Myxoma 74

Nails, examination of 29
Nausea 115
- and vomiting 115

Near vision 208
Neck
- examination of 17
- stiffness 200

Necrobiosis lipoidica diabeticorum 264
Nelson's syndrome 264
Neoplasms, testicular 236
Nephritic syndrome, acute 236
Nephrotic syndrome 236
Nervous system, examination of 155
Neurofibroma 157
Neurogenic claudication, features of 78
Neuropathy, peripheral 214
Night blindness (nyctalopia) 279
Nipple
- discharge from 18
- lesions of 18

Nitrates 321
Nitrofurantoin 308
Nocturia (frequency of urine more at night) 229
Nocturnal angina 28
Nodule 21
Non-Hodgkin's lymphoma 227
Non-inflammatory arthritis 239
Non-pitting edema 262
Noonan's syndrome 78
Normal
- apex 50
- apical impulse 49
- blood pressure 45
- breathing pattern and muscles of respiration 90
- CSF analysis 303
- height 1
- ophthalmic fundus appearance 282
- percussion of lung 100
- waves and intervals 348

Nose, examination of 17
Nuclear paralysis of 3rd, 4th and 6th cranial nerves 164
Nutritional
- assessment of 2
- status 2

Nyctalopia 279
Nystagmus 172

Obstructive emphysema 110
Occlusion of posterior cerebral artery 207
Octreotide 324
Oculocephalic reflex (doll's head movement) 271
Oliguria 231
One and half syndrome 164
Ophthalmic fundal appearance abnormal 283
Ophthalmoplegia
- painful 213
- painless 213
- types 213

Ophthalmoplegia, internuclear 164
Ophthalmoscopy 282
Optic atrophy 284
Optokinetic nystagmus 173
Oral cavity
- pain in 123
- pigmentation of 129

Oral thrush (moniliasis) 129
Orchitis 236
Organophosphorus poisoning 339
Orthopnoea 26, 84
Ortner's syndrome 70
Osler-Weber-Rendu disease 158
Osteoarthritis 243

P
- mitrale 351
- pulmonale 351
- wave 348

Pain
- abdomen 114
- in eye 278
- in oral cavity 123

Painful
- arc syndrome 245
- red eye with impairment of vision 278

Painless white eye 278
Pallor, sites to look for 4
Palmar erythema 127
Palmomental reflex 195
Pan (holosystolic) murmurs 63
Pancoast's tumour 110
Papilledema 283
Papillitis 283
Papule 21
Paralysis of 6th nerve 165
Paraplegia
- causes of 202
- in extension 203
- in flexion 203

Parkinsonian
- gait 201
- tremor 184

Parotid swelling 127
Paroxysmal
- nocturnal dyspnoea (PND) 26
- supraventricular tachycardia 353

Partial ptosis 166
Patellar clonus 194
Patent ductus arteriosus (PDA) 74
Pathogenesis of
- clubbing 7
- pretibial myxedema 264

Pathway of taste 171
Pectoral jerk 193
Pectoralis major 181
Pedal oedema 11
Pemberton's sign 265
Pen test 216
Pendular knee jerk 199
Penicillins 309
Pentalogy of Fallot 75
Percussion
- of lung apex 100
- of lung normal 100

Pericardial
- disorders 66
- effusion 76
- knock 66
- rub 66
- tamponade 76

Pericardial effusion 360
Periorbital edema 280
Peripheral
- cyanosis 5
- diagnosis 214
- general examination 214
- neuropathy 214
- types 214
- vascular disease causes of 78
- vascular system 39

Persistent vegetative state 269
Pescavus 20
- and kyphoscoliosis 158

Petechiae 22
Phases of hair growth 20
Phenobarbitone 328
Phenomenon of Gagenhalten 183
Physiological gynaecomastia 258
Pigmentation 22
- of oral cavity 129

Pink puffer 110
Pinpoint pupil 167, 273
Pioglitazone 326
PIR examination in a
- female 147
- male 147

Plaque 21
Platypnea 84
Plethoric appearance of face 15
Pleural
- effusion 107
- hemorrhagic 107
- mediastinal shift to same side 108
- left-sided 107
- right-sided 107

Pleural effusion 107
Pleural fluid
- analysis 306
- aspiration 305

Pleural rub 106
Pleurisy 107
Pleuritic pain 86
Plummer's nail 263
PND 26
- description of an attack of 26
- mechanism of 26

Pneumonic consolidation 108
Pneumothorax click (Hamman's sign) 106
Pneumothorax 107, 294
Pointing index finger 216
Polycythemia vera 225
Polymyositis 212
Polyuria 231
Posterior
- column sensations
- Wall MI 358

Post-exertional syncope 31
Post-tussive suction 106
Postural hypotension 265
Power 178

P-P interval 348
PR interval 348
Precipitancy 229
Precocious puberty 259
Precordium 49
Precordium, examination of 49
Pregnancy and heart disease 35
Pressure pain 189
Pretibial myxedema 264
  pathogenesis of 264
Primitive reflexes 195
Prinzmetal's angina 28
Prominent eyes 279
Proprioception 186
Proptosis (outward displacement of eyes) 249
  pulsating 279
Proteinuria 237
Pruritus of hepatobiliary disease 123
Pseudoathetosis 189
Pseudohypertension 45
Pseudohypertrophy 176
Psoriatic arthritis 252
Psychogenic vomiting 116
Ptosis 165
  complete 166
Puberty
  delayed 259
  in females 259
  in males 259
  precocious 259
Puddle sign 140
Pulmonary
  and pleural disorder 85
  apoplexy 32
  collapse 109
  embolism 360
  fibrosis 109
  hypertension 74
  stenosis 74
Pulsatile liver 53
Pulsating proptosis 279
Pulse
  Corrigan's or waterhammer 41
  dicrotic 42
  volume 41
Pulses
  alternans 42
  bigeminus 43
  genesis of 42
  paradoxus 42
  parvus et tardus 41
Pupil, sympathetic supply to 164
Pupillary reflexes 166
Purpura 22
Pustule 21
Pyloric obstruction 133
Pyorrhea 130
Pyrantel pamoate 329
Pyrosis 116

Q wave 348
QRS duration 356
QT interval 349
Quality of sputum 82
Quickenstedt's test 303
Quinalones 309

Radiation of pain 28
Rashes 21
Raynaud's phenomenon 79
RBC casts 361
Rebound phenomenon 198
Record syringe 347
Recording of blood pressure by cuff method 44
Rectus abdominis, divarication of 132
Red eye 278
Referred pain 114
Reflexes
  deep 192
  examination of 190
  finger flexion 196
  gag 174
  glabellar tap (Myerson's sign) 195
  grading 194
  primitive 195
  pupillary 166
  snout 195
  suckling 195
Refractory defects, different types 280
Regurgitation 115
Renal failure
  acute 237
  chronic 237
Repaglinide 325
Respiratory causes of chest pain 85
Respiratory system, examination of 89
Retina, exudates in 285
Retinal
  artery occlusion 284
  hemorrhages 284
  vein occlusion 284
Retinopathy hypertensive 284
  proliferative 285
Retrobulbar neuritis 283
Retrosternal goitre 264
Reversible ischemic neurological deficit 204
Rheumatic
  acute 76
  fever 33, 251
  nodules 244
Rheumatoid
  arthritis 244, 252
  nodules 244
Rhomboids 181
Rhonchi
  causes of 104
  different types 104
Rhythm of respiration and abnormal patterns 90
Right bundle branch block 356
Right ventricular hypertrophy 351
Right-sided heart failure 76
Rigidity 178
  types of 178
RIND (reversible ischemic neurological deficit) 204
Rinne's test 173
Rocker bottom feet 20
Roger's malady 74
Romberg's sign 188
Roth's spots 37
R-R interval 348
Rubella syndrome 78
Ryle's tube 345

S wave 348
Sacral sparing 190
Saddle anaesthesia 189
Salbutamol 322
Salivation, excessive 122
Scalp hair loss 21
Scleritis 281
Scotomas 280
Scurvy 130
Second degree AV block 355
Sengstaken-Blackemore tube 346
Sensation, cortical 190
Sensory inattention 190
Sensory pathways 186
Sensory
  examination of 186
  system 186
Serratas anterior 181
Severe
  damage to cornea 281
  MR 70
Sexual
  hair, loss of 21
  maturation, disturbances in 259
Shagreen patch 157
Shamroth's sign 7
Shawl sign 213
Shock 334
Short stature 2
Sickle cell anemia 225
Significance of Glasgow coma scale 272
Signs of liver cell failure 127
Silent mitral stenosis 69
Simple rubber catheter 344
Sinus
  arrhythmia 39, 352
  bradycardia 351
  tachycardia 352
Sister Mary Joseph nodule 132
Sites to look for jaundice 4
  pallor 4
Size of pupil, inequality in 166
Skeletal height 1
  measurement of 1
Skin
  changes in Behçet's syndrome 245
  colour, alteration of 22
  decreased pigmentation of 23
  discoloration of 121
  examination of 21
  hyperpigmentation of 23
  lesions of leprosy 23
  rash of dermatomyositis 244
  rash of SLE 244
  striae 131
Skodiac resonance 101
Skull and spine, examination of 201
SLE, skin rash of 244
Slowly progressive dyspnoea 26
Small intestinal obstruction 133
Snout reflex 195
Soft exudates 286
Somatostatin 324
Spastic paraplegia 201
Spasticity 177
  clasp knife 177
Spider naevi 127
Spinal
  cord compression 203
  cord lesion 202
  cauda equina 196
  cervical cord lesion 196
  conus medullaris 196
  Ellseberg's phenomenon 204
  extradural 203
  intramedullary 203
  multiple levels 203
Spine, examination of 250
Splenomegaly, causes of 139
Sputum, quality of 82
Squint 166
  and diplopia 166
  concomitant 166
  (strabismus) 166

ST segment 349
Stamping gait 201
Statins 321
Status epilepticus 334
Stereognosis 190
Stiffness of joints 239
Stokes-Adams attack 30
Stomach tube 342
Stool analysis 362
Strabismus 166
Straight
  back syndrome 49
  leg raising (SLR) test 251
Streptococcal tonsillitis 129
Stridor 85
Stroke
  completed 204
  in evolution 204
  in young 206
Sturge-Weber syndrome 158
Subendocardial infarction 358
Subconjunctival hemorrhage 126
Subcortical aphasias 160
Subcutaneous fat 2
Subcutaneous nodules 244
Succussion splash
  (Hippocratic splash) 106
Suckling reflex 195
Sudden
  cardiac death 335
  loss of vision 279
Sulphonylureas 340
Supinatory (brachioradialis) reflex 193
Supraspinatus 181
Supraspinatus tendinitis (painful arc
  syndrome) 245
SVC obstruction 111
Sweating, disturbance in 255
Swelling of feet 33
  swellings 236
Swellings, testicular 235
Sydenham's chorea 33
Sympathetic supply to pupil 164
Symptom analysis of an anaemic
  disorder 219
Symptoms of
  bladder and bowel dysfunction 151
  cardiovascular disease 152
  cerebellar dysfunction 151
  cranial nerve dysfunction 151
  upper respiratory illness 86
Syncope
  differential diagnosis 31
  on exertion 31
  post-exertional 31
Systolic
  hypertension 45
  murmurs 62

Tachycardia 30, 353
Tactile localisation 190
Tall stature 1
Tandem walking 199
Tapping apex 51
Taste, pathway and testing 171
Telengiectasia 157
Tenesmus 120
Testicular
  atrophy 127
  neoplasms 236
Testing the
  muscles of mastication 168
  visual acuity 279
Tests
  for 10th and 11th cranial nerves 174
  for integrity of diaphragm 98
  of hearing 173
Thalamic syndrome 208
Thalassemia
  clinical significance 3
  major 225
  minor 225
Thiabendazole 330
Thrills 53
Thrombophlebitis 77
Thumb sign 1
Thyroid
  acropachy 262
  bruit/thrill 265
  enlargement (goitre) 17
Thyroid hormones 363
  method of examination of 264
Thyrotoxic crises 339
Thyrotoxicosis 14, 256
Thyroxin 324
TIA (transient ischemic attack) 204
Tics 185
Titubation 198
To and fro murmurs 64
Tone alteration, types of 177
Tongue, enlargement of 130
Tophi 244
Torticollis (wry neck) 17
Tracheal tug 53
Tracheostomy tube 346
Transient ischemic attack 183
Traube's area 101
Trauma to head and spine 153
Tremors 184
  different types 184
Trepopnea 27
Tricuspid regurgitation 73
Trigeminal nerve (5th) 168
Triology of Fallot 75
Trochlear (4th) nerve paralysis 165
Troisier's sign 9
Trophic ulcers of the hand 20
True claw hand 247
Tuberculoid leprosy 23
Tumor markers 362
Turner's
  sign 132
  syndrome 78
Two point discrimination 190
Types
  and nature of cough 81
  of cyanosis 6
  of facial palsy 169
  of rigidity 178
  of tone alteration 177
Typical example of a case of rheumatic
  valvular disease 67

U wave 348
Ulnar
  nerve 200
  nerve lesions 246
  paradox 217
Upper
  lobe bronchial carcinoma (Pancoast's
    tumour) 110
  mimitic type of 170
  motor neuron facial palsy volitional
    type 169
  motor neuron (UMN) 175
  respiratory illness, symptoms of 86
Upper segment 1
Uremia 231
Urinary
  casts 361
  retention 230
  sediments 361
Urine analysis 361

Vagus nerve 174
Varicocoele 235
Varicose veins 77
Vas deferens 236
Vascular nevus 158
Vena caval obstruction, inferior 133
Ventricular
  fibrillation 355
  septal defect 74
  tachycardia 354
Vesicle 21
Vestibulocochlear nerve 172
Vestibulocular reflex (caloric test) 275
Vincent's angina 130
Viral hepatitis
  clinical features 144
  complications 145
Virchow's node (Troisier's sign) 9
Virilisation 260
Virilism 21
Visible veins 132
Vision
  loss of 279
  sudden loss of 279
Visual
  acuity 279
  testing 279
  field defect 262
  loss 262
Vitamin B_{12} deficiency 224
Vitiligo 23, 264
Vomiting 115
  psychogenic 116
V-sign 213
Vth nerve lesion 168

Wadding gait 201
Waist/hip ratio 3
Waldeyer's ring 9
Wasting and hypertrophy of muscles 176
Watenberg's sign 196
Waterbrash 116
Waxy casts 361
WBC casts 361
Weber's test 173
Wenckebach's phenomenon 355
Wernicke's (sensory) aphasia 159
Wheal 21
Wheeze 27, 84
Whispering pectoriloquy (WP) 105
White coat hypertension 45
Whole of cauda equina lesion 204
Whooping cough 81
William's syndrome 78
  with diurnal variation 81
  with expectoration 31, 82
Wrist sign 2
Wry neck 17

Xanthochromia of CSF 304
Xanthomas, different types, and
  (proprioception) 186

Yellowish discoloration apart from
  jaundice, causes of 4